Bone Loss and Osteoporosis: An Anthropological Perspective

Bone Loss and Osteoporosis: An Anthropological Perspective

Edited by

SABRINA C. AGARWAL
Department of Anthropology
University of Toronto

and

SAM D. STOUT
Department of Anthropology
The Ohio State University

Kluwer Academic / Plenum Publishers
New York, Boston, Dordrecht, London, Moscow

Library of Congress Cataloging-in-Publication Data

Bone loss and osteoporosis: an anthropological perspective / edited by Sabrina C. Agarwal and Samuel D. Stout.
p. cm.
Includes bibliographical references and index.
ISBN 0-306-47767-X
1. Human skeleton—Abnormalities. 2. Bones—Diseases. 3. Osteoporosis. 4. Physical anthropology. I Agarwal, Sabrina C. II. Stout, Samuel D.

GN70.B66 2003
599.9'47—dc21

2003050642

ISBN 0-306-47767-X

233 Spring Street, New York, N. Y. 10013

http://www.wkap.nl/

10 9 8 7 6 5 4 3 2 1

A C.I.P. record for this book is available from the Library of Congress

Printed in the United States of America

To Dr. Marc D. Grynpas
for teaching students about all things bone and
mineral with patience and enthusiasm, and for always leaving his
office door open.

Sabrina C. Agarwal

To Dr. Harold M. Frost
for challenging us all to think critically about what we think we know.

Sam D. Stout

Contributors

Sabrina C. Agarwal is an Assistant Professor in the Department of Anthropology at the University of Toronto. She received her B.A. and M.Sc. from the University of Toronto, and Ph.D. in 2001 from the same institution, working in both the Department of Anthropology and the Samuel Lunenfeld Research Institute of Mount Sinai Hospital. She was awarded a Social Sciences and Humanities Research Council of Canada Postdoctoral Fellowship and spent two years in the Department of Anthropology at McMaster University. Her research interests have focused broadly upon the age and sex-related changes in bone quantity and quality, and she is particularly interested in the application of biocultural and evolutionary approaches to the study of bone fragility. Her work has examined age-related changes in cortical bone microstructure, trabecular architecture, and mineral density in archaeological populations, and she is currently examining the long-term effect of parity and lactation on the human and non-human primate maternal skeleton.

Megan Brickley received her Ph.D. in 1998 from University College London, having worked jointly between the Institute of Archaeology and the Hard Tissue Research Unit (department of anatomy). She is currently a Lecturer in The Department of Ancient History and Archaeology at the University of Birmingham, UK. She has a number of publications on techniques for studying bone density and osteoporosis and has worked extensively on British post-medieval (18th–19th century) skeletal material. Publications include "Measurement of Changes in Trabecular Bone Structure with Age in an Archaeological Population," *Journal of Archaeological Science*, 1999 (with Peter Howell) and *The Cross Bones Burial Ground, Redcross Way Southwark, London*, 1999 (with Adrian Miles and Hilary Stainer). She is currently working on three post-medieval skeletal assemblages the largest of which, St. Martin's cemetery, Birmingham (875 individuals) will be published at the end of 2003. She is the chair of the British Association of Biological Anthropology and Osteoarchaeology and secretary of the British Association of Human Identification sub-committee for Forensic Anthropology.

Helen Cho is an Assistant Professor in the Department of Anthropology at Davidson College, NC. She received her B.A. in Anthropology and B.S. in Chemistry from the University of Illinois at Urbana-Champagne in 1994, M.A. and Ph.D. in Anthropology from the University of Missouri-Columbia in 1996 and 2002, respectively. She also earned a minor in Museum Studies in 1999 from the Department of Art History and Archaeology at the University of Missouri. Her academic interests include skeletal biology, bioarchaeology, and forensic anthropology.

Harold M. Frost received his B.A. degree from Dartmouth in 1943, and was awarded his M.D. degree in 1945 after attending the Dartmouth Medical School and Northwestern University School of Medicine. His career in orthopaedic medicine has spanned 5 decades. Appointments he has held include Assistant Professor of Orthopaedic Surgery, Yale University School of Medicine (1955–1957); and Henry Ford Hospital (1957–1973) where he served as attending orthopaedic surgeon, Director of the Cerebral Palsy Clinic, and Chairman of the Department of Orthopaedic Surgery, and was founder and director of its Orthopaedic Research Laboratory. In 1973, he joined the Southern Colorado Clinic, and since 1995 been "semiretired," but continues writing to pass on the benefits of his over 50 years of experience. Since 1953, Harold Frost's research history includes devising the dynamic histomorphometry for the analysis of bone tissue dynamics in health and disease that is currently used worldwide, and is also the chief architect of the Utah paradigm of skeletal physiology. His research has dealt with a wide range of important topics related to orthopaedic medicine and skeletal biology. It includes skeletal responses to drugs, hormones, mechanical influences, and other agents; metabolic bone disease; skeletal histology and pathology; skeletal biomechanics; surgical treatment of cerebral palsy; managing tennis elbow; the frozen shoulder syndrome; patellar chondromalacia; osteoarthritis; and bone healing and graft problems. His overarching goal has been to combine multidisciplinary evidence to explain the multidisciplinary determinants of skeletal health and many skeletal disorders. Harold Frost has published over 440 scientific and clinical articles, including three textbooks and eleven monographs, and contributed articles to the proceedings of many national and international conferences and symposia on skeletal disease, physiology, biomechanics, and research. He has received numerous honors and most recently was the 2001 recipient of the William Neuman Award from the American Society of Bone and Mineral Research.

Marc D. Grynpas obtained his Ph.D. degree in crystallography and biophysics at the University of London's Birkbeck College and received a post-doctoral research fellowship from the University of London's Queen Mary College. He was a researcher at the Children's Hospital, a Harvard University teaching institution where he conducted research on bone mineralization. Dr. Grynpas is currently a Professor of Laboratory Medicine and Pathobiology at the University of Toronto, and a senior scientist at the Samuel Lunenfeld Research Institute of Mount Sinai Hospital. His contributions to the study of bone have been recognized by several Canadian and international agencies. In 1992 he was offered a membership to the Space Studies Board of the National Academy of Science. Subsequently, Dr. Grynpas was invited to be the chair of the Gordon Research Conference on Calcium Phosphate Chemistry in 1994. His numerous accomplishments in the field of bone study in space were recognized with a NASA Cosmos Achievement Award in 1990, and his work in osteoporosis research by a Schering Award at the International conference on Osteoporosis (Hong Kong) in 1993. Dr. Grynpas has published more than 115 articles on bone research in peer-reviewed journals. His current research interests include the genetic determinants of bone quality, the long-term effects of drugs and trace elements on the skeleton, and bone and cartilage tissue engineering.

R. Bruce Martin received his B.S. degree in Physics from West Virginia University in 1966, and his M.S. and Ph.D. degrees in Theoretical and Applied Mechanics in 1969 and 1970, respectively. He subsequently became Director of Research in the Department of Orthopaedic Surgery at the same university. In 1984 he moved to a similar position in the Orthopaedics Department at the University of California at Davis, where he is currently Professor and Doris Linn Chair of Bone Biology, with a joint appointment in the Department of Mechanical and Aeronautical Engineering, and membership in the Biomedical Engineering Graduate Group. Dr. Martin was president of the American Society of Biomechanics in 1998–1999. He co-authored, with David Burr and Neil Sharkey, the textbook Skeletal Tissue Mechanics. In the summer he may be found somewhere along the Pacific Crest Trail, creating and removing skeletal fatigue damage and thankful that his bones, at least, are strong and light.

Dorothy A. Nelson is a Professor of Internal Medicine at Wayne State University, where she currently serves as the Director of the Department's Clinical Research Center. She also has appointments in Biomedical Engineering, Anthropology, and the Institute of Gerontology at Wayne. Dr. Nelson received her Ph.D. in Physical Anthropology from Michigan State University in 1985. Her dissertation topic was bone mass and bone loss in Native American archaeological populations. She joined the research team of the Bone and Mineral Division at Henry Ford Hospital in 1985, where she began studying ethnic differences in bone mass and risks for osteoporosis. She also investigated the accumulation of bone mass in children in a longitudinal study funded by the NIH. She moved to Wayne State University in 1993, where she expanded her interests in ethnicity and osteoporosis to include studies of bone architecture in the hip in groups from Detroit and Johannesburg, South Africa. Most recently, she has investigated the association between high bone density and an increased risk of breast cancer in White and African American women.

Michael Parfitt graduated in medicine from the University of Cambridge, England in 1954. After extensive and varied training in internal medicine, culminating in a two-year fellowship with Charles Dent, he emigrated in 1962 to an academic position in Queensland, Australia, where he practiced his recently found interest in calcium and bone metabolism as a hobby. In 1971 he moved to Henry Ford Hospital in Detroit, Michigan and devoted himself full-time to his field of special interest. In 1976 he took over Hal Frost's former laboratory; he is probably one of only two people currently active in academic medicine who have read all of his old papers, the other being Webster Jee. As an unusual feature of his academic career he undertook two Trans-Pacific sabbaticals in opposite directions, from Brisbane to Los Angeles in 1968–1969 to study renal bone disease with Chuck Kleeman, and from Detroit to Brisbane in 1988 to study disorders of parathyroid cell growth with Martyn Lloyd. In 1995 he relinquished the directorship of the Bone and Mineral Research Laboratory at Henry Ford Hospital and took up a part time position with Stavros Manolagas at the University of Arkansas for Medical Sciences in Little Rock, where he still works. In 1995 he received the Bartter award of the American Society for Bone and Mineral Research.

Alexander Robling is an Assistant Professor of Anatomy & Cell Biology at Indiana University School of Medicine. He received his Ph.D. from the University of Missouri-Columbia in 1998, after which he joined the musculoskeletal group at Indiana University for a 2-year postdoctoral fellowship. His research interests include understanding the effects of mechanical loading on bone at the organ, tissue, and cellular levels. His most recent work appears in the Journal of Bone and Mineral Research, the Journal of Experimental Biology, Bone, Medicine and Science in Sports and Exercise, Calcified Tissue International, and the Journal of Musculoskeletal and Neuronal Interaction. Dr. Robling is a member of the American Society for Bone and Mineral Research, and was awarded the New Investigator Recognition Award (NIRA) at the 2002 meeting of the Orthopaedic Research Society.

Michael Schultz is a physician, biological anthropologist, and professor of anatomy in the Zentrum Anatomie, University of Göttingen, Germany, where he has worked during most of his professional career. He holds a Dr.med. (M.D.) and a Dr.phil.nat. (Ph.D.) degree from the University of Frankfurt am Main, and a Dr.med.habil. (D.Sc.) degree from the University of Göttingen. His major research interest is in the evolution and the history of diseases and in the influence of environmental factors on prehistoric and early historic populations. He is also working on the functional and comparative anatomy of primates and in paleoanthropology. He has conducted research on diseases in archaeological human skeletal and mummified remains for 30 years. He has published more than 180 scientific articles and two monographs on microscopic research in archaeological skeletal material and non-specific inflammations in prehistoric and historic skulls. He is the editor of the two book series "Advances in Paleopathology and Osteoarchaeology" and "Beiträge zur Paläopathologie," and from 1998 to 2001, he was one of the Managing Editors of HOMO—The Journal of Comparative Human Biology. From 1996 to 2000, he was the President of the Gesellschaft für Anthropologie (GfA), and from 2001 to 2003 the President of the Paleopathology Association (PPA). Additionally, he has organized three large international scientific congresses and three international symposia. He has carried out field work in Germany, Austria, Switzerland, Italy, Slovakia, the USA, Mexico, the Union of the Soviet Socialist Republics, Turkey, Jordan, Iraq, and Egypt, and has conducted many research projects in Europe, the Near and the Middle East, USA, and Mexico. Most recently he has been engaged in developing an interdisciplinary research group for the comparative study of infectious and deficiency diseases, particularly of subadults, from prehistoric to early modern times.

William A. Stini is Professor of Anthropology, Family and Community Medicine, and Public Health at the University of Arizona. He is also a member of the Arizona Cancer Center. He has served as Editor-in-Chief of the *American Journal of Physical Anthropology*, from 1983 to 1989 and President of the American Association of Physical Anthropologists from 1989 to 1991. His research interests have been focused on various aspects of the relationship between the organism and the environment throughout the human life cycle. The questions raised in the course of his research have taken him to the Cordillera Central of Northern Colombia, where he participated in a nutritional intervention project measuring the effects of essential amino acid deficiencies on the growth of children. Subsequent laboratory experiments using domestic hogs explored the extent to which reduced intake of essential amino acids was reflected in loss of muscle fibers during early post-weaning growth and development. Returning to work with human subjects, Dr. Stini worked with women of the LaLeche League in comparing the growth and disease experience of exclusively breast-fed with those of bottle-fed infants in Southern Arizona. Later, taking advantage of the rapid growth of the retirement community in Arizona, Dr. Stini initiated a longitudinal study of the changes in bone density and other elements of body composition in aging adults. This project continued for 17 years and attracted over 5400 subjects over that period. A subsample of this population included over 500 subjects participating in a colon cancer prevention study. Additional comparative studies were also initiated in Saudi Arabia and in the State of Karnataka in southern India. The analysis of certain aspects of the data collected in these studies is still in progress.

Sam D. Stout received his Ph.D. in biological anthropology from Washington University in St. Louis, MO in 1976. He is Professor Emeritus in Department of Anthropology, University of Missouri and currently Professor in the Department of Anthropology at

The Ohio State University. His general research interests are in skeletal biology. Specifically, his research involves the microstructural analysis of bone (histomorphometry) and its applications in bioarchaeology, forensic anthropology, and paleontology. Significant publications include: Cho, H., Streeter, J. and Madsen, R.W. (2002) Population-Specific Histological Age-Estimating method: A model for known African-American and European-American skeletal remains, *Journal of Forensic Sciences*, 47(1): 12–18; Streeter, M., Stout, S.D., Trinkaus, E., Stringer, C.B., Roberts, M.B., and Parfitt, S.A. (2001) Histomorphometric Age Assessment of the Boxgrove 1 Tibial Diaphysis, *Journal of Human Evolution*, 40(4):331–338; Stout, S.D., Brunsden, B., Hildebolt, C., Commean, P., Smith, K., and Tappen, N.C. (1999) Computer assisted 3D reconstruction of serial sections of cortical bone to determine the 3D structure of osteons, *Calcified Tissue International*, 65:280–284; Robling, A. and Stout, S.D. (1999) Morphology of Drifting Osteons, *Cells, Tissues and Organs*, 164:192–204; Stout, S.D. and Lueck, R. (1995) Bone remodeling rates and maturation in three archaeological skeletal populations, *American Journal of Physical Anthropology*, 98(2):161–171; Stout, S.D. and Paine, R.R. (1992) Histological age estimation using the rib and clavicle, *American Journal of Physical Anthropology*, 87:111–115; Robling, A.G. and Stout, S.D. (2000) Methods of determining age at death using bone microstructure. In Katzenberg, M.A. and Saunders, S.R. (Eds.), *Biological Anthropology of the Human Skeleton*. New York: Wiley-Liss, pp. 187–205.

Margaret Streeter received her M.A. from the University of Missouri in 1999 and is currently enrolled in the Ph.D. program in Physical Anthropology at that same institution. Her research interests include bone biology, with special interest in histomorphometric analysis of bone as it applies to skeletal biology, paleohistology, paleopathology, forensic anthropology, and growth and development. She has worked on ancient skeletal material from Boxgrove, England; Shanidar, Iraq; Tabun and Skhul, Israel; Ajvide, Sweden; Isola Sacra, Italy; Palenque, Mexico and Sican, Peru, as well as modern forensic cases. Recent publications include "Boxgrove 1 Tibial Diaphysis" published in the *Journal of Human Evolution* (2001) (with S.D. Stout, E. Trinkaus, C.B. Stringer, M.B. Roberts, and S.A. Parfitt) and "Population-specific histological age-estimating method: A model for known African-American and European-American skeletal remains" (*Journal of Forensic Science* (2002) (with H. Cho, S.D. Stout, and R.W. Madsen). She is a member of the American Association of Physical Anthropologists and American Women in Science.

Patty Stuart-Macadam received her Ph.D. degree from Cambridge University, and was an Associate Professor in the Department of Anthropology at the University of Toronto, where she taught for ten years. Her research revolved around the health and disease of ancient human populations, with special interests in iron-deficiency anaemia, cancer, trauma, sex and gender differences, and breastfeeding. She has co-edited three books, *Diet, Demography and Disease: Changing Perspectives on Anemia* (with S. Kent), *Breast-feeding: Biocultural perspectives* (with K. Dettwyler), and *Sex and Gender in Paleopathological Perspective* (with A. Grauer). Her interests have shifted to working with living humans and she currently home-schools her four children and practices as a homoeopath, kinesiologist, and Bowen therapist in Australia.

Reinhold Vieth is an associate professor with the Department of Laboratory Medicine and Pathobiology, University of Toronto. After completing his Ph.D. at the Hospital for

Sick Children in Toronto, he completed a residency in clinical chemistry and became a Fellow of the Canadian Academy of Clinical Biochemists. Instead of heading into his expected career as a hospital service biochemist, he was hired by the Bone and Mineral Group of the University of Toronto for providing a regional service for clinical laboratory testing related to bone disease and vitamin D. This gave him the opportunity to continue with a research program that started in 1974, related to vitamin D and bone disease. In recent years, his research has shifted away from the basic science of vitamin D metabolism, toward a clinical focus aimed at re-evaluating the role of plain and simple vitamin D (what he considers to be an original "orphan drug") for the health of adults.

Marie L. Villa, M.D., is an Assistant Professor of Internal Medicine and Geriatrics at University of Washington School of Medicine, where she currently serves as an attending physician in the Long Term Care Service. Dr. Villa received her M.D. from Stanford University in 1986 with honors in Gerontology. Following training in Internal Medicine, she completed both clinical and research fellowships in Geriatrics (one year as a Hartford scholar), with a research emphasis on determinants of skeletal health in Mexican American women. She was Director of the Stanford Musculoskeletal Research Lab prior to re-locating to the University of Washington. Most recently, she is involved in issues regarding treatment of osteoporosis in nursing home settings. She also maintains an active interest in ethnic aspects of skeletal health.

Preface

With the growing incidence of fragility fractures in Europe and North America over the last three decades, bone loss and osteoporosis have become active areas of research in skeletal biology. Bone loss is associated with aging in both sexes and is accelerated in women with the onset of menopause. However, bone loss is related to a suite of complex and often synergistically related factors including genetics, pathology, nutrition, mechanical usage, and lifestyle. It is not surprising that its incidence and severity vary among populations.

There has been increasing interest to investigate bone loss and osteoporosis from an anthropological perspective that utilizes a biocultural approach. Biocultural approaches recognize the inter-relationship between biological, cultural, and environmental variables. Anthropological studies also highlight the value of evolutionary and population approaches to the study of bone loss. These approaches are particularly suited to elucidate the multifactorial etiology of bone loss.

The idea for this volume came out of a symposium organized by the editors at the 70th annual meeting of The American Association of Physical Anthropologists in Kansas City, Missouri. Many of the symposium participants, along with several additional leading scientists involved in bone and osteoporosis research, are brought together in this volume. Each chapter focuses on a different aspect of bone loss and fragility with a fresh and stimulating perspective.

The volume is divided into four parts. Part I, titled Current Concepts of Bone Loss and Osteoporosis, includes three chapters that tackle our current knowledge on the mechanisms of bone maintenance and fragility, and provides a solid foundation for the subsequent chapters. Parfitt discusses the essentials of bone remodeling, describing in detail the different types of remodeling processes that take place in structural and metabolic bone. Drawing on his own extensive work, he illustrates the cellular mechanisms of bone turnover and outlines the cellular disturbances that underlie the biological phenomenon of age-related bone loss. The second chapter by Frost, reviews the current paradigms in bone physiology. He discusses the changing perspectives on bone loss with an emphasis on the importance of mechanical influences on bone maintenance. Although, many of the newer concepts Frost discusses will spark debate, the theoretical directions he suggests will also undoubtedly continue to provide the fuel for further experimental work on the role of mechanical loading in bone biology. Grynpas discusses the important role of bone quality in bone fragility. He focuses on how qualitative elements of bone, such as bone material and composition can contribute significantly to bone strength. He draws on examples from experimental work on bone mineralization and microarchitecture that illustrate the growing realization that bone quality plays a vital role in osteoporosis independent of bone mass.

Part II includes three chapters that discuss bone mass and loss with a focus on the population level. Nelson and Villa focus on the importance of population differences in osteoporosis in their discussion of observed ethnic differences in bone mass and architecture. They discuss the geographic differences in bone mineral density and bone geometry measured by DXA using data from several large national surveys. Nelson and Villa demonstrate how varying rates of osteoporotic fracture and BMD differences amongst different populations are inextricably tied to lifestyle and other environmental factors. Stini covers the importance of bone loss and fragility in the male population. Presenting data from a longitudinal study of bone density and body composition, Stini reveals a pattern of increased bone loss in advanced aged males that appears related to the loss of lean body mass in this group. His work draws attention to the fact that age-related bone loss is a growing concern not only in women but also in men. Streeter and Stout look at bone mass in juveniles. They examine the processes of remodeling and modeling in cortical bone of sub-adult ribs, describing age-related changes in histomorphology and mass. They discuss the importance of peak bone mass achievement and timing of peak bone mass specifically in the rib, and discuss implications of this work for further studies.

Part III examines bone loss and osteoporosis from an evolutionary perspective. Agarwal and Stuart-Macadam utilize an evolutionary and historical approach to understand the role of pregnancy and lactation in bone maintenance. Although the physiological demands of reproduction have been traditionally regarded as detrimental to the maternal skeleton, the authors discuss current human and animal model data that illustrate the complex and still poorly understood effects of pregnancy and lactation on bone. Drawing valuable clues from non-human primate reproductive behaviors and patterns of bone loss and fragility in historical populations, they argue that pregnancy and lactation may even have beneficial effects on the long-term fragility of the female skeleton. Martin's provocative chapter explores the evolutionary value of bone turnover in the human skeleton. He argues that some degree of biomechanical fragility may actually have offered a selective advantage during the evolution of the human skeleton. Martin suggests that while this light skeleton may have offered an evolutionary advantage it leaves little room for additional fragility due to hormonal deficiency or pathology. Vieth discusses the importance of vitamin D in bone diseases such as osteoporosis and rickets. He provides a brief review of the metabolism and physiology of vitamin D, and further discusses the role of vitamin D deficiency in the genetic selection for skin color during human evolution. Most compelling is his argument, based on estimated concentrations of circulating 25(OH)D during human evolution and concentrations in living primates, that suggests that modern humans are chronically deprived of vitamin D with the consequence of poor bone maintenance.

Part IV, titled Bone Loss and Osteoporosis in Past Populations, deals with the theoretical and methodological issues surrounding the study of bone loss in archaeological samples. In chapter 10, Brickley and Agarwal examine the advantages and disadvantages of several techniques for the assessment of bone loss and osteoporosis in past populations. They evaluate traditional measures of bone mineral density and more recent state-of-the-art methods of microstructural measurement in archaeological samples. Schultz more closely examines the serious obstacle of diagenesis in his discussion of diagnosing bone loss in archaeological bone. He discusses various types of diagenesis as well as possible differential diagnoses of osteopenia in archaeological bone with several illustrative examples. Robling and Stout discuss the importance of mechanical loading in past populations at the microstructural level. They present a novel approach to partition systemic remodeling from mechanically induced remodeling in a dynamically loaded bone (femur) by standardization with remodeling in the rib of the same individual. Results of the application of this method on bone samples from a Precearmic site on the central Coast of Peru are presented. Cho and Stout provide an excellent example of how histomorphometric analyses can be used to provide a comparative examination of bone remodelling in archaeological and modern populations. They describe several unique patterns in rib histomorphology in an ancient urban Imperial Roman skeletal sample that suggest a reduced prevalence of osteopenia in comparison to modern urban human populations, perhaps indicative of lifestyle patterns in this group.

Each chapter highlights the multifaceted nature of bone loss and fragility. Several underlying themes are common between the chapters, particularly the value of biocultural and evolutionary perspectives in the study of bone loss and fragility. The contributors come from a variety of fields, and this volume is intended for a diverse audience including physical anthropologists, osteologists, bioengineers, and clinicians in sub-disciplines such as rheumatology, orthopedics, and general medicine. It is our hope that the interdisciplinary communication suggested by this volume can stimulate further theoretical debate and be carried to the bench towards new directions of osteoporosis research.

Sabrina C. Agarwal
Sam D. Stout
2003

Acknowledgments

We would like to thank all the contributors for their chapters and extend our sincere appreciation for their hard work, cooperation, and patience. We give special thanks to Andrea Macaluso, Life Sciences editor at Kluwer Academic Publishers, for her support and enthusiasm with this project. We also thank Felix Portnoy, Production Editor at Kluwer and his production staff for their efficiency and patience. Peter Pollard and Patrick Beauchesne are to be thanked for their meticulous editing and formatting of the final chapters.

The senior editor (S.C.A) would like to extend appreciation to several mentors. Drs. Marc Grynpas, David Begun, and Patricia Stuart-Macadam not only provided unfailing advice throughout this project, but have also offered guidance and encouragement through the years beyond the call of duty. S.C.A would also like to thank her co-editor Dr. Sam Stout for believing in her ideas and this project and taking it all on until its fruition.

The co-editor (S.D.S) would like to recognize several colleagues who have influenced his career. Drs. David J. Simmons, Steven L. Teitelbaum, Stephen Molnar, and James Gavan fostered an appreciation for the dynamic nature of bone physiology and for the importance of an anthropological perspective.

Sabrina C. Agarwal
Sam D. Stout

Contents

Part I. Current Concepts of Bone Loss and Osteoporosis

1. New Concepts of Bone Remodeling: A Unified Spatial and Temporal Model with Physiologic and Pathophysiologic Implications

A. Michael Parfitt

1. Introduction 3
2. The Purposes of Bone Remodeling 5
   2.1. The Basic Multicellular Unit as the Instrument of Bone Remodeling 6
3. Disordered Remodeling and Age Related Bone Loss 11
   References 15

2. On Changing Views about Age-Related Bone Loss

Harold M. Frost

1. Introduction 19
   1.1. On the Two Paradigms 19
      1.1.1. The 1960 Paradigm 20
      1.1.2. The Utah Paradigm 20
2. Age-Related Bone Loss 24
3. A Proposed Synthesis 26
4. Conclusions 26
   References 27
   Glossary 30

3. The Role of Bone Quality on Bone Loss and Fragility

Marc D. Grynpas

1. Introduction 33
2. Determination of Bone Quality 34
3. Aging Changes in the Skeleton 34
4. The Problem of Diagenesis 35
5. Changes in Bone Mineralization with Diseases and Treatments 36
6. What Determines Skeletal Fragility? 39
7. Conclusions 40
   References 41

Part II. Population Approaches

4. Ethnic Differences in Bone Mass and Architecture

Dorothy A. Nelson and Marie L. Villa

1. Introduction ... 47
1.1. Osteoporosis ... 47
1.2. Bone Densitometry and Assessment of Bone Architecture ... 47
1.3. Bone Density and Fracture Incidence ... 48
1.4. Use of "Race" and "Ethnicity" in Biomedical Literature on Osteoporosis ... 49
2. Bone Mass and Bone Density ... 50
2.1. Definitions of Bone Density ... 50
2.2. Ethnic Differences in Bone Density ... 50
3. Bone Quality and Bone Turnover ... 51
4. Factors Affecting Bone Mass and Bone Loss ... 51
4.1. Adjusting Bone Density for Body Size ... 51
4.2. Body Size and Composition, and Preservation of the Skeleton ... 52
4.3. Calcium Nutrition ... 53
4.4. Physical Activity ... 54
5. Bone Geometry ... 55
5.1. Hip Axis Length ... 55
5.2. Cross-Sectional Geometry ... 56
6. Fracture Incidence ... 57
7. Summary ... 58
References ... 58

5. Bone Loss, Fracture Histories, and Body Composition Characteristics of Older Males

William A. Stini

1. Background ... 63
1.1. Definition of Terms ... 63
1.2. Bone Loss in Other Primates ... 64
1.3. Population Differences ... 64
2. Risk Factors ... 65
2.1. Factors Influencing Bone Turnover ... 65
2.2. Peak Bone Mass ... 66
2.3. Endocrinological Factors ... 66
2.4. Vitamin D and Vitamin D Receptors ... 67
2.5. Body Composition and Mechanical Factors ... 68
3. The Sun City/Tucson Longitudinal Study ... 69
3.1. Objectives ... 69
3.2. Subjects ... 69
3.3. Methods ... 70
3.4. Results ... 70
4. Discussion ... 80
4.1. Observed Bone Loss ... 80
4.2. Changes in Body Composition ... 81

4.3. Nutrition, Bone Density, and Prostate Cancer 83
5. Summary and Conclusions 84
References 85

6. The Histomorphometry of the Subadult Rib: Age-Associated Changes in Bone Mass and the Creation of Peak Bone Mass

Margaret Streeter and Sam D. Stout

1. Introduction 91
1.1. Intracortical Bone Remodeling in the Subadult Rib 91
1.2. Peak Bone Mass and Age-Associated Bone Loss 92
1.3. Factors Determining Peak Bone Mass 93
2. A Study of Subadult Rib Histomorphometry 94
2.1. Cross-Sectional Areas and Bone Mass 95
2.2. Intracortical Remodeling: Osteon Population Density and Osteon Size 97
3. Summary and Conclusions 97
References 99

Part III. Evolutionary Perspectives

7. An Evolutionary and Biocultural Approach to Understanding the Effects of Reproductive Factors on the Female Skeleton

Sabrina C. Agarwal and Patricia Stuart-Macadam

1. Introduction 105
2. Pregnancy 106
3. Parity 107
4. Lactation 108
5. Animal Models 110
6. Evolutionary and Historical Evidence 111
7. Discussion 113
8. Conclusions 115
References 116

8. Functional Adaptation and Fragility of the Skeleton

R. Bruce Martin

1. Introduction 121
2. Mechanisms of Functional Adaptation 122
2.1. Effector Cells 123
2.2. Sensor Cells 123
2.3. Strain and the Mechanostat 124
2.4. The Two Poles of Adaptation 125
2.4.1. Disuse: Subnormal Loading 125
2.4.2. Overuse: Supernormal Loading 126

3. Skeletal Maintenance 126
3.1. Fatigue Damage Activates Remodeling 127
3.2. Remodeling Reduces Skeletal Weight 128
3.3. Responsive vs. Permissive Remodeling 128
3.4. The Volume Effect on Strength and Fatigue Life 129
3.5. Somatic vs. Evolutionary Adaptation 130
4. Skeletal Fragility 131
4.1. The Mechanostat and Sexual Dimorphism 132
4.2. Mechanical Priorities in Male and Female Bones 133
4.3. Estrogen and the Mechanostat Set Point 133
4.4. Menopause, the Set Point, and Postmenopausal Fragility 134
5. Summary 135
Acknowledgments 136
References 136

9. Effects of Vitamin D on Bone and Natural Selection of Skin Color: How Much Vitamin D Nutrition are We Talking About?

Reinhold Vieth

1. Introduction 139
2. Skin and Vitamin D Uptake 141
2.1. Metabolism of Vitamin D 142
3. What is Lack of Vitamin D? 142
4. "Normal" Requirements for Calcium and Vitamin D 144
5. Fur-Bearing Primates Obtain Vitamin D by Mouth 145
6. Vitamin D Deficiency Affecting Genetic Selection for Lighter Skin Color 147
7. Nutritional Implications of Vitamin D in Human Biology 149
References 151

Part IV. Bone Loss and Osteoporosis in Past Populations

10. Techniques for the Investigation of Age-Related Bone Loss and Osteoporosis in Archaeological Bone

Megan B. Brickley and Sabrina C. Agarwal

1. Introduction 157
1.1. Background 158
1.2. Problems with Diagenetic Change 158
2. Visual Examination of Complete Bones 159
3. Investigations of Cortical Bone 160
3.1. Metacarpal Radiogrammetry 160
3.2. Cortical Histomorphometry 161
4. Investigations of Trabecular Bone 162
4.1. Visual Examination of Trabecular Bone Structure 162
4.2. Singh Index 163

4.3. Image Analysis of Trabecular Architecture 163
4.4. Stereometry 164
4.5. Energy Dispersive Low Angle X-Ray Scattering (EDLAXS) 165
5. Investigative Techniques that Measure Whole Bone 165
5.1. Optical/Photo Densitometry 166
5.2. Dual Energy X-Ray Absorptiometry (DEXA) 166
6. Conclusions 168
References 168

11. Differentail Diagnoses of Intravitam and Postmortem Bone Loss at the Micro-Level

Michael Schultz

1. Introduction 173
2. Methods and Techniques Used in Histological Research of Macerated Bone Specimens 173
3. Intravitam Changes 174
3.1. Primary Osteoporosis 175
3.1.1. Idiopathic Osteoporosis 175
3.1.2. Postmenopausal Osteoporosis 175
3.1.3. Senile Osteoporosis 175
3.2. Secondary Osteoporosis 177
3.2.1. Osteoporosis due to Inactivity and Immobilization 177
3.2.2. Bone Loss Caused by Inflammatory Processes 179
3.3.3. Bone Loss Caused by Tumorous Processes 179
4. Causes of Postmortem Bone Loss 180
4.1. Soil and water 180
4.2. Plant Roots 183
4.3. Fungi, Algae, Bacteria, and Protozoa 183
4.4. Arthropods and their larvae 184
5. Conclusions and Summary 186
Acknowledgments 186
References 186

12. Histomorphology, Geometry, and Mechanical Loading in Past Populations

Alexander G. Robling and Sam D. Stout

1. Introduction 189
2. Mechanobiology Methods for Preserved Skeletal Remains 190
2.1. Interpreting Preserved Evidence of Mechanical Loading History from Bone Geometry 190
2.2. Bone Microstructure and Mechanical Loading History 192
3. Application of Geometric and Histologic Biomechanical Approaches to Past Populations: The Palomans 196
3.1. Skeletal Sample 196
3.2. Methods and Findings 197
3.3. Changes through Time at Paloma 201

4. Conclusions 203
References 203

13. Bone Remodeling and Age-Associated Bone Loss in the Past: A Histomorphometric Analysis of the Imperial Roman Skeletal Population of Isola Sacra

Helen Cho and Sam D. Stout

1. Introduction 207
2. Principles and Methodology of Bone Histomorphometry 208
2.1. Cortical Bone Sample Preparation 209
2.2. An Algorithm for Estimating Bone Remodeling rates in Ancient Skeletal Samples 210
2.3. Diagenesis 211
2.4. Age-at-Death 211
3. Previous Applications of Histomorphology in Past Populations 211
3.1. African Populations 212
3.2. European Populations 212
3.3. Native American Populations 213
3.4. Other Populations 215
4. Present Study: An Example in Histomorphology and Bioarchaeology 215
4.1. Materials 215
4.2. Methods 218
4.3. Results 218
4.3.1. Cortical Area in Isola Sacra 218
4.3.2. Bone Remodeling in Isola Sacra 220
4.3.3. Comparison of Isola Sacra with Modern samples 222
4.4. Age Associated Bone Loss in the Imperial Romans 225
5. Future Directions 225
Acknowledgments 226
References 226

Index 229

Part I

Current Concepts of Bone Loss and Osteoporosis

1

New Concepts of Bone Remodeling: A Unified Spatial and Temporal Model with Physiologic and Pathophysiologic Implications

A. Michael Parfitt

1. Introduction

For many years bone physiology has been thought of in terms of two opposing but otherwise unrelated kinds of cell, often depicted as sitting on either side of a seesaw. The assumption that osteoclasts and osteoblasts are independent still dominates the field, although it was demolished over 30 years ago by Harold Frost (1973), who recognized that the production and activity of these cells were coordinated in time and space in different modes for different biological purposes, the major modes being redistribution, repair, and replacement (Table 1.1). During growth, bone is formed in one location and soon after resorbed in a location that is different relative to the increased size and altered shape of the bone, not because there is anything wrong with it, but because it is no longer needed at that location. As bones grow in length, bone formed at the junction between the growth plate and the metaphysis is resorbed at the junction between the metaphysis and the diaphysis. As bones grow in width, bone formed beneath the periosteum is resorbed at the endosteum. At these various relative locations, resorption and formation continue with only brief interruptions for extended periods; the cells are operating in the modeling mode (Parfitt, 1997). In fracture healing, damaged bone is removed and callus in the form of woven bone is laid down; the prime consideration is speed of production while the quality of the bone is of lesser importance.

Dead bone can survive for thousands of years, but living bone gradually loses mechanical competence with increasing age and must be periodically replaced by new

---

A. Michael Parfitt • Division of Endocrinology and Center for Osteoporosis and Metabolic Bone Disease, University of Arkansas for Medical Sciences

Bone Loss and Osteoporosis: An Anthropological Perspective, edited by Sabrina C. Agarwal and Sam D. Stout. Kluwer Academic/Plenum Publishers, New York, 2003.

Table 1.1. Supracellular Organization of Bone Cells

Mode	Need
Redistribution	*Equal quality* bone
(Modeling)	In a different place
Repair	*Any* bone
(Fracture callus)	In the right place
Replacement	*Better* bone
(Remodeling)	In the same place

Table 1.2. Comparison of Two Major Modes of Supracellular Organization of Bone Cells

Feature	Modeling	Remodeling
Mode	Redistribution	Replacement
Purpose	Growth	Maintenance
Context	Youth	Maturity
Sequence	F→R	A→R→F
Timing	Continuous	Cyclical
Location	Different	Same
Coupling	Systemic	Local
Balance	Net Gain	Net Loss

Note: F—formation, R—resorption, A—activation (for explanation of different definitions of this term, see text).

bone. The replacement mechanism in the adult skeleton, in which osteoclasts and osteoblasts are cooperating for a common purpose, is referred to as remodeling. The salient features of modeling and remodeling are compared in Table 1.2. In modeling, bone is first formed and then resorbed soon after, whereas in remodeling, bone is first resorbed and then replaced. Growth is continuous but remodeling occurs infrequently; episodes lasting a few months are usually separated by several years of quiescence. In both modeling and remodeling, the rates of resorption and formation are both much higher than the differences between them, but in modeling, the processes occur on different surfaces and any matching is genetic or systemic, whereas in remodeling, the processes occur on the same surface, and there is local coupling. Modeling leads to net gain in bone mass, but remodeling usually is associated with net loss.

Modeling is the principal mode of bone cell coordination in the growing skeleton and remodeling is the principal mode in the mature skeleton, but this distinction is not absolute. The formation of secondary osteons in the long bone cortices by remodeling begins during childhood, and remodeling of cancellous bone in the central skeleton goes on throughout life (Parfitt *et al.*, 2000). After completion of longitudinal growth many bones continue to enlarge very slowly, either by maintenance at a slow rate of periosteal apposition in the modeling mode, or by very slow remodeling with prolonged interruptions (Balena *et al.*, 1992). However, remodeling is primarily a phenomenon of the endosteal envelope of the mature skeleton.

2. The Purposes of Bone Remodeling

The reasons for bone replacement depend on the function of the bone that is replaced (Parfitt, 1996b). The primary function of the bone is to resist mechanical loads; such structural bones include all cortical bone and cancellous bone in the long bone metaphyses, which transmit the loads on the synovial joints to the thick cortical bone above or below. All such bones are adjacent to yellow fatty marrow, in contrast to the red hematopoietic marrow adjacent to central cancellous bone (Parfitt, 1996b). The two kinds of marrow correspond to two kinds of cancellous bones, referred to as structural and metabolic to indicate their principal but not their only function (Table 1.3); vertebral cancellous bone is load bearing, but contributes less to compressive strength than the cortical bone surrounding it (Mazess, 1990). Note especially the difference in turnover—cortical bone in the ilium has higher turnover than cancellous bone in the extremities, so that biology trumps geometry! (Parfitt, submitted.)

As structural and metabolic bone differ in their function, they also differ in their reasons for replacement (Table 1.4). Structural bone, both cortical and cancellous, like all load bearing materials, is subject to fatigue damage after a certain number of load bearing cycles (Burr *et al.*, 1997), but unlike man-made structures, it has its own mechanism of self-repair. There may also be nontargeted remodeling to maintain bone age below some upper limit, referred to here as spare, in the sense that its abrogation will not have

Table 1.3. Significance of Marrow Composition for Cancellous Bone

Feature	Yellow marrow	Red marrow
Bone type	Structural	Metabolic
Location	Peripheral	Central
Principal	Transmit loads	Calcium homeostasis
Functions	Absorb energy	Support hematopoiesis
Cellularity	Low	High
Blood flow	Low	High
Turnover	Low	High

Table 1.4. Reasons for Bone Remodeling

Structural bone (cortical, fatty cancellous)
Replace fatigue damaged bone—Targeted
Prevent bone senescence—Spare
Metabolic bone (hematopoietic cancellous)
Replace over-mineralized bone—Targeted
Preserve osteocyte viability—? Targeted
? Release of growth factors—Spare

Spare remodeling has also been referred to as redundant, surplus, stochastic, or non-targeted (Parfitt, 2002).

immediate harmful effects, whereas the abrogation of targeted remodeling may allow fatigue damage to spread and accumulate into an overt fracture (Parfitt, 2002). The reasons for the much higher turnover of metabolic cancellous bone are less well understood. The exchange of calcium ions at the bone surface, which is an essential element of plasma calcium homeostasis (Parfitt, 1993a), is impaired by the gradual enlargement of the crystals at the expense of water, and it is likely that highly mineralized bone would need to be replaced. In the ilium, osteocyte viability declines with age in interstitial bone but not in surface bone, most likely because its aging is prevented by remodeling (Qui *et al.*, submitted). Finally, the controlled release of growth factors stored in the bone may be necessary for optimum hematopoiesis.

There are several other functions of remodeling. Bone resorption increases temporarily at night to compensate for the lack of intestinal calcium absorption (Lakatos *et al.*, 1995), most likely because existing osteoclasts work a bit harder (Parfitt, 1993a), and there must be some minimum number of osteoclasts for this mechanism to work. At times of temporary increase in calcium demand during growth, pregnancy, and lactation, there is a temporary increase in cortical porosity due to increased remodeling (Parfitt, 1980). During the adolescent growth spurt, remodeling accomplishes an increase in the thickness of trabeculae (Parfitt *et al.*, 2000), an exception to the general rule that remodeling leads only to conservation or loss of bone. Remodeling discards bone made redundant by disuse (Parfitt, 1990b), and malfunction of this mechanism may be one way in which estrogen deficiency has harmful effects (Frost, 1996). Finally, remodeling participates in primary fracture healing in cortical bone, creating dowel pins between the two fragments (Schenk and Willenegger, 1967).

2.1. The Basic Multicellular Unit as the Instrument of Bone Remodeling

All remodeling is carried out by temporary anatomic structures, first identified by Frost (1969) and named by him Basic Multicellular Units (BMU), to which, in the adult noninjured skeleton, all osteoclasts and osteoblasts belong. (See also Chapter 2, this volume.) The BMU excavates and refills a tunnel through the bone (Parfitt, 1994), leaving a new osteon in its wake (Figure 1.1). At the front is a team of multinucleated osteoclasts forming the cutting cone, behind them is a capillary that brings circulating monocytes to become pre-osteoclasts (Parfitt, 1998), surrounded by loose connective tissue, and behind that successive teams of osteoblasts forming the closing cone. During its life span of many months, the BMU while traveling through the bone maintains the same spatial and temporal relationships between its constituent cells, the osteoclasts, vascular endothelial cells, stromal connective tissue cells, and osteoblasts. Trying to understand bone remodeling while ignoring the structure of the BMU is like trying to understand endochondral ossification while ignoring the spatial and temporal relationships between the cells in the growth plate.

Histologic sections most often intercept the BMU not longitudinally, as in Figure 1.1, but transversely (Figure 1.2, see color plate facing p. 6). Each osteoblast team is assembled on the cement surface within a narrow window of time and in a narrow zone between the cutting and closing cones. Each team is like a necklace one cell deep, and about two to three new teams are formed each day. Each team refills the tunnel at a single

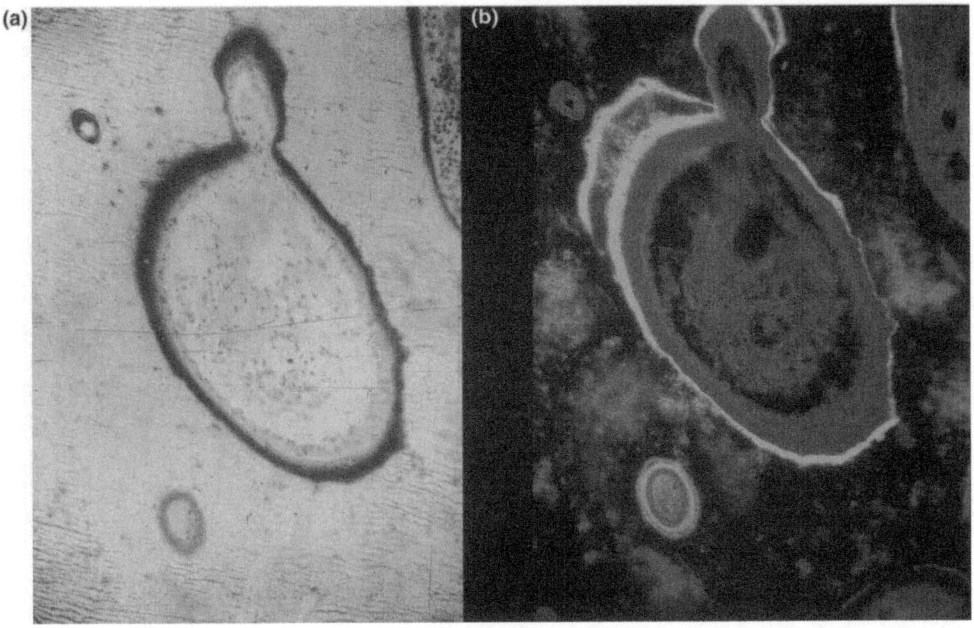

Figure 1.2. Cortical BMU in cross-section. (a) A large cavity lined by purple staining osteoid within largely unstained mineralized bone. (b) The fluorescence shows that bone formation began eccentrically, as there are two tetracycline labels in the top left corner and only one around the rest of the circumference. The osteoblasts are plump and the osteoid seen (stained purple) is wide. In the lower left is another BMU in which bone formation at this location is almost completed. The cavity is much smaller, the osteoid seam much thinner, the cells much flatter and the labels much closer together. The cutting cone of the BMU passed through the plane of section about 10 days ago in the right upper location and about 2–3 months ago in the left lower location. From the distribution of partly stained bone of low density which has been recently formed, the newer BMU has arisen adjacent to a not much older BMU in which secondary mineralization has not yet been completed, indicating a state of high bone turnover. Copyright A.M. Parfitt (2001), used with permission.

(a) (b) (c)

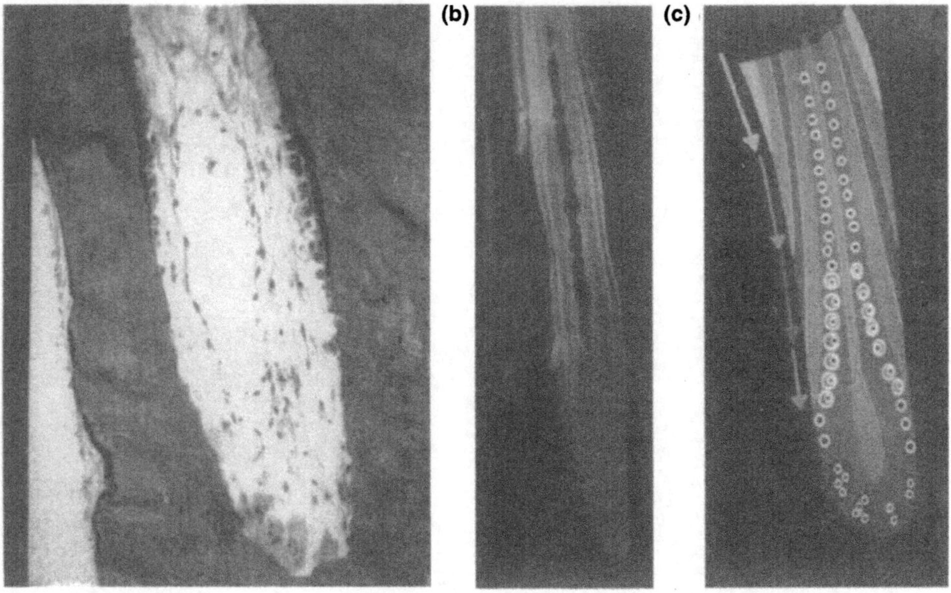

Figure 1.1. Cortical BMU in longitudinal section. (a) A typical BMU in human iliac cortical bone is shown with a team of osteoclasts at the bottom, osteoid seams (dark stain) lined with osteoblasts above, and a capillary in between. The entire structure, which is approximately 1–2 mm long and 0.2–0.4 mm wide, is traveling downward at a rate which can be measured by the longitudinal distance between the (b) tetracycline labels and which in humans is about 25 μm per day (Parfitt, 1994) (c) Schematic of coordinated movement. (b) and (c) are reproduced by courtesy of Dr. Robert Schenk.

cross-sectional location as completely as possible. New osteoblasts can join the team only while it is being assembled, not after it has begun to deposit new bone matrix (Parfitt, 1990a). As one goes further back, the teams were born earlier and so are closer to completing their task (Figure 1.1c). As it moves through tissue space, the BMU creates and leaves behind successive cross-sectional cycles of remodeling, each one slightly out of step with the one before, and at each cross-sectional location resorption moves centrifugally until the cavity is the right size, and formation moves centripetally until refilling of the cavity has been completed at that location.

Until recently it was widely believed that the three-dimensional organization of the BMU just described applied only to cortical bone, but it is now clear that a similar organization applies to cancellous bone (Parfitt, 1994). A cancellous BMU shows the same relationship between the osteoclastic cutting hemicone in front and the osteoblastic closing hemicone following behind (Figure 1.3). Such structures are rarely observed since this requires precise orientation of the randomly generated section in three orthogonal planes. However, considerable indirect evidence, reviewed in detail elsewhere (Parfitt, 1994), indicates that this is the normal, characteristic, manner of cancellous bone remodeling, referred to as hemiosteonal because the BMU excavates a trench across the surface of the bone, rather than a tunnel through the bone, leaving in its wake what may be termed, with some geometrical latitude, a hemiosteon rather than an osteon. Both osteonal and

(a)

(b)

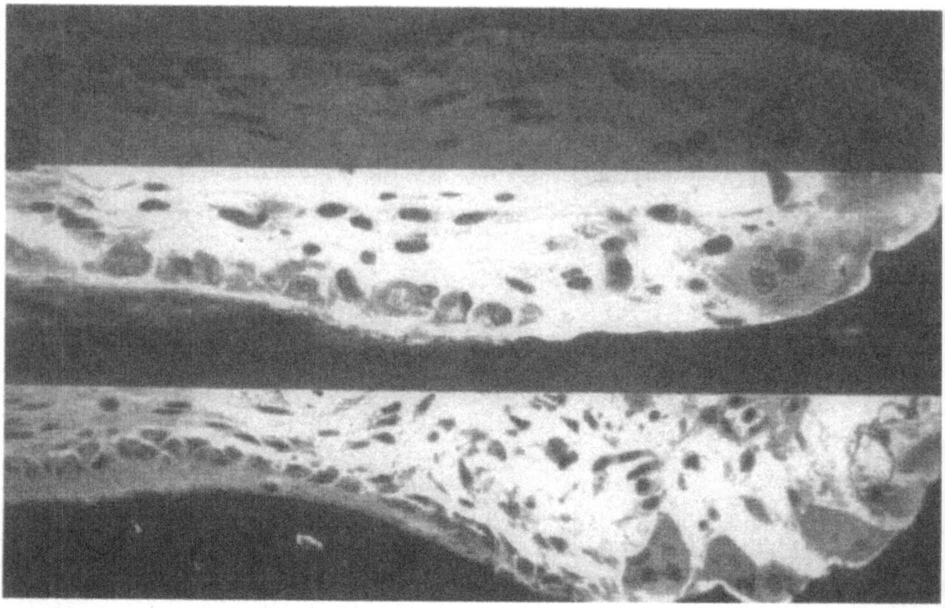

Figure 1.3. Osteonal and hemi-osteonal remodeling. (a) A representative cortical BMU in the dog, with the upper half shaded. (b) A cancellous BMU in a patient with secondary hyperparathyroidism, in which the spatial organization resembles the bottom half of (a). Although it is possible that the appearance is specific to the particular disease state in which it was observed, reasons are given in Parfitt (1994) and in the text for believing that the structure is characteristic of cancellous bone remodeling in general, but is more likely to be observed when bone turnover is very high because the necessary circumstances will otherwise rarely occur. Called to author's attention by Dr. David Baylink. Original provided by Dr. Robert Schenk, and reproduced with permission.

hemiosteonal remodeling display the same relationships between cells that are maintained during BMU progression, the same localization of osteoblast assembly to the narrow zone between the cutting and closing cones or hemicones, and the same dependence on the circulation (Parfitt, 2000, 2001), providing a source for osteoclast precursors and a conduit for ion exchange and intercellular signaling.

Frost (1983) has drawn attention to interesting analogies between the BMU and the nephron, representing the intermediary organization of their respective organs, although whole nephrons are easier to dissect from the kidney than whole BMUs are from the bone! Calcium removed from the bone by osteoclasts is analogous to calcium removed from the extracellular fluid via glomerular filtration. Calcium returned to the bone by osteoblasts is analogous to calcium returned to the extracellular fluid by tubular reabsorption. In the BMU, hydrogen ions move in the opposite direction, since they must be removed from sites of mineralization and supplied to osteoclasts to support mineral dissolution. These ionic movements are likely mediated by local microcirculation, which is probably also involved in cellular communication. In the kidney, glomerulo-tubular balance is a property of the nephron, not of the whole kidney, and in much the same way bone balance is a property of the BMU, not of the whole bone.

As the BMU exists and moves in three-dimensional space, it has a beginning (called origination), a middle (called progression), and an end (called termination). Each BMU begins on a quiescent surface in response to a target, which is a region of bone in need of replacement (Parfitt, 1996b, 2002). The site of origination must be reasonably close to a blood vessel, and in most cases it will be some distance from the target, to which the BMU must progress by excavating a trench in cancellous, or a tunnel in cortical bone. Once the target has been reached, it will take some time for the machinery which has been cranked up to be cranked down again, so that the BMU will often progress for some distance beyond the target (Figure 1.4). Such post-target progression provides a convenient basis for spare remodeling, and the distance traveled will depend on the availability of circulating osteoclast precursors, which are produced in the bone marrow under hormonal control, forming a pool whose size depends on the concentration in the blood (Parfitt, 1998). During origination, only osteoclasts are needed and during termination, only osteoblasts are needed, but during progression, which is much the longest phase, both osteoclasts and osteoblasts are needed at the same time, but at different locations.

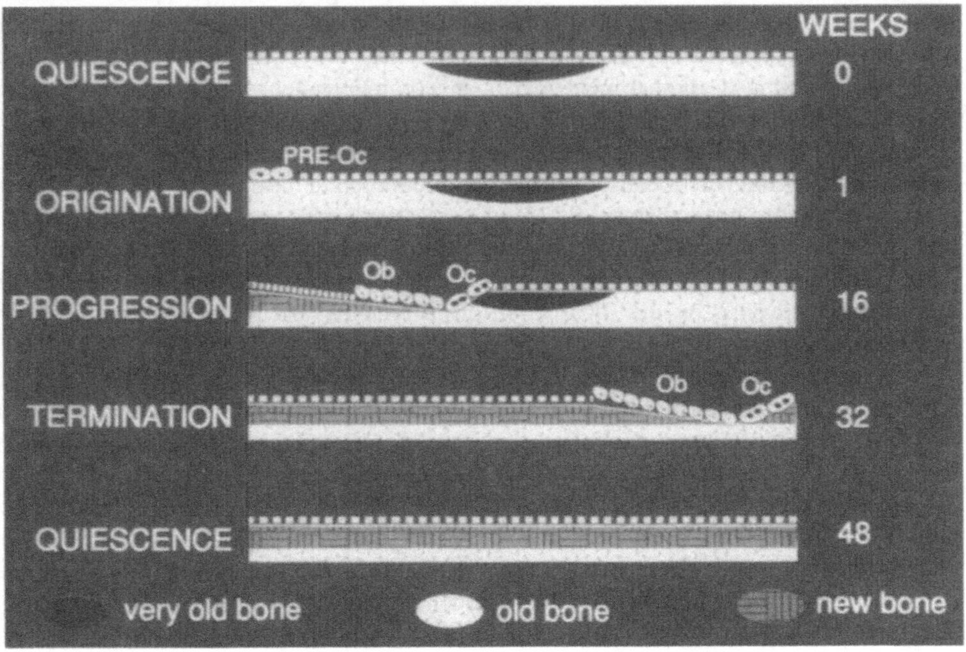

Figure 1.4. Cancellous bone remodeling. Evolution of a single BMU through successive stages. BMU is shown as traveling from left to right, excavating a trench across the surface. It originates where a blood vessel arborizes over the bone surface (location denoted by vertical line on left), and is directed to remove a region of bone that is too old to carry out its function, whether this function is primarily mechanical, as in the metaphyses of the long bones, or primarily metabolic, as in the axial skeleton (Parfitt, 1996b). The BMU progresses beyond this target as part of the stochastic or spare component of remodeling. Progression is sustained by the continued recruitment of new preosteoclasts (Pre.Oc.), which need to be precisely targeted to the apex of the cutting hemicone, adjacent to the lining cells that cover the bone that is about to be resorbed. Termination occurs when the supply of Pre.Oc. is turned off, but osteoblast recruitment continues until the trench is refilled. For further details see text. Copyright A.M. Parfitt (1995), used with permission.

How a new BMU gets started is still only dimly understood. The first step must be to recognize that some bone needs replacement. For fatigue microdamage, the necessary targeting is probably mediated by local death of osteocytes by apoptosis (Verborgt *et al.*, 2000), although the signals involved are unknown. How, or even whether, targeting is achieved in metabolic bone is unknown (Parfitt, 2002). Frost (1973) originally defined activation as a stimulus to precursor cells to proliferate. It is now often stated that the first step in remodeling is the activation of osteoclasts, but in the normal adult skeleton there are no osteoclasts waiting to be activated. Bone lining cells must be involved in site selection and it is these cells that are activated, to remove the thin endosteal membrane that normally separates them from the mineralized bone, and to retract, providing a foothold for the future BMU (Parfitt, 1994). A new vessel then grows toward the site to allow access to circulating mononuclear precursors (Parfitt, 1998), which are presumably attracted by chemotaxis and fuse to form the first new osteoclasts (Parfitt *et al.*, 1996), which begin resorbing in the right direction toward the target.

In order for a BMU to progress through the bone or across the surface of the bone, several conditions must be satisfied. First, access for circulating preosteoclasts must be maintained. In cortical bone this is achieved by neoangiogenesis, the central capillary keeping up with the cutting cone (Parfitt, 2000), but in cancellous bone it is more likely achieved by vasculogenic mimicry, by lining cells that persist as a canopy over the remodeling site, forming a compartment that is in communication with a marrow sinusoid (Parfitt, 2001). Second, signals for the arrival of new preosteoclasts must persist, analogous to the continued recruitment of leukocytes to sites of inflammation (Parfitt *et al.*, 1996). Third, the precursor cells that leave the circulation to form new osteoclasts must be replaced from the bone marrow. If all of these conditions are met, new transversely oriented cycles of remodeling will continue to be generated. The number of such cycles, corresponding to the histomorphometric index called activation frequency, determines the total distance traveled by the BMU both toward and beyond its target (Parfitt, 1996b; Parfitt *et al.*, 1996).

Activation frequency, which is a two-dimensional concept, is the best histologic index of the overall intensity of bone remodeling, but it is not a measure of the birth rate of new BMU, which is a three-dimensional concept. For example, one BMU that progresses for nine units of distance will have exactly the same effect on all histologic, radiokinetic, and biochemical indices of bone turnover as three BMUs that each progress for only three units of distance (Parfitt, 1996b; Parfitt *et al.*, 1996), but the biological significance will be quite different. The former represents a low demand for remodeling with a large surplus component, the latter a high demand for remodeling that is efficiently satisfied. Endocrine abnormalities such as estrogen deficiency, or parathyroid or thyroid hormone excess, that increase the availability of osteoclasts can increase the extent of post-target progression without increasing BMU origination, if the demand for remodeling has not changed (Parfitt, 1996a). Hormones are indifferent to bone structure and have no means of specifying where a new BMU will be formed.

Bone remodeling resembles hematopoiesis in several respects. Both are examples of bone marrow cell renewal, in which changes in the number of functioning cells are more important than changes in individual cell activity. In both, the executive cells have a short life span and need to be continually replaced. In both, a basal rate of cell production can be increased on demand; in both, cell number depends not only on cell production but on the timing of cell death, which determines cell life span; and in both, dysregulation of cell number will lead to disease. The life span of the BMU comprising separate stages of origination, progression, and termination, is measured in months, but the life span of osteoblasts while they are making bone is measured in weeks, and the life span of osteoclast nuclei is measured in days. All cells that originate in the marrow die after a rather short time, and all osteoclasts die by apoptosis. (Parfitt *et al.*, 1996), while osteoblasts, derived from local stromal cells, have a more complex fate. A high proportion die fairly soon by apoptosis, a few become lining cells, and many become osteocytes (Parfitt, 1990a). These may survive for decades, but eventually will either be removed as the bone is remodeled or themselves die by apoptosis (Qui *et al.*, submitted).

3. Disordered Remodeling and Age-Related Bone Loss

Age-related bone loss is a near universal characteristic of the human species, from which no group is known to be exempt. But whatever the proximate causes such as physical inactivity, altered nutrition, or sex hormone deficiency, and whatever the genetic susceptibilities or molecular mechanisms, all bone loss must be accountable in terms of disordered remodeling. But first the distinction between its reversible and irreversible components must be clarified.

Reversible bone loss is an inevitable consequence of an increase in bone remodeling, most clearly exemplified by the changes in rib cortical porosity during the antler growth cycle in deer, referred to as cyclic physiologic osteoporosis (Banks *et al.*, 1968; Parfitt, 1981). Some of the calcium needed for the antlers is borrowed from the skeleton by starting up a large number of new BMUs, and when they have run their course, the debt is fully repaid. The aggregate volume of all the new holes is the remodeling space, but the reversible deficit also includes unmineralized bone matrix or osteoid, which has a short life span, and incompletely mineralized matrix in young recently formed bone, which has a long life span (Parfitt, 1980). Because completion of mineralization takes a long time, mineral density increases steadily with the age of the bone. Increased remodeling reduces mean bone age and mean mineral density (Figure 1.2) with converse changes when normal remodeling is restored. All three components of the reversible deficit contribute to temporary calcium needs during growth, pregnancy, and lactation (Parfitt, 1981).

It is useful to consider the mechanisms of irreversible bone loss in terms of the sequential changes at a single cross-sectional location that are initiated by a BMU as it travels perpendicular to the plane of section, even though this is an inaccurate description of the bone remodeling process in three-dimensions (Figure 1.5). The cycle begins with a quiescent surface covered by flat lining cells, continues with activation of the lining cells and recruitment of preosteoclasts, resorption to a certain depth, the reversal phase after the termination of resorption, osteoblast recruitment and bone formation, and in the ideal situation in a young healthy adult, complete refilling of the cavity and restoration of the bone surface to its previous location (Parfitt, 1993b). Because of the perpendicular movement of the bone surface, I call this the down and up model. In terms of this model, all irreversible bone loss is the result of focal imbalance between the depth of a resorption cavity and the depth of the new bone deposited within the cavity, which corresponds to the histologic measurement of wall thickness (Figure 1.6). This focal imbalance can result either because

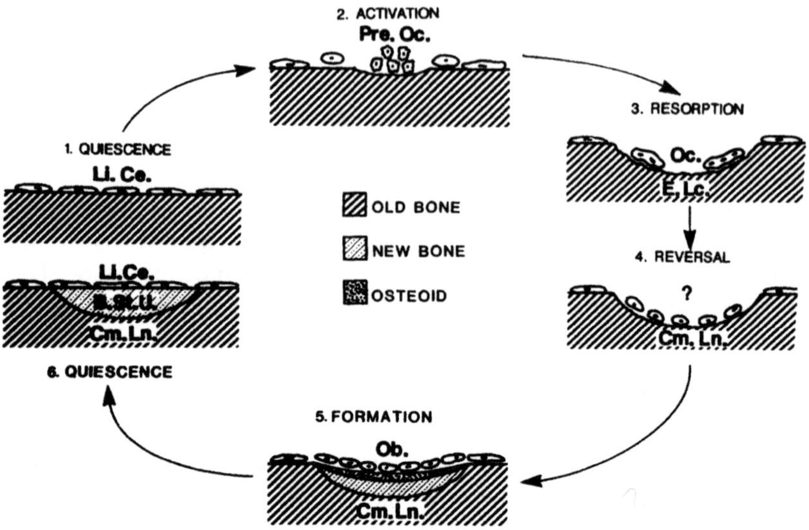

Figure 1.5. Diagrammatic representation of the remodeling cycle in cancellous bone. Successive stages of quiescence, activation, resorption, reversal, formation, and back to quiescence at a single cross-sectional location generated by the movement of the BMU perpendicular to the plane of section are depicted, the so-called down and up model. Li.Ce. = lining cell; Pre.Oc. = preosteoclast; Oc. = osteoclast; E.Lc. = eroded lacuna; Cm.Ln. = cement line; Ob. = osteoblast; B.St.U. = bone structural unit (hemiosteon). Refilling is assumed to be complete, and bone marrow lying above the lining cells is omitted for clarity. Reproduced from Parfitt (1993b) with permission of the publisher.

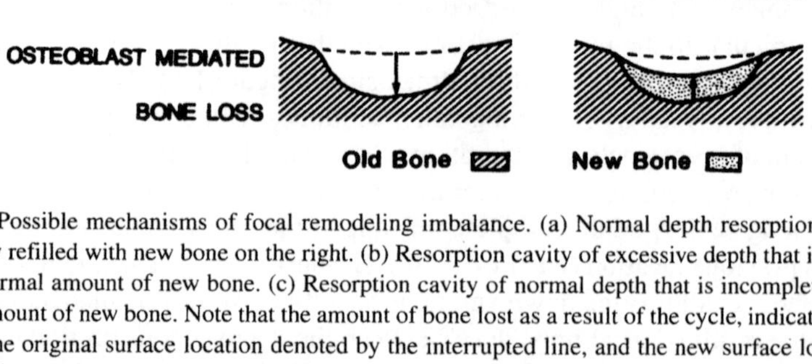

Figure 1.6. Possible mechanisms of focal remodeling imbalance. (a) Normal depth resorption cavity on the left, completely refilled with new bone on the right. (b) Resorption cavity of excessive depth that is incompletely refilled by a normal amount of new bone. (c) Resorption cavity of normal depth that is incompletely refilled by a subnormal amount of new bone. Note that the amount of bone lost as a result of the cycle, indicated by the clear area between the original surface location denoted by the interrupted line, and the new surface location, can be the same even though the cellular mechanism is quite different. Modified from Parfitt (1988) with permission of the publisher.

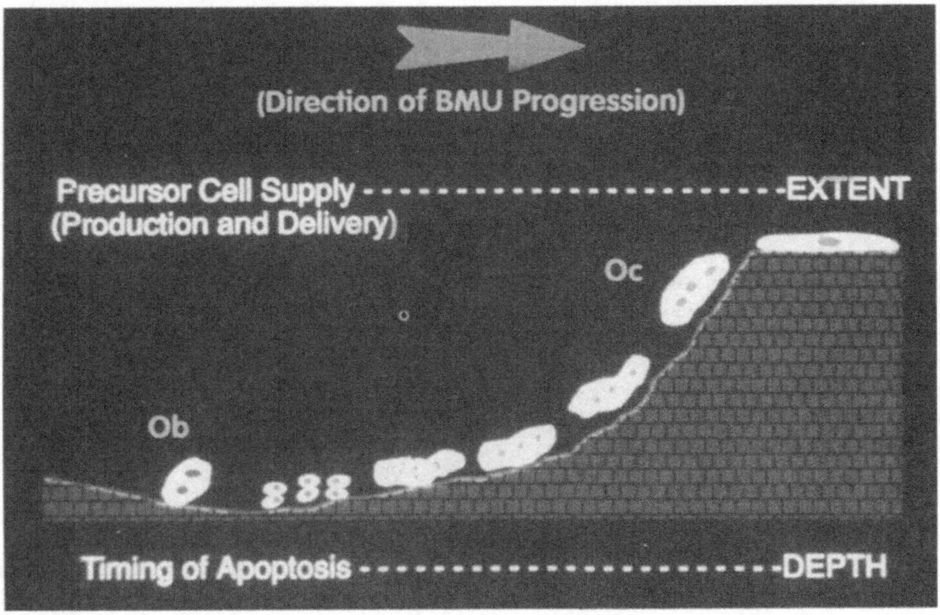

Figure 1.7. Two aspects of bone resorption. A BMU is traveling across the cancellous surface from left to right. At the apex, the youngest osteoclast abuts the lining cell covering the surface that is about to be resorbed. The *extent* of resorption in the direction of progression depends on maintaining the supply of mononuclear osteoclast precursors, which are produced in the bone marrow and delivered to the resorption site by the circulation. The depth of resorption, which determines the magnitude of the task set for the osteoblasts, depends on the timing of apoptosis. Copyright A.M. Parfitt (2001), used with permission.

the cavity is too deep or because the new bone is too shallow. The bone loss is irreversible because each cycle of remodeling, representing events within a two-dimensional slice of bone generated by the movement of the BMU in three dimensions, constitutes a transaction that once completed cannot be revoked.

Due to the three-dimensional organization of the BMU, bone resorption can be partitioned into horizontal and vertical components (Figure 1.7). The horizontal component is the distance traveled by the BMU across the surface, which depends on the supply of osteoclast precursor cells, both production in the marrow and delivery by the circulation. The vertical component is the depth of the cavity, of which the main determinant is the timing of osteoclast apoptosis. Earlier apoptosis means a shallower cavity, later apoptosis a deeper cavity, with consequent perforation of trabecular plates and cancellization of the inner third of the cortex (Parfitt, 1988). The timing of apoptosis is independent of birth rate, since delayed apoptosis can occur in the early stages of estrogen deficiency, in which osteoclast production is increased (Manolagas, 2000) or in glucocorticoid excess, in which it is decreased (Weinstein *et al.*, 1998). Unlike bone resorption, bone formation has only a vertical component, but like bone resorption, it is influenced by cell death as well as by cell birth. At each cross-sectional location, new osteoblasts assemble on the cement surface at the floor of the resorption cavity. They are columnar in shape and closely packed, and become progressively fewer, flatter, and less active until those remaining

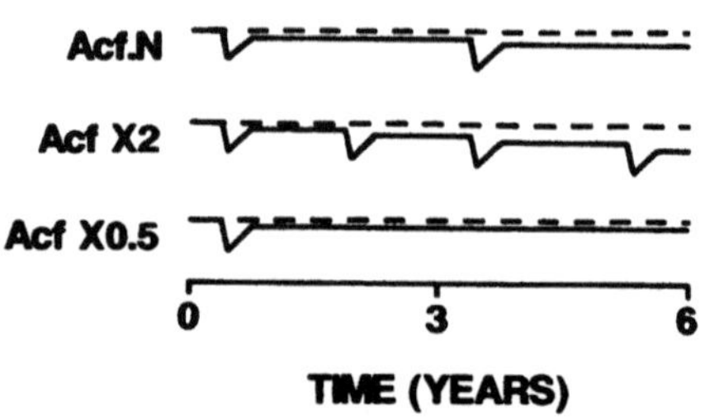

Figure 1.8. Remodeling determinants of bone loss. (a) In normal adult human cancellous bone, one cycle occurs about once every 3 years. (b) If the activation frequency is doubled, there will be four cycles in 6 years instead of two, and (c) if it is halved, there will be only one cycle, with corresponding differences in the cumulative bone loss, indicated by the distances between the interrupted and solid lines after 6 years, even if the amount lost in each cycle remains constant. Differences in the magnitude of focal imbalance will lead to proportional differences in the rate of bone loss if there is no change in activation frequency. Copyright A.M. Parfitt (2001), used with permission.

become lining cells (Figure 1.2). In the elderly, each team of osteoblasts on the cancellous surface makes less bone, partly because there are fewer initial members of the team and partly because some die sooner, which leads to trabecular and cortical thinning (Parfitt, 1988). This can be the result of physical inactivity, estrogen deficiency, glucocorticoid excess, or aging per se.

All bone loss occurs from an internal surface, one of the three subdivisions of the endosteal envelope, in contrast to the periosteal envelope which may slowly gain bone, so that the decline in total bone mass is always smaller than the amount lost (Duan *et al.*, 2001). The absolute rate of bone loss from a surface, expressed as volume of bone per unit surface per unit time, depends on the average amount lost in each cycle of remodeling and how often the cycles occur (Figure 1.8), which is why there is a general relationship between the rate of bone loss and the rate of bone turnover (Garnero and Delmas, 2001). The rate of loss expressed as a percentage of the initial amount also depends on the surface-to-volume ratio, which is why the relative rate is slower in cortical than in cancellous bone, even though the absolute amount lost is greater (Han *et al.*, 1996). The absolute amount lost from a *bone* depends also on the absolute extent of surface, which declines with age in cancellous bone because whole structural elements are removed, and increases with age in cortical bone because subendocortical cavities become larger (Martin, 1972; Parfitt, 1988), which is why the fractional rate of loss tends to fall with age in cancellous bone but may increase with age in cortical bone (Ensrud *et al.*, 1995).

A remarkable feature of age-related bone loss is its universality, affecting not only almost every person, but almost every bone. Although different skeletal sites may lose bone at different rates in the short term, the wider the age range over which the data collected, the more similar the rates become. For both central and peripheral sites, comprising various proportions of cortical and cancellous bone, the long-term rates of bone loss measured cross-sectionally are in the range of 1–1.5%/y (Parfitt, 1996b). Most bone lost with age is cortical and cortical thinning is mainly the result of increased resorption depth (Parfitt, 1990c; Han *et al.*, 1997), which is the two-dimensional reflection of deeper penetration by endocortical BMUs. Because the rates of fractional loss are so similar, the increase in resorption depth at different sites must be inversely related to the customary rate of turnover and positively related to the usual thickness of cortical bone at each site (Parfitt, 1996b). When bone loss is both generalized and sustained, as in normal aging, it appears that resorption depth at different sites increases to the extent necessary to bring about much the same rates of fractional bone loss, and to adjust for differences in bone turnover contingent on differences in marrow composition and for differences in local bone structure and geometry (Parfitt, 1996b). The only conceivable kind of explanation for such a phenomenon is biomechanical.

All mechanical influences on bone remodeling are mediated by strain, the technical term for relative deformation of a structural material as the result of load bearing. Similar fractional rates of bone loss throughout the skeleton will produce similar proportional changes in the strains that occur in different bones as the result of the same pattern and intensity of physical activity. The recruitment and activity of osteoclasts and osteoblasts are orchestrated by the mechanostat in such a way that strain is maintained within an acceptable range (Frost, 1996). As a result of the sedentary lifestyle made possible by economic development, aging is in most persons accompanied by a progressive reduction in physical activity and muscle strength, of earlier onset and greater severity than is biologically mandated (Frost, 1997). The risk of fracture should not be increased, as the reduced bone mass would remain appropriate to the reduced level of activity, but this does not take into account the age-related increase in the liability to falls, to which the mechanostat is blind. It this were the sole explanation for age-related bone loss, its magnitude should have been less in more physically active populations, but perhaps the mechanostat is reset, so that the bones respond not to actual but to erroneously perceived disuse (Frost, 1996), either because of estrogen deficiency, or as a consequence of the aging process itself (Parfitt, 1996b).

References

Balena, R., Shih, M.-S., and Parfitt, A.M. (1992). Bone resorption and formation on the periosteal envelope of the ilium: A histomorphometric study in healthy women. *J. Bone Miner. Res.*, **7**, 1475–1482.

Banks, W.J., Epling, G.P., Kainer, R.A., and Davis, R.W. (1968). Antler growth and osteoporosis. I. Morphological and morphometric changes in the costal compacta during the antler growth cycle. *Anatom. Record.*, **162**, 387–398.

Burr, D.B., Forwood, M.R., Fyhrie, D.P., Martin, R.B., Schaffler, M.B., and Turner, C.H. (1997). Bone microdamage and skeletal fragility in osteoporotic and stress fractures. *J. Bone Miner. Res.*, **12**, 6–15.

Duan, Y., Turner, C.H., Kim, B.T., and Seeman, E. (2001). Sexual dimorphism in vertebral fragility is more the result of gender differences in age-related bone gain than bone loss. *Bone Miner. Res.*, **16**, 2267–2275.

Ensrud, K.E., Palermo, L., Black, D.M., Cauley, J., Jergas, M., Orwoll, E.S., Nevin, M.C., Fox, K.M., and Cummings, S.R. (1995). Hip and calcaneal bone loss increase with advancing age: Longitudinal results from the study of osteoporotic fractures. *J. Bone Miner. Res.*, **10**, 1778–1787.

Frost, H.M. (1969). Tetracycline-based histological analysis of bone remodeling. *Calc. Tiss. Res.*, **3**, 211–237.

Frost, H.M. (1973). *Remodeling and its Relationship to Metabolic Bone Diseases*. Springfield: Charles C. Thomas.

Frost, H.M. (1983). The skeletal intermediary organization. *Metab. Bone Dis. Rel. Res.*, **4**, 281–290.

Frost, H.M. (1996). Perspectives: A proposed general model of the "mechanostat." *Anatom. Record*, **244**, 139–147.

Frost, H.M. (1997). On our age-related bone loss: Insights from a new paradigm. *J. Bone Miner. Res.*, **12**, 1539–1546.

Garnero, P. and Delmas, P.D. (2001). Biochemical markers of bone turnover in osteoporosis. In R. Marcus, D. Feldman, and J. Kelsey (eds), *Osteoporosis*, 2nd edn, Academic Press, New York, pp. 459–477.

Han, Z.-H., Palnitkar, S., Rao, D.S., Nelson, D., and Parfitt, A.M. (1996). Effect of ethnicity and age or menopause on the structure and geometry of iliac bone. *J. Bone Miner. Res.*, **11**, 1967–1975.

Han, Z.-H., Palnitkar, S., Rao, D.S., Sudhaker, Nelson, D., and Parfitt, A.M. (1997). Effects of ethnicity and age or menopause on the remodeling and turnover of iliac bone: Implications for mechanisms of bone loss *J. Bone Miner. Res.*, **12**, 498–508.

Lakatos, P., Blumsohn, A., Eastell, R., Tarjan, G., Shinoda, H., and Stern, P.H. (1995). Circadian rhythm of in vitro bone-resorbing activity in human serum. *J. Clin. Endo. Metab.*, **80**, 3185–3190.

Manolagas, S.C. (2000). Birth and death of bone cells: Basic regulatory mechanisms and implications for the pathogenesis and treatment of osteoporosis. *Endo. Rev.*, **21**, 115–137.

Martin, R.B. (1972). The effects of geometric feedback in the development of osteoporosis. *J. Biomech.*, **5** 447–455.

Mazess, R.B. (1990). Fracture risk: A role for compact bone. *Calcif. Tissue Int.*, **47**, 191–193.

Parfitt, A.M. (1980). Morphologic basis of bone mineral measurements. Transient and steady state effects of treatment in osteoporosis (Editorial). *Miner. Electrolyte Metab.*, **4**, 273–287.

Parfitt, A.M. (1981). Integration of skeletal and mineral homeostasis. In H.F. Deluca, H.M. Frost, W. Jee C. Johnston, and A.M. Parfitt (eds), *Osteoporosis: Recent Advances in Pathogenesis and Treatment* University Park Press, Baltimore, pp. 115–126.

Parfitt, A.M. (1988). Bone remodeling: Relationship to the amount and structure of bone and the pathogenesis and prevention of fractures. In B.L. Riggs and L.J. Melton (eds), *Osteoporosis-Etiology, Diagnosis and Management*. Raven Press, New York, pp. 45–94.

Parfitt, A.M. (1990a). Bone-forming cells in clinical conditions. In B.K. Hall (ed.), *Bone: A Treatise*, Vol. 1, Telford Press, Caldwell, NJ, pp. 351–429.

Parfitt, A.M. (1990b). Pharmacologic manipulation of bone remodelling and calcium homeostasis. In J.A. Kanis (ed.), *Progress in Basic and Clinical Pharmacology, Vol. 4, Calcium Metabolism*. Karger, Basel, pp. 1–27.

Parfitt, A.M. (1990c). The three organizational levels of bone remodeling: Implications for the interpretation of biochemical markers and the mechanisms of bone loss. In C. Christiansen and K. Overgaard (eds), *Osteoporosis. Proc. 3rd Int. Symp.* Osteopress ApS, Denmark, pp. 429–434.

Parfitt, A.M. (1993a). Calcium homeostasis. In T.J. Martin (ed.), *Handbook of Experimental Pharmacology*, Vol. 107. Springer-Verlag, Heidelberg, pp. 1–65.

Parfitt, A.M. (1993b). Morphometry of bone resorption: Introduction and overview. *Bone*, **14**, 435–441.

Parfitt, A.M. (1994). Osteonal and hemi-osteonal remodeling: The spatial and temporal framework for signal traffic in adult human bone. *J. Cell. Biochem.*, **55**, 273–286.

Parfitt, A.M. (1996a). Hormonal influences on bone remodeling and bone loss—application to the management of primary hyperparathyroidism. *Ann. Intern. Med.*, **125**, 413–415.

Parfitt, A.M. (1996b). Skeletal heterogeneity and the purposes of bone remodeling: Implications for the understanding of osteoporosis. In R. Marcus, D. Feldman, and J. Kelsey (eds), *Osteoporosis*. Academic Press, San Diego, pp. 315–329.

Parfitt, A.M. (1997). Genetic effects on bone mass and turnover-relevance to black/white differences. *J. Amer. Coll. Nutr.*, **16**, 325–333.

Parfitt, A.M. (1998). Mini-review—osteoclast precursors as leucocytes: Importance of the area code. *Bone*, **23**, 491–494.

Parfitt, A.M. (2000). Mini-review—the mechanism of coupling—A role for the vasculature. *Bone*, **26**, 319–323.

Parfitt, A.M. (2001). The bone remodeling compartment: A circulatory function for bone lining cells. *J. Bone Miner. Res.*, **16**, 1583–1585.

Parfitt, A.M. (2002). Targeted and non-targeted bone remodeling: Relationship to BMU origination and progression. *Bone*, **30**, 1, 5–7.

Parfitt, A.M. (2002). Misconceptions (2): Turnover is always higher in cancellous than in cortical bone. *Bone*, **30**, 6, 807–809.

Parfitt, A.M., Mundy, G.R., Roodman, G.D., Hughes, D.E., and Boyce, B. (1996). A new model for the regulation of bone resorption, with particular reference to the effects of bisphosphonates. *J. Bone Miner. Res.*, **11**, 150–159.

Parfitt, A.M., Travers, R., Rauch, F., and Glorieux, F.H. (2000). Structural and cellular changes during bone growth in healthy children. *Bone*, **27**, 487–494.

Qui, S., Rao, D.S., Palnitkar, S., and Parfitt, A.M. (2002). Age and distance from the surface but not menopause reduce osteocyte density in human iliac cancellous bone. *Bone*, **31**, 2, 313–318.

Schenk, R. and Willenegger, H. (1967). Morphological findings in primary fracture healing. *Symp. Biol. Hung.*, **7**, 75–86.

Verborgt, O., Gibson, G.J., and Schaffler, M.B. (2000). Loss of osteocyte integrity in association with microdamage and bone remodeling after fatigue in vivo. *J. Bone Miner. Res.*, **15**, 60–67.

Weinstein, R.S., Jilka, R.J., Parfitt, A.M., and Manolagas, S.C. (1998). Inhibition of osteoblastogenesis and promotion of apoptosis of osteoblasts and osteocytes by glucocorticoids. Potential mechanisms of their deleterious effects on bone. *J. Clin. Invest.*, **102**, 274–282.

2

On Changing Views about Age-Related Bone Loss

Harold M. Frost

"...between muscle and bone there can be no change in the one but it is correlated with changes in the other...." (D'Arcy Thompson, 1942).

1. Introduction

Age-related bone loss interests anthropologists and physiologists as well as gerontologists and clinicians concerned with "osteoporosis." Changing views about the nature and causes of bone loss depend mainly on adding later evidence and ideas to a 1960 paradigm of skeletal physiology. *Ca* 1995 those additions led to a new paradigm of skeletal physiology, the Utah paradigm, of which it was recently said, "*all musculoskeletal biologists should be aware of the Utah paradigm of skeletal physiology*" (Jee and Yao, 2001).

This chapter shares with readers some evidence and concepts on which the Utah paradigm's alternative view of the nature and causes of age-related bone loss stand. It is concerned with what facts mean more than their validity, which is not in serious dispute. Therefore it will merely state those facts on which the synthesis presented in the chapter depends, which would seem to fit Schermer's statement (2001) that "*...facts...must be interpreted through the colored lenses of ideas...*," as well as related statements by Evans (1987), Gorski (1997), Mayr (1961), and Polanyi (1968). This chapter concerns the physiology of mammalian load-bearing bones with an emphasis on lamellar bone and humans. It does not concern problems associated with longitudinal bone growth, neoplasms, trauma, and infections. It includes a brief Glossary.

1.1. On the Two Paradigms

Because the past can help to understand the present (deMenocal, 2001) a brief review of the Utah paradigm's origins follows.

Harold M. Frost • Department of Orthopaedic Surgery, Southern Colarado Clinic.

Bone Loss and Osteoporosis: An Anthropological Perspective, edited by Sabrina C. Agarwal and Sam D. Stout. Kluwer Academic/Plenum Publishers, New York, 2003.

1.1.1. The 1960 Paradigm (Luck, 1950; Weinmann and Sicher, 1955; McLean and Urist, 1961; Putschar, 1960)

This paradigm began to gel *ca* 1900 when it was already known that osteoblasts make bone and osteoclasts resorb it (Lewis, 1906). However no tissue-level functions in bone were recognized as such before 1963, which helps to explain the development by 1960 of five erroneous assumptions about bone physiology. These assumptions were not consciously made, and thus not verbalized or printed. The first is that osteoblasts and osteoclasts (bone's "effector cells") worked and were controlled independently of each other. As a result of this assumption, it was believed that continually stimulating only osteoclasts, or continually depressing only osteoblasts, would cause continually progressing bone loss and decreasing whole-bone strength, and thus a progressing osteopenia. It was also assumed that bone lacked important tissue-level mechanisms and functions, and that mechanical factors and muscle had little or no important effects on whole-bone strength and bone "mass." And finally, after birth, chiefly genetic and humoral factors controlled bone's effector cells and their effects on bone strength, bone loss, and the bone bank.

Those hidden assumptions went wholly unchallenged before 1964. They still linger (Favus, 1999) and led to the following assumptions relating to age-related bone loss: (a) Excessive osteoclastic activity, or depressed osteoblastic activity, or some combination of those supposedly independently working and controlled features, caused it without any tissue-level intermediary. (b) Chiefly genetic and/or humoral effects and some effects of aging all exerted directly on osteoblasts or/and osteoclasts, caused it. (c) Only increased osteoblastic activity could increase, and only increased osteoclastic activity could reduce, the bone bank. (Here and below, bone bank is used in place of the term bone mass.) (d) No nephron-equivalent mechanisms and functions were recognized. (e) Biomechanics and muscle contributed little or nothing to the cause of age-related bone loss. (f) Evaluating the bone bank evaluated bone health too (Kanis, 1994).

1.1.2. The Utah Paradigm (Jee, 1995, 2000, 2001a,b; Takahashi, 1995; Schönau, 1996; Martin *et al.*, 1998; Frost, 2000a,b, 2001a,b)

Supplementing the 1960 paradigm with evidence produced or recognized after 1960, along with newer meanings inferred from accumulated evidence, led to the Utah paradigm. It gelled mainly at the University of Utah's Hard Tissue Workshops (Jee, 2001), and also includes all evidence on which the 1960 paradigm stood, but it rejects the latter's false hidden assumptions. While the Utah paradigm concerns cartilage, joints, ligaments and tendons, as well as bone and bones, its features that concern age-related bone loss follow.

Similar to the livers and kidneys, bones do have tissue-level nephron-equivalent mechanisms (Frost, 2000a). These include bone *modeling* by separate formation and resorption drifts (Figure 2.1), and bone *remodeling* by BMUs (Basic Multicellular Units; Figure 2.2) (Jee, 1989).

Each mechanism uses both osteoblasts and osteoclasts to do its work. At present histologists view them as the same kinds of cells in each mechanism (Jee, 1989). Yet while the blood carries the same humoral agents to all effector cells in bones, and while all those

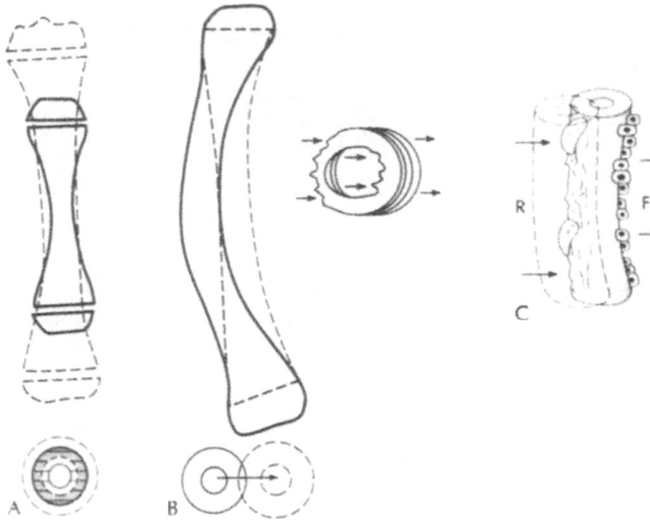

Figure 2.1. Bone modeling by drifts. (A) diagrams an infant's long bone with its original size and shape in solid line. To keep its shape as it grows in length and diameter, drifts move its surfaces in tissue space as the dashed lines suggest. *Formation drifts* make and control new osteoblasts to build some surfaces up. *Resorption drifts* make and control new osteoclasts to remove bone from other surfaces. (B) A different drift pattern can correct the fracture malunion in a child shown in solid line. The cross section view to the right shows the endocortical as well as the periosteal drifts that do that. (C) shows how the drifts in (B) would move the whole segment to the right. Changing the bone architecture in that way reduces the bone's bending moments. Drifts are created when and where they are needed, and include capillaries, precursor and "supporting" cells, and some leukocytes. They are multicellular entities in the same sense as renal nephrons (reproduced by permission: Frost, H.M. (1997). Strain and other mechanical influences on bone strength and maintenance. *Current Opinion in Orthopaedics* **8**, 60–70).

cells have the same genome, in the same bone at the same time the osteoblastic and osteoclastic activities associated with modeling can decrease or stop, while those associated with BMU-based remodeling can increase (Jee and Li, 1990; Li *et al.*, 1990; Jee *et al.*, 1991; Li and Jee, 1991; Frost, 1992; Chen *et al.*, 1995; Jee, 1995; Yeh *et al.*, 1995).

Bone modeling (not osteoblasts alone) provides nature's chief mechanism for increasing whole-bone strength and the bone bank. Similarly, it is the disuse-mode remodeling described below (not osteoclasts alone) that provides nature's chief way to reduce that strength and the bone bank. Seldom if ever does either mechanism provide the other's function.

Strain-dependent signals caused by mechanical loads on bones help to control those modeling and remodeling functions (Martin *et al.*, 1998; Martin, 2000). Where strains exceed a range called the *modeling threshold*, modeling turns on to increase local bone strength. Otherwise mechanically-controlled modeling stays off.

BMU-based remodeling can function in two modes. In its "conservation mode" *completed* BMUs make and resorb equal amounts of bone, which does not cause permanent bone gain or loss. But when bone strains stay below a lower range called the *remodeling threshold*, "disuse-mode" remodeling usually turns on. In this mode completed BMUs make less bone than they resorb, resulting in permanent bone losses. However,

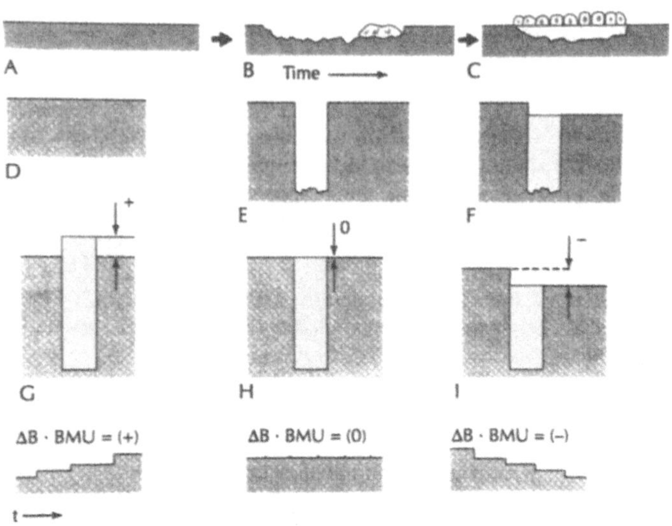

Figure 2.2. Bone remodeling BMUs. Top row: An activation event on a bone surface at (A) causes a packet of bone resorption at (B), and then replacement of the resorbed bone by osteoblasts at (C) on the right. The BMU makes and controls the new osteoclasts and osteoblasts that do this. *Second row*: This emphasizes the *amounts* of bone resorbed (E) and formed (F) by *completed* BMUs. *Third row*: In these "BMU graphs" (after the author) (G) shows a small excess of formation over resorption. (H) shows equalized resorption and formation as on haversian surfaces and in "conservation-mode" remodeling. (I) shows a net deficit of formation, as in "disuse-mode" remodeling of endocortical and trabecular bone. *Bottom row*: These "stair graphs" (after P.J. Meunier) show the effects of a series of BMUs of the kind immediately above on the local bone "bank." BMUs are created when and where they are needed, and include a capillary, precursor and "supporting" cells, and some leukocytes. They are multicellular entities in the same sense as renal nephrons (reproduced by permission: Frost, H.M. (1997). Strain and other mechanical influences on bone strength and maintenance. *Current Opinion in Orthopaedics* **8**, 60–70).

disuse-mode bone remodeling only affects bone touching or close to marrow, so the resulting permanent bone losses mainly affect trabecular and endocortical bone (Jee and Li, 1990; Li *et al.*, 1990; Jee *et al.*, 1991; Li and Jee, 1991; Frost, 1966). When strains exceed the remodeling threshold, mechanically-controlled remodeling begins to switch to its conservation mode. The increased remodeling space that accompanies increased bone turnover causes a transient or temporary instead of a permanent bone loss (Jaworski, 1984; Heaney, 1994).

The different modeling and remodeling strain thresholds make the largest bone strains, and thus the largest bone loads, control mechanical influences on bone modeling and remodeling, whole-bone strength, and the bone bank (Figure 2.3). Because a bone's largest voluntary loads and strains come from muscle forces instead of body weight (Crowninshield *et al.*, 1978; Currey, 1984; Burr, 1997; Martin *et al.*, 1998), *muscle strength* should and does strongly influence postnatal whole-bone strength and the bone bank (Schiessl *et al.*, 1998a; 1999; Schiessl and Willnecker, 1998; Heinonen *et al.*, 2000; Schönau *et al.*, 2000, 2001; Beck *et al.*, 2001; Hasegawa *et al.*, 2001). The relative importance of strain magnitude, rate, kind, frequency, accumulated numbers, and duration to this process is under study (Martin *et al.*, 1998; Martin, 2000; Robling *et al.*, 2001); so are the involved signaling mechanisms (Marotti, 2000).

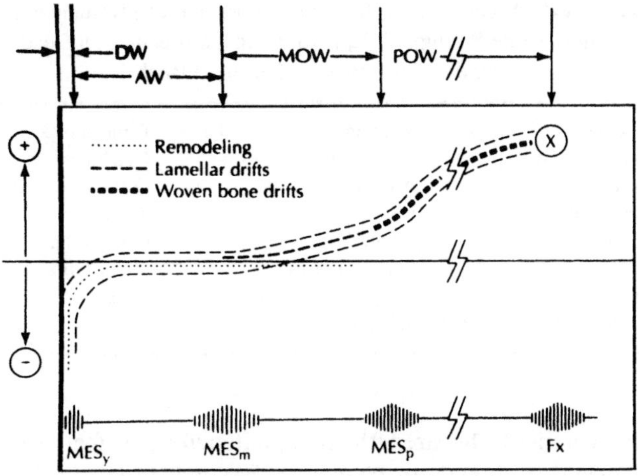

Figure 2.3. Combined modeling and remodeling effects on bone strength and the bone bank. The horizontal line at the bottom suggests typical peak bone strains from zero on the left, to the fracture strain on the right (Fx), plus the locations of the bone remodeling, modeling, and microdamage thresholds (MESr, MESm, MESp respectively; microdamage is not discussed in this article). The horizontal axis represents no net gains or losses of whole-bone strength. The *lower dotted line* curve suggests how remodeling would remove bone next to marrow when strains stay below the MESr range, but otherwise would tend to keep existing bone. The *upper dashed line* curve suggests how modeling drifts would begin to increase bone strength and the bone bank where strains exceed the MESm range. The *dashed outlines* suggest the combined modeling and remodeling effects on a bone's strength and the bone bank. D.H. Carter originally suggested such a curve (Carter, 1984). Fx=the fracture strain range centered near 25,000 microstrain. At the top, DW= disuse window; AW = adapted window as in normally adapted young adults; MOW = mild overload window as in healthy growing mammals; POW = pathologic overload window (Frost, 1992).

The remodeling and modeling thresholds would make the mechanostat make whole-bone strength keep peak bone strains within the adapted window (reproduced by permission: Frost, H.M. (1997). Strain and other mechanical influences on bone strength and maintenance. *Current Opinion in Orthopaedics* **8**, 60–70).

All the above features combine to form a negative feedback system called the *mechanostat*. It would control the *relationship* between a load-bearing bone's architecture and strength on the one hand, and the size of the loads on it on the other hand, as in Figure 2.3 (Frost, 1996; Martin *et al.*, 1998; Gasser, 1999). Nonmechanical factors like those in Table 2.1 might help or modulate how this mechanostat affects such a bone's strength (Martin *et al.*, 1998), but as JL Ferretti noted (personal communication, 1999) they cannot duplicate or replace the mechanostat's control of modeling and remodeling in time and anatomical space. Aided by the modeling and remodeling thresholds, this mechanostat could tell if, when, and where a bone or trabecula needs more strength or has too much. Then it would make modeling or remodeling respectively correct the error (Frost, 2001a).

This model could help to explain why in healthy mammals strong muscles always accompany strong load-bearing bones, and persistently weak muscles always (nearly always?) accompany weak load-bearing bones (Frost, 1999). D'Arcy Thompson may have had that in mind when he quoted what is mentioned in this article's Introductory epigraph (Thompson, 1942). Of the mechanostat hypothesis A.M. Parfitt recently said, "*How the mechanostat works is the most important unsolved problem in bone biology...*" (Parfitt, 2000). (For further discussion of the bone remodeling process in time and space,

Table 2.1. Some Nonmechanical Factors that can Influence how Whole-Bone Strength Adapts to Postnatal Mechanical Loads and could Influence the Bone Bank

Hormones	Vitamins	D metabolites
Dietary calcium	Other minerals	Cytokines
Paracrine effects	Autocrine effects	Cell–cell interactions
Amino acids	Lipids	The genome
Gene expression	Ethnic origin	Occupation
Gender	Some diseases	Malnutrition
Aging	Apoptosis	Ligands
Medications and Other Artificial Agents		

see Chapter 1, this volume.) The strength and architecture of some weakly-loaded cranial bones may not depend on bone's mechanostat. Examples include the turbinates, nasal bones, ethmoids, wing of the sphenoid, frontal and parietal bones, and inner ear ossicles (Frost, 1987).

By the time of birth expression of genetic information *in utero* has created the basic anatomy of bones and features that constitute bone's *baseline conditions* (Frost, 2001b). It is the above biologic "machinery" that can adapt them to postnatal mechanical and nonmechanical challenges. At any time after birth the *differences* between bones in congenitally or neonatally totally paralyzed limbs and in the contralateral normal limbs should show the adaptations to mechanical usage in the normal limbs. Bones in the totally paralyzed limbs should show genetic and postnatal humoral influences on the baseline conditions but no normal mechanical usage effects. Bones never disappear completely in total-permanent disuse (Frost, 1999), and the persisting part could represent the baseline conditions part.

2. Age-Related Bone Loss

Most age-related bone loss comes from bone next to marrow, not from subperiosteal or intracortical bone, so it chiefly affects hollow bones (Epker and Frost, 1964; Sedlin, 1964; Smith and Walker, 1964; Frost, 1966, 1969; Garn, 1970; Smith and Gilligan, 1989; Marotti, 1996). Bone loss mainly next to marrow also characterizes the osteopenias found in situations like those in Table 2.2 (Riggs and Melton, 1995; Marcus *et al.*, 1996). In all such adult-acquired "disuse-pattern" osteopenias on earth, and in "microgravity" existence in space, the marrow space is enlarged, some trabecular and endocortical bone removed, and cortical thickness decreased. Outside bone diameter does not decrease and might even increase slightly, and permanent (steady state) intracortical porosity changes relatively little (Frost, 1969). Such osteopenias weaken bones so injuries can fracture them more easily.

The excellent study by Bousson *et al.* (2001) reported values of ≈20% cortical porosity in endocortical regions of the anterior midfemoral cortex in 16 subjects over 80 years of age. That differs from the ≈7% value found in rib cortex of over 40 subjects at similar ages by Frost (1969). However, unlike Frost's study, the French study was not confined to

Table 2.2. Situations Usually Accompanied by a Disuse-Pattern Osteopenia in Humans

Loss of estrogen in females, and of androgens in males
Prolonged treatment with adrenalcortical steroid hormone analogs
Chronic muscle weakness
Malnutrition
Starvation
Chronic debilitating illnesses such as cardiac, pulmonary, hepatic and renal failure, asthma
Cystic fibrosis
Polyarthritis
Stroke
Life in microgravity situations
Alcoholism
AIDs
Aging
Turner's syndrome
Osteogenesis imperfecta
Idiopathic juvenile osteoporosis
Advanced multiple sclerosis
Paraplegia and other chronic paralyses or pareses

healthy subjects who died suddenly and unexpectedly, mostly from trauma. Accordingly a transiently increased remodeling space associated with terminal medical disorders could have affected many or even most subjects in the French study.

In principle bone loss can occur on four "envelopes": the periosteal, haversian, endocortical, and trabecular surfaces (Sedlin, 1964). Pathologic observations show that even in people of advanced age abundant precursor and effector cells can appear on all those envelopes in response to varied needs. Ergo, a lack of such cells on periosteal and haversian envelopes cannot explain the facts above, or the characteristics of various osteopenias. Some kind of *mediator mechanism in marrow* (Frost, 1966, 1998) should help to control the switching between conservation-mode and disuse-mode remodeling of bone next to marrow.

Usually human muscle strength and mass peak in young adults around 20–30 years of age and then decline slowly, so less than half the young-adult muscle strength can remain by 75 years of age, a phenomenon called sarcopenia (Burr, 1997). Corresponding disuse-pattern osteopenias usually accompany that sarcopenia. Other causes of persistent loss of muscle strength, among them those in Table 2.2, also usually associate with corresponding disuse-pattern osteopenias. Because aging adults who keep doing hard physical labor can keep at least most of their young-adult muscle and bone strength and bone bank (Riggs and Melton, 1995; Burr, 1997), aging itself should not be the chief cause of age-related bone loss.

Muscle weakness due to factors like deficiencies of androgens, calcium, and vitamin D (Glerup *et al.*, 2000) could also cause a corresponding disuse-pattern osteopenia (Rittweger and Rauch, 2001). Loss of estrogen and testosterone in aging females and males respectively is usually associated with loss of bone next to marrow so they usually lead to disuse-pattern osteopenias (Marcus *et al.*, 1996; Yao *et al.*, 2000, 2001; Schoenau *et al.*, 2001).

The most important function of load-bearing bones could constitute providing only enough strength (Carter *et al.*, 1996) to keep voluntary loads from fracturing them, whether those loads are persistently subnormal, normal, or supranormal in size (Frost, 2000b). While bone mineral density (BMD) or bone mineral content (BMC) values determined by DEXA (dual energy X-ray absorptiometry) usually evaluated bone bank deposits in the past (Marcus *et al.*, 1996), they do not reliably indicate whole-bone strength too, and BMD values provide particularly unreliable indicators of it (Augat *et al.*, 1996; Ferretti *et al.*, 1996; Banu *et al.*, 1999; Jiang *et al.*, 1999; Banu *et al.*, 1999; Rittweger *et al.*, 2000; Hasegawa *et al.*, 2001). As an extreme example, healthy mouse and horse femurs would have similar volumetric BMD values, yet their strengths differ more than 1,000 times. Bone strength indices (BSIs), usually obtained at present by quantitative computed tomography, provide much better such indicators (Ferretti *et al.*, 1992, 1996, 2001; Banu *et al.*, 1999; Ferretti, 1999; Jiang *et al.*, 1999; Wilhelm *et al.*, 1999; Rauch and Schoenau, 2001). The observation's significance lies in the fact that architectural factors can make bones like a femur with lower BMD values than another femur still be the stronger bone (Ferretti, 1999; Schoenau *et al.*, 2001). Such factors may relate to apparent contradictory findings for bone mass and fracture risk when different populations are compared. (For further discussion of population differences in bone mass and architecture, see Chapter 4, this volume.)

3. A Proposed Synthesis

Most age-related bone loss should stem from the effects of age-related muscle weakness, plus age-related declines in estrogen and androgen effects, on a marrow mediator mechanism that helps to control removal of bone next to marrow by disuse-mode remodeling. Bone loss can but need not always decrease whole-bone strength too. If aging and/or genetic factors have separate effects on that loss—which seems possible—to the knowledge of this author, the studies needed to prove it have not been done. In this synthesis age-related declines in the responsiveness of the bone-biologic mechanisms, while possible, would not be the chief cause of age-related bone loss, and neither would biochemical, humoral, and cell and molecular biologic influences exerted directly on osteoblasts or osteoclasts. The idea that independently working and controlled osteoclasts (or osteoblasts) cause bone loss was logical in terms of 1960s' knowledge, but in 2001 it seems too simplistic (Brown and Haglund, 1995; Parfitt, 1995, 2000).

Future studies of this matter might rank the importance of age-related loss of whole-bone *strength* above age-related decreases in BMD, BMC, or the bone bank. Comparing the nature and magnitudes of such losses in bones with and without marrow cavities might help to resolve the differences in assumptions between the 1960 and Utah paradigms.

4. Conclusions

Past explanations of age-related bone loss in terms of the 1960 paradigm seem to ignore all features of the Utah paradigm presented here. The 1960 paradigm's chief mechanisms included genetic and humoral effects on bone's effector cells, and more recently on their precursor cells. Today its adherents emphasize things like cellular and molecular biology, ligands, cell receptors, endocrinology, biochemistry, apoptosis, diet, cytokines, chemokines, etc. One can understand why advocates of long-accepted wisdom about this matter could have reservations about the synthesis suggested here, but two comments about such reservations might deserve some thought. To wit: "*The history of plate tectonics should remind all of us that accepted wisdom can be wrong*" (Gingrich, 2000); also, "*...the temptation to assume that the key players are those that are currently known (is) ever present*" (Bird, 1999).

Still, in 2001 the above synthesis and the views it would compete with are hypotheses, and in logic no hypothesis can invalidate any other. Only facts can do that. Accordingly further facts and better interdisciplinary communication in skeletal science must reveal which is the better hypothesis. I strongly favor the above synthesis but respect those who would reserve judgment.

As for poor interdisciplinary communication, early recognition of its harmful effects, and of the existence of tissue-level mechanisms and mechanical and neuromuscular roles in skeletal physiology, led W.S.S. Jee to begin organizing the University of Utah's famous Hard Tissue Workshops in 1965 (Jee, 2001). For similar reasons, these topics are starting to be addressed and shared within an international association (Frost, 2000a). The collection of papers in this volume by experts from a diversity of disciplines is a contribution to interdisciplinary communication. It is hoped that readers can agree that supplementing former facts and views in skeletal physiology with newer ones could lead to building better things with their sum.

References

Augat, P., Reeb, H., and Claes, L. (1996). Prediction of fracture load at different skeletal sites by geometrical properties of the cortical shell. *J. Bone Miner. Res.* **11**, 1356–1363.

Banu, M.J., Orhii, P.B., Mejia, W., McCarter, R.J.M., Mosekilde, L., Thomsen, J.S., and Kalu, D.N. (1999). Analysis of the effects of growth hormone, voluntary exercise, and food restriction on diaphyseal bone in female F344 rats. *Bone* **25**, 479–480.

Beck, T.J., Oreskovic, T.L., Stone, K.L., Ruff, C.B., Ensrud, K., Nevitt, M.C., Genant, H.K., and Cummings, S.R. (2001). Structural adaptation to changing mechanical load in the progression toward hip fragility: The study of osteoporotic fractures. *J. Bone Miner. Res.* **16**, 1108–1119.

Bird, A. (1999). DNA methylaation de novo. *Science* **286**, 2287–2288.

Bousson, V., Meunier, A., Bergot, C., Vicaut, E., Rocha, M.A., Morais, M.H., Laval-Jeantet, A.-M., and Laredo, J.G. (2001). Distribution of intracortical porosity in human midfemoral cortex by age and gender. *J. Bone Min. Res.* **16**, 1308–1317.

Brown, W., and Haglund, K. (1995). Landmarks. *J. NIH. Res.* **7**, 54–59.

Burr, D.B. (1997). Muscle strength, bone mass, and age-related bone loss. *J. Bone Miner. Res.* **12**, 1547–1551.

Carter, D.R. (1984). Mechanical loading histories and cortical bone remodeling. *Calc. Tiss. Int. Suppl.* **36**, 19–24.

Carter, D.R., van der Meulen, M.C.H., and Beaupre, G.S. (1996). Skeletal development. Mechanical consequences of growth, aging and disease. In R. Marcus, D. Feldman and J. Kelsey (eds) *Osteoporosis*. Academic Press, San Diego, pp. 333–350.

Chen, M.-M., Yeh, J.K., and Aloia, J.F. (1995). Skeletal alterations in hypophysectomized rats: II. A histomorphometric study on tibial cortical bone. *Anat. Rec.* **241**, 513–518.

Crowninshield, R.D., Johnston, R.C., Andrews, J.G., and Brand, R.A. (1978). A biomechanical investigation of the human hip. *J. Biomech.* **11**, 75–85.

Currey, J.D. (1984). *The Mechanical Adaptations of Bones*. Princeton University Press, Princeton.

deMenocal, P.B. (2001). Cultural responses to climate change during the late Holcene. *Science* **292**, 667–673.

Epker, B.N., and Frost, H.M. (1964). The parabolic index: A proposed index of the degree of osteoporosis in ribs *J. Gerontol.* **19**, 469–473.

Evans, R.A. (1987). Is there a need for whole body physiology? *Bone and Min.* **2**, 243–244.

Favus, M.J. (ed.) (1999). *Primer on the Metabolic Bone Diseases and Disorders of Mineral Metabolism* 4th edn Lippincott-Williams and Wilkins, Philadelphia, PA.

Ferretti, J.L., Spiaggi, E.P., Capozza, R., Cointry, G., and Zanchetta, J.R. (1992). Interrelationships between geometric and mechanical properties of long bones from three rodent species with very different biomass Phylogenetic implications. *J. Bone Min. Res.* **7**(Suppl 2), 423–425.

Ferretti, J.L., Capozza, R.F., and Zanchetta, A.R. (1996). Mechanical validation of a tomographic (pQCT) index for the noninvasive assessment of rat femur bending strength. *Bone* **18**, 97–102.

Ferretti, J.L. (1999). Peripheral, quantitative computed tomography (pQCT) for evaluating structural and mechanical properties of small bone. In Y.H. An and R.A. Draughn (eds) *Practical Guide for Mechanical Testing of Bone*. CRC Press, Boca Raton, FL, pp. 1–25.

Ferretti, J.L., Cointry, J.R., Capozza, R.F., Capiglioni, R., and Chiappe, M.A. (2001). Analysis of biomechanical effects on bone and on the muscle-bone interactions in small animal models. *J. Musculoskel Neuron Interact.* **1**, 263–274.

Frost, H.M. (1966). *Bone Dynamics in Osteoporosis and Osteomalacia*. Charles C. Thomas, Springfield.

Frost, H.M. (1987). Secondary osteon population densities: An algorithm for estimating the missing osteons *Yearb. Phys. Anthropol.* **30**, 239–254.

Frost, H.M. (1992). Perspectives: Bone's mechanical usage windows. *Bone and Min.* **19**, 257–271.

Frost, H.M. (1996). Perspectives: A proposed general model of the mechanostat (suggestions from a new paradigm). *Anat. Rec.* **244**, 139–147.

Frost, H.M. (1998). On rho, a marrow mediator and estrogen: Their roles in bone strength and "mass" in human females, osteopenias and osteoporoses (insights from a new paradigm). *J. Bone Miner. Metab.* **16**, 113–123

Frost, H.M. (1999). The author's personal observation(s) during 50 years as an orthopaedic surgeon, teacher researcher and amateur pathologist, and of a matter others must have observed too so it need not be original to the author. However it did not previously seem important or relevant enough to deserve formal study and publication.

Frost, H.M. (2000a). Why the ISMNI and the Utah paradigm? Their role in skeletal and extraskeletal disorders *J. Musculoskel. Neuron. Interact.* **1**, 29–30.

Frost, H.M. (2000b). The Utah paradigm of skeletal physiology: An overview of its insights for bone, cartilage and collagenous tissue organs. *J. Bone Miner. Metab.* **18**, 305–316.

Frost, H.M. (2001a). From Wolff's Law to the Utah paradigm: Insights about bone physiology and its clinical applications. *Anat. Rec.* **262**, 398–419.

Frost, H.M. (2001b). Cybernetic aspects of bone modeling and remodeling, with special reference to osteoporosis and whole-bone strength. *J. Hum. Biol.* **13**, 235–248.

Garn, S. (1970). *The Earlier Gain and Later Loss of Cortical Bone*. Charles C. Thomas, Springfield.

Gasser, J.A. (1999). Modulation of strain sensing: A new approach for the treatment of osteoporosis. In G.P. Lyritis (ed.) *Musculoskeletal Interactions*, Vol II. Hylonome Editions, Athens, pp. 77–82.

Gingrich, N. (2000). An opportunities-based science budget. *Science* **290**, 1303.

Glerup, H., Mikkelsen, K., Poulsen, L., Hass, E., Overbeck, S., Andersen, H., Charles, P., and Eriksen, E.F. (2000). Hypovitaminosis D myopathy without biochemical signs of osteomalcic bone involvement. *Calc. Tiss. Int.* **60**, 419–424.

Gorski, J. (1997). Do we need new paradigms? *Endocr. News* **22**, 4, 12.

Hasegawa, Y., Schneider, P., and Reiners, C. (2001). Age, sex, and grip strength determine architectural bone parameters assessed by peripheral quantitative computed tomography (pQCT) at the human radius. *J. Biomech.* **34**, 497–503.

Heaney, R.P. (1994). The bone-remodeling transient: Implications for the interpretation of clinical studies of bone mass change. *J. Bone Miner. Res.* **9**, 10, 1515–1523.

Heinonen, A., Sievanen, H., Kannus, P., Oja, P., Pasanen, M., and Vuori, I. (2000). High impact exercise and bones of growing girls: A 9-month controlled trial. *Osteopor. Inter.* **11**, 1010–1017.

Jaworski, Z.F.G. (1984). Lamellar bone turnover system and its effector organ. *Calc. Tiss. Int. Suppl.* **36**, 46–55.

Jee, W.S.S. (1989). The skeletal tissues. In L. Weiss (ed.) *Cell and Tissue Biology. A Textbook of Histology*. Urban and Schwartzenberg, Baltimore, pp. 211–259.

Jee, W.S.S., and Li, X.J. (1990). Adaptation of cancellous bone to overloading in the adult rat: A single photon absorptiometry and histomorphometry study. *Anat. Rec.* **227**, 418–426.

Jee, W.S.S., Li, X.J., and Schaffler, M.B. (1991). Adaptation of diaphyseal structure with aging and increased mechanical usage in the adult rat. A histomorphometrical and biomechanical study. *Anat. Rec.* **230**, 332–338.

Jee, W.S.S. (ed.) (1995). Proceedings of the International Conference on Animal Models in the Prevention and Treatment of Osteopenia. *Bone* **17**(Suppl), 1–466.

Jee, W.S. (2000). Principles in bone physiology. *J. Musculoskeletal Interactions* **1**, 9–11.

Jee, W.S.S., and Yao, W. (2001). Animal models of bone diseases. *J. Musculoskel. Neuron. Interact.* **1**, 183–184.

Jee, W.S.S. (2001a). Integrated bone tissue physiology: Anatomy and physiology. In S.C. Cowin (ed.) *Bone Mechanics Handbook* (2nd ed). CRC Press, Boca Raton, pp. 1–68.

Jee, W.S.S. (2001b). The Hard Tissue Workshops organized annually since 1965 by Prof Jee provided a uniquely seminal multidisciplinary forum for presenting and discussing new methods, evidence and ideas about human skeletal physiology and disorders. Hundreds of international authorities in many disciplines participated in them, the University of Utah sponsored them, and private and federal funds supported them. They probably had more effect on how people think about and study skeletal disorders than any other meetings in the past century. The Utah paradigm had its genesis at these Workshops; hence its name.

Jiang, Y., Zhao, J., Rosen, C., Gensens, P., and Genant, H. (1999). Perspectives on bone mechanical properties and adaptive response to mechanical loading. *J. Clin. Densitom.* **2**, 422–433.

Kanis, J.A. (1994). Assessment of fracture risk and its application to screening for postmenopausal osteoporosis: Synopsis of a WHO report. *Osteoporosis Int.* **4**, 368–381.

Lewis, F.T. (1906). *Stohr's Histology* (ed.) (6th U.S. edn.) Blakiston's Son, Philadelphia.

Li, X.J., Jee, W.S.S., Chow, S.-Y., and Woodbury, D.M. (1990). Adaptation of cancellous bone to aging and immobilization in the rat. A single photon absorptiometry and histomorphometry study. *Anat. Rec.* **227**, 12–24.

Li, X.J., and Jee, W.S.S. (1991). Adaptation of diaphyseal structure to aging and decreased mechanical loading in the adult rat. A densitometric and histomorphometric study. *Anat. Rec.* **229**, 291–297.

Luck, J.V. (1950). *Bone and Joint Diseases.* Charles C. Thomas, Springfield.

Marotti, G. (1996). The structure of bone tissues and the cellular control of their deposition. *Ital. J. Anata. Embryol.*, 101–179.

Marotti, G. (2000). The osteocyte as a wiring transmission system. *J. Musculskel. Neuron. Interact.* **1**, 133–136.

Martin, R.B., Burr, D.B., and Sharkey, N.A. (1998). *Skeletal Tissue Mechanics.* Springer-Verlag, New York.

Martin, R.B. (2000). Towards a unifying theory of bone remodeling. *Bone* **26**, 1–6.

Marcus, R., Feldman, D., and Kelsey, J. (eds) (1996). Osteoporosis. Academic Press, Orlando, Fl.

Mayr, E. (1961). Cause and effect in biology. *Science* **134**, 1501–1506.

McLean, F.C., and Urist, M.R. (1961). *Bone* (2nd edn.). University of Chicago Press, Chicago.

Parfitt, A.M. (1995). Problems in the application of *in vitro* systems to the study of human bone remodeling. *Calcif. Tiss. Int.* **56**(Suppl 1), S5–S7.

Parfitt, A.M. (2000). Osteoporosis: 50 years of change, mostly in the right direction. In J. Compston and S. Ralston (eds) *Osteoporosis and Bone Biology*. International Medical Press, pp. 1–13.

Pirok, D., Ramser, J.R., Takahashi, H., Villanueva, A.R., and Frost, H.M. (1966). Normal histologic, tetracycline, and dynamic parameters in human mineralized bone sections. *Henry Ford Hosp. Med. Bull.* **14**, 195–218.

Polanyi, M. (1968). Life's irreducible structure. *Science* **160**, 1308–1312.

Putschar, W.G.J. (1960). General pathology of the musculoskeletal system. In F. Buchner, E. Letterer and F. Roulet (eds) Handbuch der Allgemeinen Pathologie. Springer-Verlag, Berlin, pp. 361–488.

Rauch, F., and Schoenau, E. (2001). Changes in bone density during childhood and adolescence: An approach based on bone's biological organization. *J. Bone Miner. Res.* **16**, 597–604.

Riggs, B.L., and Melton, L.J. III (eds) (1995). Osteoporosis. Etiology, Diagnosis and Treatment (2nd edn.) Lippincott-Raven Publishers, Hagerstown, MD.

Rittweger, J., Beller, G., Ehrig, J., Jung, C., Koch, U., Ramolla, J., Schimdt, F., Newitt, D., Majumdar, S., Schiessl, H., and Felsenberg, D. (2000). Bone-muscle strength indices of the human lower leg. *Bone* **27**, 319–326.

Rittweger, J., and Rauch, F. (2001). What is new in musculo-skeletal interactions? *J. Musculoskel. Neuron. Interact.* **1**, 171–176.

Robling, A.G., Burr, D.B., and Turner, C.H. (2001). Skeletal loading in animals. *J. Musculoskel. Nueron. Interact.* **1**, 263–274.

Schermer, M. (2001). Colorful pebbles and Darwin's dictum. *Scientific American* **284**, 38.

Schiessl, H., Ferreti, J.L., Tysarczyk-Niemeyer, G., Willnecker, J., and Wilhelm, G. (1998a). The role of muscles to the mechanical adaptation of bone. In G.P. Lyritis (ed.) *Advances in Osteoporosis*. Vol I. Hylonome Editions, Athens, Greece, pp. 53–62.

Schiessl, H., and Willnecker, J. (1998b). New insights about the relationship between bone strength and muscle strength. In E. Schönau and V. Matkovic (eds) *Paediatric Osteology. Prevention of Osteoporosis—a Paediatric task*? Excerpta Medica, Amsterdam, pp. 33–39.

Schiessl, H., and Willnecker, J. (1999). Muscle cross sectional area and bone cross sectional area in the lower leg measured with peripheral computed tomography. In G.P. Lyritis (ed.) *Musculoskeletal Interactions* (vol II). Hylonome Editions, Athens, pp. 47–52.

Schönau, E. (1996). *Paediatric Osteology. New Trends and Diagnostic Possibilities* Elsevier Science, Amsterdam.

Schoenau, E., Neu, C.M., Rauch, F., and Manz, F. (2001). The development of bone strength at the proximal radius during childhood and adolescence. *J. Clin. Endocrinol. Metab.* **86**, 613–618.

Schönau, E., Neu, C.M., Mokov, E., Wassmer, G., and Manz, F. (2000). Influence of puberty on muscle area and cortical bone area of the forearm in boys and girls. *J. Clin. Endocrinol. Metab.* **85**, 1–4.

Sedlin, E.D. (1964). Uses of bone as a model system in the study of aging. In H.M. Frost (ed.) *Bone Biodynamics*. Little-Brown Co, Boston, pp. 655–666.

Smith, R.R., and Walker, R.R. (1964). Femoral expansion in aging women: Implications for osteoporoses and fractures. *Science* **145**, 156–157.

Smith, E.L., and Gilligan, C. (1989). Mechanical forces and bone. *Bone and Min. Res.* **6**, 139–173.

Takahashi, H.E. (ed.) (1995). *Spinal Disorders in Growth and Aging*. Springer-Verlag, Tokyo.

Thompson, D.W. (1942). *On Growth and Form*. The Complete Revised Edition. Dover Publications Inc, NY, p. 1019.

Weinmann, J.P., and Sicher, H. (1955). *Bone and Bones*, 2nd Ed. CV Mosby Co, St Louis.

Wilhelm, G., Felsenberg, D., Bogusch, G., Willnecker, J., Thaten, I., and Gummert, P. (1999). Biomechanical examinations for validation of the Bone Strength Strain Index SSI, calculated by peripheral quantitative computed tomography. In GP Lyritis (ed.) *Musculoskeletal Interactions* (vol II). Holonome Edtions, Athens, pp. 105–110.

Yao, W., Jee, W.S.S., Chen, J., Liu, H., Ta, C.S., Cui, L., Zhou, H., Setterberg, R.B., and Frost, H.M. (2000). Making rats rise to erect bipedal stance for feeding partially prevented orchidectomy-induced bone loss and added bone to intact rats. *J. Bone Min. Res.* **15**, 1158–1168.

Yao, W., Jee, W.S.S., Chen, J.L., Li, C.-Y., and Frost, H.M. (2001). A novel method to "exercise" rats: Making rats rise to erect bipedal stance for feeding—raised cage model. *J. Musculoskel. Neuron. Interact.* **1**, 241–247.

Yeh, J.K., Chen, M.M., and Aloia, J.F. (1995). Skeletal alterations in hypophysectomized rats: I. A histomorphometric study in tibial cancellous bone. *Anat. Rec.* **241**, 505–512.

Glossary

Because some terms have different meanings in the literature this Glossary defines their meanings in this article.

BMU: Basic Multicellular Unit of bone remodeling. In ≈4 months and in a biologically-coupled sequence of activation, resorption, and formation or ARF sequence, it turns over ≈0.05 mm^3 of bone (Figure 2.2). When a BMU makes less bone than it resorbs, this tends to remove bone permanently. Adult humans may create about 3 million new BMUs annually, and about a million may function at any moment in the whole skeleton. Creating a new BMU involves creation by precursor cells of new local osteoclasts, osteoblasts, supporting cells, and a nourishing capillary. A new BMU is a separate tissue-level mechanism with its own functions in the same sense as nephrons in kidneys.

Bone bank: The amount of bone tissue in an intact bone or whole skeleton, best thought of as a volume instead of a true mass. A common equivalent term: bone "mass," where "mass" does not mean the same thing as it does in physics.

Drift: see "modeling" below.

Effector cells: here and in bone these cells would be the osteoblasts and osteoclasts that actually make and resorb bone respectively. The term would exclude precursor cells, osteocytes, "supporting," and other cells.

Mechanostat: the putative mechanism that controls the adaptations of bone architecture, strength, and the bone bank to voluntary mechanical usage to let bones endure that usage for life. It would use the modeling threshold to "decide" where and if more bone was needed for mechanical reasons, and the remodeling threshold to "decide" when bone was no longer needed for those reasons. It would have the same role in bone physiology as the steering wheel, brakes, and accelerator in driving a car. Mechanical usage would analogize the car's "driver."

Modeling: the biologic processes that produce functionally and biomechanically efficient sizes, shapes, and strength to bones. Mostly independent resorption and formation modeling drifts do it (Figure 2.1). Bone modeling normally adjusts a bone's strength to keep its strains from exceeding its modeling threshold. Modeling (not osteoblasts alone) normally controls additions of bone strength. Creating a new modeling drift involves the creation by precursor cells of one or more new capillaries to nourish the drift, as well as its osteoblasts or osteoclasts and its supporting and other cells. A modeling drift is a separate tissue-level mechanism with its own special functions, so it is analogous to a renal nephron.

Modeling threshold (MESm in Figure 2.3): a range of bone strains (or equivalent mechanical stimulus) within or above which modeling turns on to increase bone strength. Where strains stay below it, mechanically-controlled modeling would switch off. This range may center near 1,000 microstrain in healthy young adults. "MES" stands for Minimum Effective Strain or other Signal.

Muscle strength: a muscle's maximum *momentary* contractile force can be measured as the peak torque produced across joints like the hip, elbow, knee, and fingers. That differs from *endurance*, which concerns how long and often submaximal muscle forces can be exerted, as in marathon running, walking, and long distance swimming. It differs from mechanical work or *energy*, which can be expressed in Newton-meters, Joules, or kilowatt-hours. It differs from muscle *power*, which concerns how rapidly mechanical work is done and is usually expressed in Newton-meters/sec, Joules/sec, or watts (one Joule/sec = one watt). Since bones seem to adapt their strength to the typical peak momentary loads they carry, accounting for these distinctions can minimize errors in interpreting mechanical usage effects on whole-bone strength and the bone bank.

Osteopenia: here, less bone and less whole-bone strength than usual for most healthy people of the same age, height, weight, sex, and race. Also less bone and/or whole-bone strength than before in the same individual. It would be a disorder in the statistical sense but need not always represent a disease too.

Remodeling: turnover of bone in small packets by BMUs (see above). Pre-1964 literature lumped modeling and remodeling together as "remodeling." In remodeling's disuse mode completed BMUs make less bone than they resorb. In its conservation mode completed BMUs tend to equalize their bone resorption and formation. Knowing that osteoblasts make bone and osteoclasts resorb it can no longer introduce basic bone physiology adequately. BMU-based remodeling (not osteoclasts alone) normally controls conservation and losses of bone strength.

Remodeling space: increased BMU creations increase the number of temporary holes in a bone and excavations on its surfaces. That causes a temporary bone loss called the remodeling space. It is temporary because when BMU creations return to normal the existing holes refill with bone, because of the ARF sequence in BMUs. Substantial increases in cortical porosity usually represent transient remodeling space effects (Jaworski, 1984).

Remodeling threshold (MESr in Figure 2.3): a strain range (or equivalent mechanical stimulus) such that when strains stay below it, disuse-mode remodeling removes bone next to marrow, thereby reducing bone strength and the bone bank deposits. When strains stay above it, remodeling begins to conserve both bone strength and the bone bank deposits. It could center in the region of 50–100 microstrain. For comparison, bone's fracture strain in healthy young adults lies in the 25,000 microstrain range.

Strain: the deformation or change in dimensions and/or shape caused by a load on any bone. Special gages can measure bone strains in the laboratory and *in vivo*. Loads always cause strains, even if very small ones, and they include tension, compression, and shear. Biomechanicians often express strain in microstrain units, where 1,000 microstrain in compression would shorten a bone by 0.1% of its original length, 10,000 microstrain would shorten it by 1% of that length, and 100,000 microstrain would shorten it by 10% of that length (and break it).

Strength: the load, strain, or stress that, when applied once, will fracture a bone. "Whole-bone strength" distinguishes the strength of intact bones from the strength of bone as a tissue or material.

3

The Role of Bone Quality on Bone Loss and Bone Fragility

Marc D. Grynpas

1. Introduction

Normal bone mass in humans, after growth has ceased, is maintained by the balance between bone formation by osteoblasts and bone resorption by osteoclasts. With age, starting around the third decade of life, after peak bone mass has been reached there is a slow and steady loss of bone. A similar age related loss of bone occurs in all mammalian species. Osteoporosis is a multifactorial, age-related metabolic bone disease characterized by low bone mineral density and the deterioration of the microarchitecture of cancellous bone. The resulting changes in the material properties of bone lead to enhanced bone fragility and to a consequent increase in the risk of fracture (Wasnich, 1996). There are two types of osteoporosis, each with their own characteristics. Type I osteoporosis, also called post-menopausal osteoporosis, is characterized by an increase in bone turnover and an accelerated loss of cancellous bone leading to vertebral fracture. It affects mainly post-menopausal women. Type II osteoporosis, also called age-related osteoporosis, affects older women and men and is not accompanied by increased bone turnover, but leads to hip fracture and has a greater mortality and morbidity than type I osteoporosis. The risk factors for osteoporosis are age, gender, genetic, environmental (nutrition, physical activity, medication, smoking, etc.), hormonal deficiency, reproductive history, chronic diseases, and physical characteristics of bone. While osteoporosis is a complex disease that leads to fracture, there is no way to measure the strength of bone in humans to predict fracture risk. Bone mineral density (BMD) as measured by dual energy x-ray absorptiometry (DEXA) has become the main way to assess the risk of fracture even if it is only a surrogate measure of bone strength. Osteoporosis is diagnosed (by the WHO criteria) when the value for BMD is 2.5 standard deviations or more below the mean of the young adult reference range (Kanis, 1994).

However, while bone mass correlates to a certain degree with the risk of fracture, there are other parameters which are very important in predicting bone strength and which

---

Marc D. Grynpas • Department of Laboratory Medicine and Pathobiology, University of Toronto, and the SLRI of Mount Sinai Hospital, Toronto.

Bone Loss and Osteoporosis: An Anthropological Perspective, edited by Sabrina C. Agarwal and Sam D. Stout. Kluwer Academic/Plenum Publishers, New York, 2003.

are not reflected in bone mass measurements. These parameters, known collectively as bone quality, are bone microarchitecture, bone mineralization, and bone mechanical properties. Therefore the risk of fracture in osteoporotic patients is determined in part by their BMD and in part by the quality of their bone, and it is this latter component of bone fragility that we will examine in this chapter.

2. Determination of Bone Quality

Bone quality can be determined by examining the mechanical properties, the architecture, the degree of mineralization of the bone matrix, the chemistry and structure of bone mineral crystals, and the remodeling of bone (as shown in Figure 3.1). Both ovariectomy and menopause are thought to result in a loss of bone structure, but no alteration in the bone material itself is believed to occur. Along with aging changes in mineralization a number of therapies (such as fluoride and the bisphosphonates) are known to affect the degree of mineralization of bone, which would result in a change in the material properties of bone. These changes can be assessed by a number of methods. Mineralization profile histograms of the density of the bone can be established by either direct determination (density fractionation), or by the use of back-scattered electron (BSE) imaging, or by microradiography. In the former, bone powder is successively suspended and centrifuged in liquids of calibrated density, resulting in pellets of bone powder that fall within specified density ranges (Grynpas *et al.*, 1994). Similarly, the brightness of an area on a BSE image is related to the average molecular weight (and therefore to the degree of mineralization) and a histogram of the area of bone in each brightness range produces a mineralization profile (Grynpas *et al.*, 1994). The latter is only semi-quantitative, but it is adequate to detect changes as a result of treatment. It is equivalent to microradiography where the distribution of mineral in thin slices of bone (100 μm) is studied using the absorption of x-rays (Amprino and Engstrom, 1952). In the density fractionation technique, the varying densities reflect the distribution of mineral in a unit volume of finely powdered bone and therefore the packing of the mineral crystals in the bone tissue. Finally, an average degree of mineralization (rather than a profile) can be determined by using microhardness testing. This technique involves indenting the surface of a material with a diamond-shaped indenter. The hardness of the material is a measure of the amount of resistance to deformation, and is related to the size of the resulting indentation. This, in turn, is closely correlated to the degree of mineralization of the local region, which determines bone material properties. Both bisphosphonate and fluoride therapies have been shown to increase bone mineral density and alter mechanical properties (Grynpas *et al.*, 1994a; Grynpas *et al.*, 1994b).

3. Aging Changes in the Skeleton

Using histological techniques, an increase in intracortical porosity with aging has been demonstrated in the human skeleton. This increase is secondary to an increase in the number and mean diameter of haversian systems. The inner cortex is more affected than the outer cortex (Martin *et al.*, 1980) and Wolff's law has been invoked to explain this effect. Laval-Jeantet *et al.* (1983) hypothesized that an increase in porosity would lead to a decrease in

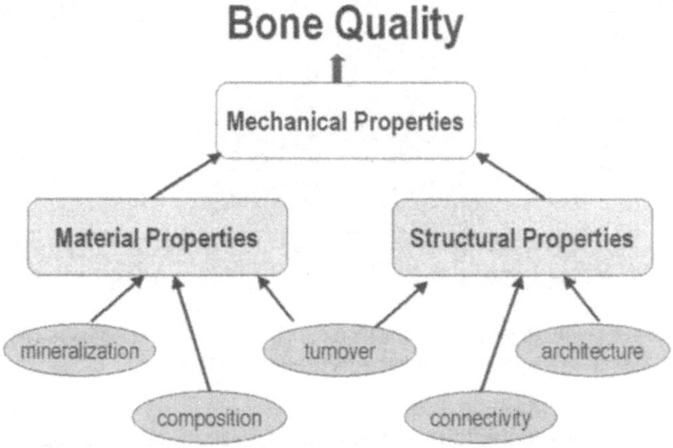

Figure 3.1. Diagram of bone quality.

macroscopic mineral density, but others have found an increase in mineral density with age in males (Lindahl and Lindgren, 1967). Decrease in cross sectional area of long bones with age has also been documented (Dequeker, 1975; Thompson, 1980), however it remains controversial (Laval-Jeantet *et al.*, 1983). Microradiographic studies by Sharpe (1979) and Jowsey *et al.* (1974) confirmed the histological findings of more variably mineralized bone, with hyper and hypo-mineralized osteons and more fragmented osteons with plugged caniculi with aging. Portigliatti Barbos *et al.* (1983) developed a classification of osteons based on degree of mineralization: an initial stage, two intermediate stages, and a final stage of full mineralization. These findings correspond to the concept of bone mineral being laid down very quickly to reach 65% of final mineralization (primary mineralization) followed by a period of maturation during which the remainder of the mineral is gradually deposited over a period of months (secondary mineralization). Microradiography has also been used to try and determine the rate of intra-osteonal (Lacroix and Dhem, 1967; Pankovich *et al.*, 1974; Trotter and Hixon, 1974) remodelling by comparing single and double osteons (type II). Double osteons are the result of intra-osteonal remodelling, their number increases with age while the number of single osteons decreased at a rate of 2.5% per decade after the age of 30. An increase in the number of incomplete osteons with age was also found. Coupled with the fact that the outermost lamellae in double osteons were nearly always highly mineralized it suggests that remodelling favors older more highly mineralized osteons. In most studies it is also suggested that net bone loss begins in normal aging only after the third or fourth decade of life and takes place at different rates in trabecular and cortical bone (Atkinson, 1969; Mazess, 1982; Riggs *et al.*, 1982).

4. The Problem of Diagenesis

The desire to determine the state of health in ancient populations through chemical or morphological analysis of their recovered skeletons has led to numerous investigations by archaeologists and physical anthropologists. However, the problem of diagenesis—the

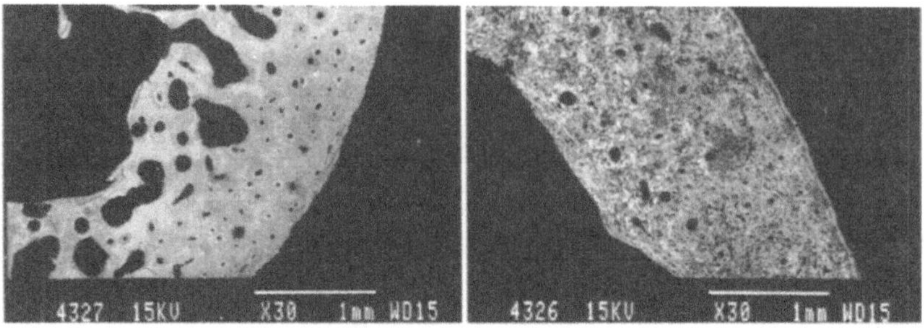

Figure 3.2. Scanning electron micrograph from sections of human ribs (a) 1 modern bone (b) archeological bone showing signs of diagenesis. Images courtesy of Dr. Sabrina Agarwal.

addition and removal of elements in the soil due to chemical exchanges and reactions—needs to be carefully evaluated before any meaningful conclusions can be drawn. (See also the chapter by Schultz in this volume.) A confounding factor is that, while profound chemical changes occur in the fabric of the bone mineral, often the morphological shape of the bone remains intact. This is illustrated in Figure 3.2.

Many studies have used trace element analysis of archeological bones in the hope of reconstructing ancient diet (Bratter *et al.*, 1977; Lambert *et al.*, 1979; Geidel, 1982; Gilbert, 1982; Nelson and Sauer, 1984; Kyle, 1986; Grupe, 1987; Runia, 1987; Antoine *et al.*, 1988; Lambert and Liang, 1988), and while a number of these have discussed diagenesis, few have compared their findings to the trace elements contents of modern bones. Others (Grynpas *et al.*, 1987; Hancock *et al.*, 1987, 1989) have shown a wide variation in the chemical composition of bones from mummies of different periods and different origin. In addition they have shown an enormous variation in the chemical composition of different bones from a single archaeological site that implies that cortical and trabecular bones are affected differentially by chemical diagenesis. Unless it can be demonstrated that changes in the bone mineral preceded death, the validity of the chemical analysis of ancient bones, including bone mineral density, will remain doubtful.

5. Changes in Bone Mineralization with Diseases and Treatments

Many human diseases and pathological conditions result in changes in bone tissue that affect the rate of bone deposition, resorption, or turnover. This will affect bone mineral and the distribution of domains of bone containing various amounts of mineral within the tissue. These changes in bone tissue are usually studied by bone density measurements (DEXA) or by histology and histomorphometry. However, changes in mineralization patterns cannot be detected by these methods making it difficult to distinguish between normal age related bone loss and osteoporosis.

Using the density fractionation techniques, Chantraine *et al.* (1986) showed that following the onset of traumatic paraplegia cortical and cancellous bone mineralization profiles were shifted to lower mineral densities compared to normal. However, when investigated after 2 years the mineralization profile of paraplegics approach that of normal subjects.

Therefore, we can say in this case that high turnover bone loss induced hypomineralization of the bone. Grynpas *et al.* (1991) have also shown this in the case of subchondral bone of patients with osteoarthritis. In this case, the phenomenon was probably local, but it resulted in the near disappearance of the heaviest bone mineral fraction, while the amount of subchondral bone increased. Whether this is due to enhanced repair of microfracture or to an incomplete mineralization of the newly formed bone remains to be determined.

Because no mammalian species, other than humans, fracture when it loses bone there is no recognized animal model of spontaneous osteoporosis. Therefore, various manipulations have been used in experimental animals to induce excessive bone loss in order to produce a model for osteoporosis. However, very few attempts have been made to verify that in these models the bone, which remained was indeed more fragile. Various procedures have been used to induce bone loss in animal models such as immobilization by plaster casting, nerve or tendon sectioning (Burkhart and Jowsey, 1967; Utoff and Jaworski, 1978). Ovariectomy induces bone loss in the rat in an age-dependent manner (Wronsk and Yen, 1991) as well as in the dog and other large mammalian species. Various dietary manipulations such as calcium deficiency, high protein diet, high phosphate diet, and acid loading can also induce severe bone loss (Jowsey *et al.*, 1974; Barzel, 1975; Whiting and Draper, 1980) . Some drugs can cause excessive bone loss such as corticosteroids or heparin (Thompson, 1973). Inflammation can cause localized or generalized bone loss (Bauss *et al.*, 1985). We must mention here that the lack of gravity induced by space travel changes the mineralization profile of bone in a manner that is different from ground-based disuse models (Simmons *et al.*, 1986). Finally, we must point out that not all changes in mineralization profiles in disease are simply caused by changes in turnover. Dickson and Kodicek (1979) have shown that vitamin D deficiency caused a shifting to lower mineral density in the chick due to decreased mineral formation. This mineralization defect is accompanied by abnormal mineral chemistry (Bonar *et al.*, 1983). However not all bone disorders lead to bone loss. In the case of osteoporosis, in the incisor absent rat, Boskey and Marks (1985) have shown that a shift in mineralization profile towards higher mineralization was due to lack of resorption. This leads to an increase in crystal size compared to normal littermates, which is due to a continual accretion of new mineral on pre-existing crystals.

Trace elements have been shown to have a profound influence on the chemistry and solubility of bone mineral as the skeleton is the target organ for many heavy metals. Chemical changes with age in bone have received little attention. To show the effect of trace elements on bone mineralization, we will concentrate on two elements which are present in the food chain but have also been used as drugs and which are toxic if taken in excess. The first element is fluoride (F), which has been at the center of many controversies. Fluoride is known to have biological effects on osteoblasts at moderate to high doses but we will concentrate on the chemical effects of fluoride on bone mineral, which occurs at all doses (Bonar *et al.*, 1985). F has been used to prevent cavities and treat patients with osteoporosis (Harrison *et al.*, 1986). It is generally accepted that F substitutes for OH in the apatite lattice, making the lattice more stable and less soluble (Grynpas, 1990). It is incorporated mainly in the mineral of bones and teeth where it increases the crystallinity of the bone mineral and reduces its specific surface area. F influences the chemistry of the bone mineral decreasing the citrate content and may change the carbonate and magnesium content of bones. F affects bone crystal size by inducing no change in crystal length, and an increase in crystal thickness (Posner *et al.*, 1963; Chachra *et al.*, 1999). While F has been shown to increase the turnover of bone by increasing formation, studies on bone mineralization using density fractionation (Grynpas *et al.*, 1986) have shown a shift of the mineralization profile towards heavier mineral density. This may also explain why F reduces the solubility of bone mineral (Grynpas and Cheng, 1988).

These data also concur with data showing that rats fed a high F diet were more resistant to bone loss during periods of dietary calcium deficiency than control rats (Ericsson and Kberg, 1975). It has also been shown that F does not accumulate uniformly (Bang, 1978) in bone. When F is taken in excess, it can create bone, which is structurally disorganized and hypermineralized in certain areas. This may explain the findings of Turner *et al.* (1992) that, an increase in bone F, first increases and then decreases mechanical strength of rat bone above a given threshold.

Strontium (Sr), in both its stable and radioactive forms, is a bone seeking ion that is readily exchanged for calcium in the apatite lattice (LeGeros *et al.*, 1979). Increasing the Sr content in the food increases the amount of Sr in bone mineral (Skoryna, 1981). Sr in low doses has also been used to remineralize bone lesions in humans (Skoryna, 1984) and to augment bone mass in the rat (Marie *et al.*, 1985a, 1985b). At high doses Sr produces rickets in experimental animals (Matsumoto, 1976). Grynpas and Marie (1990) have shown that when stable Sr is given in doses that increase bone mass the mineralization profile of that bone is shifted to lower mineral densities. This is accompanied by a decrease in crystal size and a decrease in the CO_3 content of bone mineral proportional to the increase in bone Sr content. Sr does not appear to be preferentially incorporated into any mineral pool and its effect is to decrease bone crystallinity (Johnson, 1973). Therefore, Sr appears to increase bone mass by decreasing bone mineralization straining the apatite lattice by replacement of Ca by larger Sr ions and increasing bone mineral solubility.

Many other trace elements such as lead (Pb), copper (Cu), manganese (Mn), etc., have a profound influence on the skeleton, but their effect on bone mineralization has not been studied. Aluminium (Al) has been shown to induce osteomalacia in patients with chronic renal failure (Ott *et al.*, 1982). Al ions have been shown to interfere in a concentration-dependent manner with the formation of hydroxyapatite (Blumenthal and Posner, 1984). In this way, Al induces a mineralization defect similar to osteomalacia. Finally, some drugs can also induce shifts in mineralization. The bisphosphonates are a class of drugs, which have been developed in the last decades to prevent bone resorption (Francis and Martodam, 1983). They are characterized by their P-C-P bond, which makes them analogues of pyrophosphates. They bind strongly to hydroxyapatite crystals. This binding has been shown *in vitro* to inhibit both crystal formation and dissolution (Jung *et al.*, 1973). Their mode of action *in vivo* is still a matter of controversy, but they accumulate in the skeleton because of their apatite-binding ability. Both inhibition of calcification and the effect on bone resorption are highly dependent on the chemistry of the specific bisphosphonate (Shinoda *et al.*, 1983). The interaction of bisphosphonates with apatite crystals accounts for their binding to bone but not for their ability to inhibit bone resorption. Grynpas *et al.* (1992) have shown using the bisphosphonate disodium APD on dogs that the mineralization profile of bone treated with APD was significantly shifted to greater mineral densities in a dose-related manner. There was no change in the bone chemistry, but a decrease in the crystal size was also dose-related. The mechanism of this shift in mineralization could be due to both the inhibition of resorption and to the crystal poison effect of bisphosphonates.

6. What Determines Skeletal Fragility?

While the risk of fracture increases with decreasing bone mass, Heaney (1992) has even asked the question whether rapid bone loss is the consequence rather than the cause of osteoporosis. This is based on observations obtained during a multicenter study using ultrasound (Heaney *et al.*, 1989) and showing a nearly complete overlap between "mild osteoporotic" and "normal" measurements with respect to spinal bone mass; while "severe osteoporotic" measurements had a 50% overlap. Melton *et al.* (1989) also found a nearly complete overlap in the bone mass distribution of community samples of osteoporotic and normal subjects. Hui *et al.* (1988) have also shown that for a given bone mass the risk of fracture increases with age. They have shown that for a given bone density of 0.70–0.79 g/cm the risk of fracture in a 75-year-old woman is 7-fold higher than in a 45-year-old woman. All these observations led us to believe that there is a qualitative change in bone material properties, which is an important factor in human osteoporosis. Osteoporotic bone fractures result from a failure of the bone structure to sustain normal load bearing or minimal falls. In order to understand the causes of these fractures we have to know what the mechanical properties of bone are. The parameters measured on a load-deformation curve are the stiffness, maximum load, and maximum deformation a bone can sustain. When these parameters are normalized to the cross-section on which the force is applied they become the elastic modulus, the maximum stress or strength, the maximum strain and the toughness or energy needed to break a bone (Turner and Burr, 1993). There is considerable literature showing a loss of mechanical properties in bone with age. Burstein *et al.* (1976) have shown that while the elastic modulus of human femora decreases by 8%, their toughness decreases by 42% between the ages of 20 and 90. This indicates that the energy needed to fracture cortical bone, which is the relevant clinical factor, decreases at a much faster rate than its elastic modulus. Wall *et al.* (1979) have shown the non-linear relationship between bone density and bone strength by demonstrating that a 2.6% decrease in femora cortical density results in a 20% loss of strength. Mosekilde (1990) has shown that while the density of the human vertebral body declines 35–40% between the ages of 20 and 80 years its strength decreases by 60–65%. The reason why trabecular bone is lost faster than cortical bone is that trabecular bone turnover is much greater than cortical turnover due to the much greater number of bone cells and to the greater surface area of trabecular bone. The elastic modulus and toughness of vertebrae also decrease faster than their bone mass (Mosekilde, 1993). It has also been shown that for a similar bone mass the risk of fracture increases dramatically with age (Mosekilde, 1989). There are various factors, which influence bone mechanical strength such as bone architecture especially in trabecular bone. Anisotropy defined as the ratio of length in vertical versus horizontal trabeculae in vertebrae increases significantly between 20 and 80 years of age, which is the result of loss of horizontal trabeculae leading to loss of connectivity and strength independent of bone volume or mass (Mosekilde, 1989). It is now accepted that one of the roles of remodeling is to repair microdamage accumulated in everyday activities. However microcracks, which can be detected histologically, have been shown to accumulate with age in an exponential fashion in cortical bone after the age of 40 (Schaffler *et al.*, 1995). This phenomenon is associated with a decrease in cortical osteocyte lacunar density (Vashishth *et al.*, 2000). Burr *et al.* (1997) have suggested that microdamage accumulation and the failure to repair it properly may render osteoporotic bone more prone to fracture.

As we can see the remodeling process tends to become less effective at repairing damaged bone with age, which may be due to osteocyte death. Another factor is the paradox that while bone density decreases with age the bone that remains behind is becoming more mineralized (Grynpas, 1993). This in turn may increase the stiffness of bone while decreasing its toughness, and thus the amount of energy needed for bone to fracture (Currey, 1984). The increased bone turnover induced by menopause reduces bone mass and bone strength but the increased porosity can also affect bone toughness. Usually microcracks accumulate in the interstitial bone that is becoming more mineralized with age; if this bone is very porous the resorption cavities can act as stress concentrators (Currey, 1962). When microcracks accumulate, bone may fail in fatigue, which means that the bone will fail in smaller number of cycles than predicted by its strength. Zioupos *et al* (1996) have shown that bones in older women have a lower fatigue strength due to increased porosity and reduced bone mass. However bone strength can be partially preserved by continual new periosteal bone apposition, which occurs throughout life in long bones, especially in males (Martin *et al.*, 1980). This phenomenon also occurs in the cortical shell of vertebrae of males but not females (Mosekilde, 1993), which may in part explain why vertebral fractures are more common in women. Finally, local factors may play an important role in preserving the strength of certain bones as has been shown recently by Verna *et al.* (1999) in their comparison of remodeling parameters in mandibular versus iliac crest bone.

7. Conclusions

In determining the fracture risk in older bone, bone mass or BMD is only one of the factors to take into consideration. Bone quality, which includes bone architecture, bone mineralization, and bone mechanical properties, is very important in predicting bone fragility. These parameters are dependent on bone remodeling and can be modified by drugs and trace elements. For bone trabecular architecture, which is essential in the vertebrae, loss of connectivity will be a determinant factor in predicting crush fracture. In long bones, bone mineralization, porosity, and the distribution of bone tissue in cross-section will determine the mechanical properties. The most important of these mechanical properties is bone toughness, which determines the amount of energy needed to break a bone. Microcrack accumulation may also reduce the fatigue strength of bone. From these observations we can conclude that the properties of bone, both mechanical and homeostatic, are dependent on its mineral component and on the relation between the mineral and the organic matrix. In every piece of bone there is a distribution of mineral particles with varying mineral content. The shape of that distribution (mineralization profile) and its changes with aging and disease will, in turn, influence the material properties of bone, its role as a mechanical support and as an ion reservoir, and its ability to affect acid-base balance in the body. The size, orientation, chemistry, and solubility of the apatite crystals of bone and the way they pack to create a composite material with the collagen and noncollagenous proteins will determine not only the static properties of bone as a tissue but also the dynamics of change induced by bone cells in this tissue. It may very well be that hypermineralized bone is harder to resorb and to repair and that hypomineralized bone is more susceptible to resorption and more malleable.

References

Amprino, E., and Engstrom, A. (1952). Studies on X-ray absorption and diffraction of bone tissues. *Acta. Anat.* **15**, 1–22.

Antoine, S.E., Pollard, A.M., Desser, P.Q., and Whittle, A.W.R. (1988). Bone chemistry and dietary ctreconstruction in prehistoric Britain:Examples from Neolithic Orkney. In R.M. Faruhar, R.G.V. Hancock and L.A. Pavlish (eds) *Proceeding of the 26th Archaeometry Symposium.* pp. 101–106.

Atkinson, P.J. (1969). Structural aspects of ageing bone. *Gerontologia* **15**(2), 171–173.

Bang, S. (1978). Effects of fluoride on the chemical composition of inorganic bone substance. B. Courvoisier, A. Donath and C.A. Baud. Bern, Hans Huber: 56–61.

Barzel, U.S. (1975). Studies in osteoporosis: The long-term effect of oophorectomy and of ammonium chloride ingestion on the bone of mature rats. *Endocrinology* **96**(5), 1304–1306.

Bauss, F., Minne, H.W., Sterz, H., Weng, U., Wesch, H., and Ziegler, R. (1985). Comparative bone analysis via inflammation-mediated osteopenia (IMO) in the rat. *Calcif. Tissue Int.* **37**(5), 539–546.

Blumenthal, N.C., and Posner, A.S. (1984). In vitro model of aluminum-induced osteomalacia: Inhibition of hydroxyapatite formation and growth. *Calcif. Tissue Int.* **36**(4), 439–441.

Bonar, L.C., Grynpas, M.D., Roberts, J.E., Griffin, R.G., and Glimcher, M.J. (1985). Physical and chemical characterization of the development and maturation of bone mineral. In W.T. Butler (ed.) *The chemistry and biology of mineralized tissues.* pp. 226–233.

Bonar, L.C., Roufosse, A.H., Sabine, W.K., Grynpas, M.D., and Glimcher, M.J. (1983). X-ray diffraction studies of the crystallinity of bone mineral in newly synthesized and density fractionated bone. *Calcif. Tissue Int.* **35**(2), 202–209.

Boskey, A.L., and Marks, S.C., Jr. (1985). Mineral and matrix alterations in the bones of incisors-absent (ia/ia) osteopetrotic rats. *Calcif. Tissue Int.* **37**(3), 287–292.

Bratter, P., Gwlik, D.L., and Rosick, U. (1977). On the distribution of trace elements in human skeletons. *J. Radioanal. Chem.* **37**, 393–403.

Burkhart, J.M., and Jowsey, J. (1967). Parathyroid and thyroid hormones in the development of immobilization osteoporosis. *Endocrinology* **81**(5), 1053–1062.

Burr, D.B., Forwood, M.R., Fyhrie, D.P., Martin, R.B., Schaffler, M.B., and Turner, C.H. (1997). Bone microdamage and skeletal fragility in osteoporotic and stress fractures. *J. Bone Miner. Res.* **12**(1), 6–15.

Burstein, A.H., Reilly, D.T., and Martens, M. (1976). Aging of bone tissue: Mechanical properties. *J. Bone Joint Surg. [Am.]* **58**(1), 82–86.

Chachra, D., Turner, C.H., Dunipace, A.J., and Grynpas, M.D. (1999). The effect of fluoride treatment on bone mineral in rabbits. *Calcif. Tissue Int.* **64**(4), 345–351.

Chantraine, A., Nusgens, B., and Lapiere, C.M. (1986). Bone remodeling during the development of osteoporosis in paraplegia. *Calcif. Tissue Int.* **38**(6), 323–327.

Currey, J. (1984). The mechanical adaptations of bones. In J. Currey (ed.) *The mechanical adaptations of bones.* Princeton University Press, Princeton, NJ, pp. 88–97.

Currey, J.D. (1962). Stress concentration in bone. *J. Microscop. Sci.* **103**, 111–133.

Dequeker, J. (1975). Bone and ageing. *Ann. Rheum. Dis.* **34**(1), 100–115.

Dickson, I.R., and Kodicek, E. (1979). Effect of vitamin D deficiency on bone formation in the chick. *Biochem. J.* **182**(2), 429–435.

Ericsson, Y., and Kberg, O. (1975). Dietetically provoked general and alveolar osteopenia in rats and its prevention or cure by calcium and fluoride. *Periodontal Res.* **10**, 56–69.

Francis, M.D., and Martodam, R.R. (1983). Chemical, biochemical and medicinal properties of the disphosphonates. In R.L. Hildebrand (ed.) *The role of phosphonates in living systems.* CRC Press, Boca Raton, pp. 55–96.

Geidel, R. (1982). Trace element studies for Mississipian skeletal remains:Findings from neutron activation analysis. *MASCA. J.* **2**, 13–16.

Gilbert Jr., R. (1982). Trace elements in human hair and bone, in hair, trace elements and human illness (eds. A.C.Brown and FR.G.Crounse). *Praeger*, 35–44.

Grupe, G. (1987). Impact of the choice of bone samples on trace element data in cavated human skeletons. *J. Archaeol. Sci.* **15**, 123–129.

Grynpas, M. (1993). Age and disease-related changes in the mineral of bone. *Calcif. Tissue Int.* **53**(Suppl 1), S57–S64.

Grynpas, M.D. (1990). Fluoride effects on bone crystals. *J. Bone Miner. Res.* **5**(1), S169–S175.

Grynpas, M.D., Acito, A., Dimitriu, M., Mertz, B.P., and Very, J.M. (1992). Changes in bone mineralization, architecture and mechanical properties due to long-term (1 year) administration of pamidronate (APD) to adult dogs. *Osteoporos. Int.* **2**(2), 74–81.

Grynpas, M.D., Alpert, B., Katz, I., Lieberman, I., and Pritzker, K.P. (1991). Subchondral bone in osteoarthritis. *Calcif. Tissue Int.* **49**(1), 20–26.

Grynpas, M.D., and Cheng, P.T. (1988). Fluoride reduces the rate of dissolution of bone. *Bone Miner.* **5**(1), 1–9.

Grynpas, M.D., Holmyard, D., and Pritzker, K.P. (1994a). Bone mineralization and histomorphometry in biopsies of patients treated with fluoride. *Cells Mater.* **4**(3), 287–297.

Grynpas, M.D., Kasra, M., Dumitriu, M., Nespeca, R., Very, J.M., and Mertz, B.P. (1994b). Recovery from pamidronate (APD): A two-year study in the dog. *Calcif. Tissue Int.* **55**(4), 288–294.

Grynpas, M.D., and Marie, P.J. (1990). Effects of low doses of strontium on bone quality and quantity in rats. *Bone* **11**(5), 313–319.

Grynpas, M.D., Pritzker, K.P., and Hancock, R.G. (1987). Neutron activation of bulk and selected trace elements in bones using a low flux slowpoke reactor. *Biol. Trace Elem. Res.* **13**, 333–344.

Grynpas, M.D., Pritzker, K.P., Simmons, E.D., Hancock, R.G., and Harrison, J.E. (1986). Is fluoridated bone different from non-fluoridated bone? In Y. Ali (ed.) *Cell-mediated calcification nad. matrix vesicles.* Elsevier Science, New York. pp. 409–414.

Hancock, R., Grynpas, M., and Alpert, B. (1987). Are archaeological bones similar to modern bones? An archaeological assessment. *J. Radioanl.Nucl.Chem.* **110**, 283–291.

Hancock, R., Grynpas, M., and Pritzker, P. (1989). The abuse of bone analyses for archaeological dietary studies. *Archaeometry* **31**(2), 169–179.

Harrison, J.E., Bayley, T.A., Josse, R.G., Murray, T.M., Sturtridge, W., Williams, C., Goodwin, S., Tam, C. *et al.* (1986). The relationship between fluoride effects on bone histology and on bone mass in patients with postmenopausal osteoporosis. *Bone Miner.* **1**(4), 321–333.

Heaney, R.P. (1992). The natural history of vertebral osteoporosis. Is low bone mass an epiphenomenon? *Bone* **13**(Suppl 2), S23–S26.

Heaney, R.P., Avioli, L.V., Chesnut, C.H., Lappe, J., Recker, R.R., and Brandenburger, G.H. (1989). Osteoporotic bone fragility. Detection by ultrasound transmission velocity. *Jama.* **261**(20), 2986–2990.

Hui, S.L., Slemenda, C.W., and Johnston, C.C., Jr. (1988). Age and bone mass as predictors of fracture in a prospective study. *J. Clin. Invest.* **81**(6), 1804–1809.

Johnson, A.R. (1973). The influence of strontium on characteristic factors of bone. *Calcif. Tissue Res.* **11**(3), 215–221.

Jowsey, J., Reiss, E., and Canterbury, J.M. (1974). Long-term effects of high phosphate intake on parathyroid hormone levels and bone metabolism. *Acta. Orthop. Scand.* **45**(6), 801–808.

Jung, A., Bisaz, S., Bartholdi, P., and Fleisch, H. (1973). Influence of pyrophosphate on the exchange of calcium and phosphate ions on hydroxyapatite. *Calcif. Tissue Res.* **13**(1), 27–40.

Kanis, J.A. (1994). Assessment of fracture risk and its application to screening for postmenopausal osteoporosis: Synopsis of a WHO report. *Osteoporos. Int.* **4**(6), 368–381.

Kyle, J.H. (1986). Effect of post-burial conditions on the concentrations of major and minor elements in human bones and teeth-the implications of palaeodietary research. *J. Archaeol. Sci.* **13**, 403–416.

Lacroix, P., and Dhem A., (1967). Aging of the bones. A microradiographic study of compact bone. *Acta. Orthop. Belg.* **33**(4), 745–760.

Lambert, J., and Liang, X. (1988). Diet and excavatated bone. In R.M. Farquhar, R.G.V. Hancock and A. Pavlish (eds) *Proceedings of the 26th Archaeometry Symposium.* pp.107–109.

Lambert, J., Szpunar, C., and Buikstra, J. (1979). Chemical analysis of excavated human bone from middle and late woodlan sites. *Archaeometry* (21), 115–29.

Laval-Jeantet, A.M., Bergot, C., Carroll, R., and Garcia-Schaefer, F. (1983). Cortical bone senescence and mineral bone density of the humerus. *Calcif. Tissue Int.* **35**(3), 268–272.

LeGeros, R.Z., Quirologico, G., and LeGeros, J.P. (1979). Incorporation of strontium in apatite: Effect of pH. *J. Dent. Res.* **58(A)**, 169 abstract.

Lindahl, O., and Lindgren, A.G. (1967). Cortical bone in man. 1. Variation of the amount and density with age and sex. *Acta. Orthop. Scand.* **38**(2), 133–140.

Marie, P.J., Garba, M.T., Hott, M., and Miravet, L. (1985a). Effect of low doses of stable strontium on bone metabolism in rats. *Miner. Electrolyte Metab.* **11**(1), 5–13.

Marie, P.J., Hott, M., and Garba, M.T. (1985b). Contrasting effects of 1,25-dihydroxyvitamin D3 on bone matrix and mineral appositional rates in the mouse. *Metabolism* **34**(8), 777–783.

Martin, R.B., Pickett, J.C., and Zinaich, S. (1980). Studies of skeletal remodeling in aging men. *Clin. Orthop.*(149), 268–282.

Matsumoto, A. (1976). Effect of strontium on the epiphyseal cartilage plate of rat tibiae—histological and radiographic studies. *Jpn. J. Pharmacol.* **26**(6), 675–681.

Mazess, R.B. (1982). On aging bone loss. *Clin. Orthop.*(165), 239–252.

Melton, L.J., Kan, S.H., Frye, M.A., Wahner, H.W., O'Fallon, W.M., and Riggs, B.L. (1989). Epidemiology of vertebral fractures in women. *Am. J. Epidemiol.* **129**(5), 1000–1011.

Mosekilde, L. (1989). Sex differences in age-related loss of vertebral trabecular bone mass and structure—biomechanical consequences. *Bone* **10**(6), 425–432.

Mosekilde, L. (1990). Sex differences in age-related changes in vertebral body size, density and biomechanical competence in normal individuals. *Bone* **11**(2), 67–73.

Mosekilde, L. (1993). Normal age-related changes in bone mass, structure, and strength—consequences of the remodelling process. *Dan. Med. Bull.* **40**(1), 65–83.

Nelson, D., and Sauer, N. (1984). An evaluation of post-depositional changes in the trace element content of human bone. *Amer. Antiquity* **49**, 141–147.

Ott, S.M., Maloney, N.A., Coburn, J.W., Alfrey, A.C., and Sherrard, D.J. (1982). The prevalence of bone aluminum deposition in renal osteodystrophy and its relation to the response to calcitriol therapy. *N. Engl. J. Med.* **307**(12), 709–713.

Pankovich, A.M., Simmons, D.J., and Kulkarni, V.V. (1974). Zonal osteons in cortical bone. *Clin. Orthop.* **100**(0), 356–363.

Portigliatti Barbos, M., Bianco, P., and Ascenzi, A. (1983). Distribution of osteonic and interstitial components in the human femoral shaft with reference to structure, calcification and mechanical properties. *Acta. Anat. (Basel)* **115**(2), 178–186.

Posner, A.S., Eanes, E.D., and Harper, R.A. (1963). X-ray diffraction analysis of the effect of fluoride on human bone apatite. *Arch. Oral Biol.* **8**, 549–570.

Riggs, B.L., Seeman, E., Hodgson, S.F., Taves, D.R., and O'Fallon, W.M. (1982). Effect of the fluoride/calcium regimen on vertebral fracture occurrence in postmenopausal osteoporosis. Comparison with conventional therapy. *N. Engl. J. Med.* **306**(8), 446–450.

Runia, L.T. (1987). Analysis of bone from the Bronze age site Bovenkarspel-Het Valkje. The Netherlands: A preliminary report. *Archaeometry* **29**, 221–223.

Schaffler, M.B., Choi, K., and Milgrom, C. (1995). Aging and matrix microdamage accumulation in human compact bone. *Bone* **17**(6), 521–525.

Sharpe, W.D. (1979). Age changes in human bone: An overview. *Bull. N. Y. Acad. Med.* **55**(8), 757–773.

Shinoda, H., Adamek, G., Felix, R., Fleisch, H., Schenk, R., and Hagan, P. (1983). Structure-activity relationships of various bisphosphonates. *Calcif. Tissue Int.* **35**(1), 87–99.

Simmons, D.J., Russell, J.E., and Grynpas, M.D. (1986). Bone maturation and quality of bone material in rats flown on the space shuttle 'Spacelab-3 Mission.' *Bone Miner.* **1**(6), 485–493.

Skoryna, S.C. (1981). Effects of oral supplementation with stable strontium. *Can. Med. Assoc. J.* **125**(7), 703–712.

Skoryna, S.C. (1984). Metabolic aspects of ht epharmacologic use of trace elements in human subjects with specific reference to stable strontium. *Trace Subst. Environ. Health* **18**, 3–23.

Thompson, D.D. (1980). Age changes in bone mineralization, cortical thickness, and haversian canal area. *Calcif. Tissue Int.* **31**(1), 5–11.

Thompson, R., Jr. (1973). Heparin osteoporosis. An experimental model using rats. *Bone Joint Surg. Am.* **55**, 606–612.

Trotter, M., and Hixon, B.B. (1974). Sequential changes in weight, density, and percentage ash weight of human skeletons from an early fetal period through old age. *Anat. Rec.* **179**(1), 1–18.

Turner, C.H., Akhter, M.P., and Heaney, R.P. (1992). The effects of fluoridated water on bone strength. *J. Orthop. Res.* **10**(4), 581–587.

Turner, C.H., and Burr, D.B. (1993). Basic biomechanical measurements of bone: A tutorial. *Bone* **14**(4), 595–608.

Utoff, H.K., and Jaworski, Z.F. (1978). Bone loss in response to long-term immobilization. *J. Bone Joint Surg.* **60**(8), 420–429.

Vashishth, D., Verborgt, O., Divine, G., Schaffler, M.B., and Fyhrie, D.P. (2000). Decline in osteocyte lacunar density in human cortical bone is associated with accumulation of microcracks with age. *Bone* **26**(4), 375–380.

Verna, C., Melsen, B., and Melsen, F. (1999). Differences in static cortical bone remodeling parameters in human mandible and iliac crest. *Bone* **25**(5), 577–583.

Wall, J.C., Chatterji, S.K., and Jeffery, J.W. (1979). Age-related changes in the density and tensile strength of human femoral cortical bone. *Calcif. Tissue Int.* **27**(2), 105–108.

Wasnich, R.D. (1996). Epidemiology of osteoporosis. In M.J. Favus (ed.) *Primer on the metabolic bone diseases and disorders of mineral metabolism.* Lippincott-Raven, Philadelphia. pp. 249–251.

Whiting, S.J., and Draper, H.H. (1980). The role of sulfate in the calciuria of high protein diets in adult rats. *J. Nutr.* **110**(2), 212–222.

Wronski, R., and Yen, C. (1991). The ovariectomized rat as an animal model for postmenopausal bone loss. *Cells Mater.* **1**(Suppl), 69–74.

Zioupos, P., Wang, X.T., and Currey, J.D. (1996). Experimental and theoretical quantification of the development of damage in fatigue tests of bone and antler. *J. Biomech.* **29**(8), 989–1002.

Part II

Population Approaches

4

Ethnic Differences in Bone Mass and Bone Architecture

Dorothy A. Nelson and Marie L. Villa

1. Introduction

1.1. Osteoporosis

The term "osteoporosis" refers to a systemic skeletal condition that predisposes individuals to fragility fractures. Osteoporosis is characterized by a low bone mass, architectural deterioration of the bone tissue, and an increased fracture risk (Consensus Development Conference, 1991). It is well known that bone loss after middle age (menopause in women, some years later in men) is a universal phenomenon. However, the amount of peak bone mass achieved in young adulthood contributes to the likelihood of developing osteoporosis, since the effect of age-related bone loss will be different in individuals who start with high bone mass compared with those with a lower peak bone mass. Sex and ethnic differences in peak bone mass partially explain sex and ethnic differences in osteoporosis and fracture risk.

1.2. Bone Densitometry and Assessment of Bone Architecture

Advances in methods of bone densitometry have allowed the assessment of bone mass, or bone mineral density (BMD), in a variety of geographic areas and ethnic groups. The most commonly used bone densitometry method is dual-energy x-ray absorptiometry (DEXA) which measures several different skeletal sites quickly and noninvasively (Figure 4.1). The usual measurement sites are skeletal regions where the most common osteoporotic fractures occur, particularly the spine, hip, and wrist.

In-vivo assessment of bone architecture is more problematic, but DEXA data can be used to measure several features of bone geometry. These include a simple measure of hip axis length, done by hand on the image that is produced, or using automated software from the manufacturer. Additionally, it is possible to reconstruct cross-sectional bone geometry from the raw data, with the use of specialized programs not provided by the manufacturer.

Dorothy A. Nelson • Wayne State University School of Medicine, Detroit, Michigan.
Marie L. Villa • University of Washington School of Medicine, Seattle, Washington.

Bone Loss and Osteoporosis: An Anthropological Perspective, edited by Sabrina C. Agarwal and Sam D. Stout. Kluwer Academic/Plenum Publishers, New York, 2003.

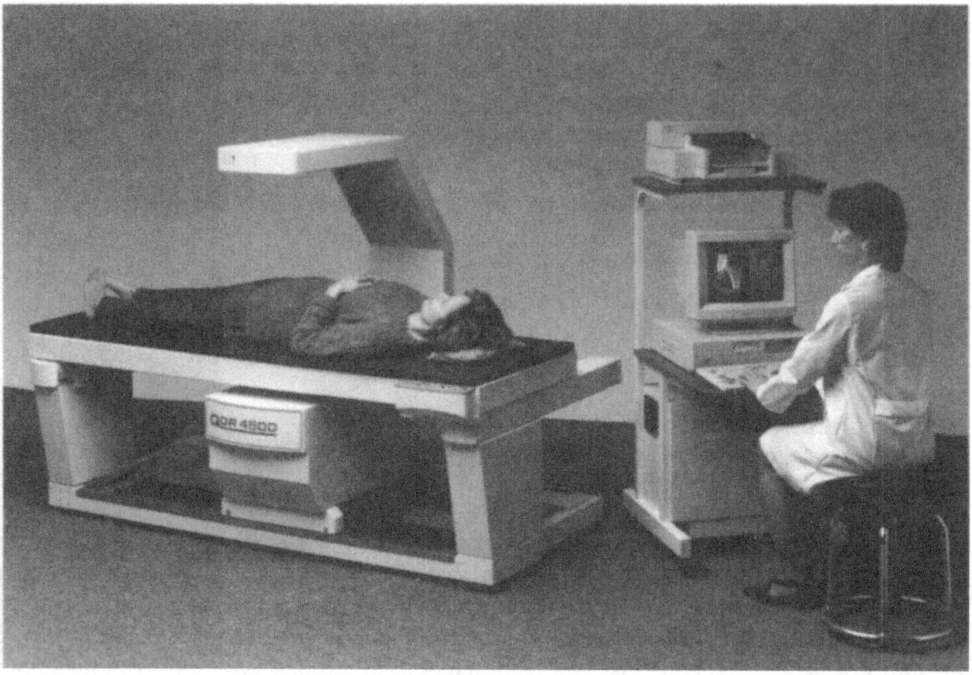

Figure 4.1. Example of bone densitometry instrument that utilizes dual-energy x-ray absorptiometry (DEXA): Hologic QDR 4500 (Waltham, MA).

1.3. Bone Density and Fracture Incidence

Fracture incidence has been reported for a variety of populations. However, estimates are variable for many types of fracture and are affected by the source of data. Hip fracture incidence rates are perhaps easiest to document since they almost always result in hospital admission and therefore produce a record of the event. Available data on fracture incidence show a wide variation among populations.

The relationship between decreasing BMD and increasing fracture risk has been well documented in populations of European ancestry in the United States and much of Europe. The Study of Osteoporotic Fractures (SOF) (Cummings SR *et al.*, 1990) has resulted in estimates of the relative risk of fractures per standard deviation decrease in bone density at a variety of skeletal sites, ranging from 1.5–2.6 (Figure 4.2). This large study, often referred to as "SOF," comprises 9,704 women over age 65 who were recruited for a longitudinal study of osteoporosis and fractures. Unfortunately, SOF enrolled only White women, and there are no comparable data for other ethnic groups. However, sufficient data have been amassed in a number of other groups that some comparisons can be made across geographic and cultural groups. While it appears that the relationship between BMD and fracture risk holds in most populations, there are some exceptions. The positive relationship between high bone mass and low incidence of hip fracture is seen in New Zealand Polynesians (Stott *et al.*, 1980; Reid *et al.*, 1986). However, Hispanics have hip fracture incidence rates comparable to those of African Americans, yet have bone mass values

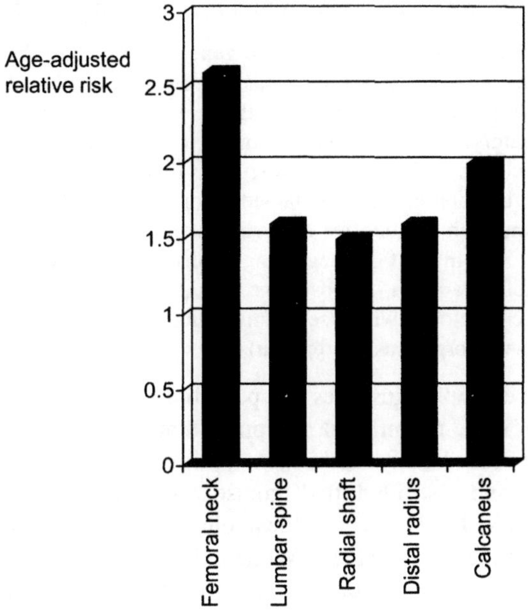

Figure 4.2. Age-adjusted relative risk for hip fracture for each standard deviation decrease in bone mineral density at five skeletal sites. (Adapted from Cummings *et al.*, 1993.)

closer to those of non-Hispanic Whites (Looker *et al.*, 1995; Villa *et al.*, 1995; Haddock *et al.*, 1996). Asian Americans demonstrate a similar relationship (Yano *et al.*, 1984; Hagiwara *et al.*, 1989; Russell-Aulet *et al.*, 1991; Lauderdale *et al.*, 1997). One South American ethnic group in Vilcabamba, Ecuador enjoys an extremely low rate of hip fracture despite BMD values much lower than that of non-Hispanic Whites (Mazess, 1978). There are a few published studies investigating bone health in extant Native American groups (Mazess and Mather, 1974; Harper *et al.*, 1984; McHugh *et al.*, 1993; Perry *et al.*, 1998). Unfortunately, hip fracture studies entirely exclude this group so that relationships between bone mass and fracture risk cannot be drawn.

Bone mass may not be the factor that best predicts fracture risk in many ethnic groups. It has been hypothesized that features of bone architecture may play a very important role in fracture risk, and that such factors are different in different populations.

1.4. Use of "Race" and "Ethnicity" in Biomedical Literature on Osteoporosis

In biomedical publications reporting osteoporosis rates and fracture incidence, population differences are usually referred to as "racial" differences. One notable exception is an editorial by Marie Luz Villa (1994) that examined the limitation of the race concept, and the importance of cultural determinants, in bone research. While many if not most anthropologists have recognized these issues for decades, in 1998 the American Anthropological Association's (AAA) Executive Board adopted an official statement of the AAA's position on "race." Excerpts from this statement appear below:

> In the United States both scholars and the general public have been conditioned to viewing human races as natural and separate divisions within the human species based on visible physical differences. With the vast expansion of scientific knowledge in this century, however, it has become clear that human populations are not unambiguous, clearly demarcated, biologically distinct groups .... The continued sharing of genetic materials has maintained all of humankind as a single species .... At the end of the 20th century, we now understand that human cultural behavior is learned, conditioned into infants beginning at birth, and always subject to modification .... Our temperaments, dispositions, and personalities, regardless of genetic propensities, are developed within sets of meanings and values that we call "culture." (www.ameranthassn.org/stmts/racepp.htm)

The following example illustrates one potential pitfall of utilizing simplistic "racial" categories instead of more meaningful groupings that reflect the ethnic identification of a group. In a study of bone density in children, a large subgroup of the subjects considered themselves "White" and also identified themselves as Chaldean, an Iraqi ethnic group (Nelson and Barondess, 1997). The Chaldean children's whole body bone mass was significantly higher than the non-Chaldean White children, and was not different from other study subjects who considered themselves Black/African American. Since Middle Easterners are included in the U.S. Census category "White/Caucasian," such a difference would not have been detected if a model based on "race" had been used. That is, the Chaldean children would have been included with the non-Chaldean White children and the interesting and possibly very important ethnic difference in bone mass would not have been detected. In this chapter, the term "ethnicity" rather than "race" is used to reflect cultural, religious, dietary, geographic, and other group characteristics that might contribute to population differences in osteoporosis risk.

2. Bone Mass and Bone Density

2.1. Definitions of Bone Density

The term bone mass can refer to a variety of measurements, including bone mineral content (BMC in g), areal BMD (BMD in g/cm^2), and volumetric or true bone density (BMD in g/cm^3). Bone densitometry based on DEXA results in a measurement of "areal" BMD in g/cm^2 while quantitative computed tomography (QCT) provides BMD in g/cm^3. The magnitude of ethnic differences in bone mass reported by various investigators varies with the measurement used as well as other factors.

2.2. Ethnic Differences in Bone Density

African Americans have significantly greater areal BMD than Whites (Liel *et al.*, 1988; Luckey *et al.*, 1989; Kleerekoper *et al.*, 1994b; Looker *et al.*, 1995; Nelson *et al.*, 1995; Barondess *et al.*, 1997), which is thought to contribute to their lower rate of hip fracture. Kleerekoper *et al.* (1994a) have shown that volumetric BMD measured by QCT is 40% higher in African American women compared with White women, considerably greater than the 5–15% difference in areal BMD generally reported for African American versus White adults.

Most studies based on absorptiometry (such as DEXA) find higher bone mass among African Americans throughout childhood (Li *et al.*, 1989; Laraque *et al.*, 1990; Bell *et al.*, 1991; Nelson *et al.*, 1997). However, Gilsanz and colleagues (1991) examined volumetric bone density (g/cm^3), based on QCT, in African American and White children at different stages of sexual development. In contrast to the findings with DEXA, these investigators found that significant ethnic differences did not occur until late puberty.

It has been hypothesized (or assumed) that the higher bone mass seen in African Americans stems in part from genetic factors. Therefore, it might be assumed that any population of African origin would have a high bone mass similar to African Americans, but this has not been borne out. Investigations of Blacks in South Africa (Solomon 1979; Patel *et al.*, 1992; Daniels *et al.*, 1995) and Gambia (Prentice *et al.*, 1990; Aspray *et al.*, 1996) show that their bone mass does not exceed, and in some cases is even lower than that of age-matched Whites living in Africa. These data illustrate the difficulty in generalizing about a "racial" group, when obviously ethnic gradations in bone mass exist within people of African descent, with further differences introduced by admixture and acculturation in areas to which Black Africans migrated.

3. Bone Quality and Bone Turnover

Risk for osteoporotic fracture depends not only upon the mass of bone, but its quality as well. The rate and efficiency of bone turnover (affected by many factors, including reproductive hormone status, body composition, vitamin D/calcium nutriture, and physical activity) impacts bone architecture, which is an essential component of skeletal strength.

Low bone turnover in African American adults may partially explain their greater lifelong bone mass and lower fracture risk than American Whites. Some studies found biochemical evidence that African Americans have lower rates of bone turnover than non-Hispanic Whites (Meier *et al.*, 1992; Kleerekoper *et al.*, 1994b; Han *et al.*, 1997). In addition, histomorphometric studies showed mean rates of bone formation in African Americans to be significantly lower than that of Whites (Weinstein and Bell, 1988; Han *et al.*, 1997). These authors conclude that most if not all ethnic differences observed in bone cell function could be the result of differences in bone accumulation during growth: higher bone mass would result in less fatigue damage and less need for repair by directed bone remodeling.

However, studies comparing South African Blacks and Whites suggested higher bone turnover in Blacks, which was hypothesized to lead to fewer fractures because of better trabecular bone quality and less skeletal fragility (Schnitzler *et al.*, 1990; Schnitzler 1993). These contrasting studies again highlight the pitfalls associated with assuming that subgroups (such as geographically different populations) of a "racial" group will be biologically similar.

4. Factors Affecting Bone Mass and Bone Loss

4.1. Adjusting Bone Density for Body Size

Body size appears to be an independent contributor to variance in BMD. However, BMD as measured by DEXA controls only partially for bone size (area rather than volume).

Therefore, use of a mathematical correction for differences in densitometric bone size (Katzman *et al.*, 1991) from one population to another might correct for differences in body habitus and shed some light on the seeming discrepancies between bone mass and fracture risk across ethnic groups. In a multisite study of hormone replacement and its effects on bone mass in postmenopausal women, it was noted that although African Americans had the highest measured bone mass, when adjustments were made for bone size, the ethnic differences in bone density were significantly attenuated (Marcus *et al.*, 1994). Analysis of Inuit ("Eskimo") bone mineral content shows it to be lower than that of non-Hispanic Whites, but their low rate of fracture is thought to be due to relatively larger bone size (Harper *et al.* 1984). Despite the widely accepted axiom that Asians have lower bone mass than Whites a recent comparison of closely matched non-Hispanic White and Chinese women found slightly higher bone mass in the Chinese when height and weight (and theoretically differences in bone size) were controlled (Russell-Aulet *et al.*, 1993). Recent data suggest that differences in bone accumulation in multi-ethnic populations of adolescents may predominantly reflect bone size (Bhudhikanok *et al.*, 1996; Wang *et al.*, 1997).

4.2. Body Size and Composition, and Preservation of the Skeleton

Body weight factors heavily in the maintenance of bone density, and thinness is an important risk factor for hip fracture in African American, White, and Asian women (Pruzansky *et al.*, 1989; Lau *et al.*, 1993; Grisso *et al.*, 1994). However, it appears that both fat and lean body mass contribute to preservation of the skeleton (Aloia *et al.*, 1991; Reid *et al.*, 1992), perhaps due in part to peripheral aromatization of androgen to estrogen that occurs in adipose tissue and skeletal muscle (Matsumine *et al.*, 1986). Serum estrone levels relate positively to degree of obesity, and bone mass correlates positively with body weight in both African American and White women (DeSimone *et al.*, 1989). However, differences in body weight does not explain all of the differences in bone mass between these groups (Nelson *et al.*, 1988).

Epidemiologic studies indicate that African American women are classified as overweight twice as frequently as non-Hispanic White women (Kumanyika, 1987). Obesity classification typically depends upon self-report of weight and height, with subsequent computation of body mass index (BMI), which is conventionally expressed as weight/height^2. Obesity has been defined in the recent past as BMI $>$ 27.3 kg/m^2 (Najjar and Rowland, 1987). This definition is based upon statistics from the second National Health and Nutrition Examination Survey (NHANES II), using the 85th percentile of BMI for 20–29 year-old non-Hispanic Whites as an obesity cutoff point. More recent guidelines were established by the World Health Organization in 1997, using a BMI of 25 kg/m^2 as the lower limit of obesity (Report of a WHO Consultation on Obesity, 1997). Application of the older definition for obesity has not been race- or ethnicity-adjusted in the majority of studies. Lopez and Mâsse (1992) compared anthropometric data from NHANES II to data acquired during the 1982–1984 Hispanic Health and Nutrition Examination Survey (HHANES). They found that use of the NHANES II obesity cutoff consistently labeled 12–14% more Puerto Rican and Mexican American women as obese than if ethnicity-specific cutoff data from HHANES were used (Lopez and Masse, 1992). BMIs of Cuban American women reflected those of NHANES II data, suggesting that a "Hispanic"-specific cut-off is of limited use because there are differences in height and weight distribution among Hispanic ethnic groups.

A recent study of a northern Indian population reported that the current conventional cutoff for obesity (BMI = 25 kg/m^2) did not accurately identify subjects who were overweight in this sample (Dudeja *et al.*, 2001). These investigators found that a lower cutoff value (21.5 kg/m^2 for men and 19 kg/m^2 for women) showed the best sensitivity and specificity for classifying individuals who were above or below a sex-specific body fat standard. Not surprisingly, the body fat norms for this northern Indian population were very different than those that have been reported for other major ethnic groups (Dudeja *et al.*, 2001).

It is clear that the optimal formula for a BMI varies among populations. If the purpose of using a weight for height index is to minimize the effect of height on body mass, then one approach to identifying an appropriate index is to find the exponent for the denominator that minimizes the correlation between weight and height (such that $r = 0$) in a given population (Lee *et al.*, 1981). Kleerekoper *et al.* (1994c) applied this approach to 201 White and 77 African American postmenopausal women participating in a longitudinal study of bone mass and biochemical markers of bone remodeling. The African American women had a significantly greater BMI based on the conventional formula. However, the formula that best provided a height(m)-free measure of weight(kg) was different for the White (weight/height 1.17) and the African American women (weight/height 1.30) (Kleerekoper *et al.*, 1994c). When BMI was calculated using these population-specific formulae, there was no significant difference between the two groups, suggesting that these African American women were not more "obese." This underscores the need to consider population-specific approaches to studying human biologic phenomena.

Although BMI is often used to estimate degree of obesity, body composition is much more complex. The simplest model uses bone, fat, and lean body mass as the three major components. Since bone and lean body mass are closely related (Ellis and Cohn, 1975), it stands to reason that groups with increased muscle mass, such as African Americans and Polynesians (Cohn *et al.*, 1977; Reid *et al.*, 1990), will have higher bone mass. Therefore, total body weight will be greater in those with higher bone mass, not necessarily because of obesity but also due to the contribution of bone and muscle weight. Body composition comparisons made between African American and White women demonstrate consistently greater muscle and bone mass in the former (Aloia *et al.*, 2000), underscoring the importance of using population-specific reference populations when interpreting body habitus data.

4.3. Calcium Nutrition

Calcium intake affects attainment of peak bone mass as well as ability to preserve skeletal calcium throughout life (Heaney, 1999). In an early study, Matkovic and colleagues (1979) demonstrated that hip fracture rates differed significantly within an ethnic group living in two regions of Croatia with divergent levels of dietary calcium intake, and concluded that these differences were due to differences in attainment of peak bone mass. Gradations in bone mass related to calcium intake are also observed in other ethnic groups. Hu and collaborators (1993), in an excellent dietary study of Chinese women with similar ethnic backgrounds, demonstrated a wide range in BMD depending upon dietary calcium intake (Hu *et al.*, 1993). In this group, although the women with higher calcium intake had higher BMD, the rate of bone loss with age was not affected by dietary calcium, supporting the hypothesis that the differences in bone mass observed in older women were realized earlier in life. Calcium nutriture may contribute to differences in the bone mass of Japanese and Japanese American groups as well (Fujita *et al.*, 1977; Yano *et al.*, 1985), and calcium supplementation has been shown to reduce bone loss in elderly Chinese women (Lau *et al.*, 1992). However, calcium is only one dietary component that contributes to skeletal health, and is not sufficient by itself to ensure adequate bone mass at all ages and life stages (Heaney, 1999). Calcium interacts with other nutrients, physical activity levels, body size and compositon, age, general health status, and other biocultural variables (Nelson, 1996). In an anthropological review of low bone mass in various populations, Pfeiffer and Lazenby (1994) concluded that evolutionary models of skeletal health must consider the synergism among calcium and other nutritional factors.

When analyzing HHANES and NHANES II data, Looker and co-workers found that calcium intakes in Hispanic diets paralleled those of non-Hispanic Whites, and were somewhat higher than those of African Americans (Looker *et al.*, 1993). Striking differences existed in the dietary sources of calcium for the three Hispanic groups, although total calcium intakes did not vary significantly. Milk was the single greatest contributor for all three, but corn tortillas were second in importance for Mexican Americans alone. A listing of the top ten contributors to dietary calcium for Mexican Americans also included flour tortillas and pinto beans, whereas for Cuban Americans and Puerto Ricans, pizza and rice were major sources. The bioavailability of calcium may vary widely among these diverse foods. For some, such as pinto beans, calcium absorbability is less than that of milk (Heaney and Weaver, 1992), but the total intake of calcium from all sources may be sufficient to exceed gastrointestinal and renal losses. Questionnaire assessment of dietary calcium intake should therefore be tailored to include ethnic foods in order to collect representative data.

Ethnic differences in the absorption and excretion of calcium may affect overall calcium balance. One study conducted under conditions of severe calcium restriction found African Americans to have low vitamin D levels and compensatory hypersecretion of parathyroid hormone, theoretically maximizing urinary retention of calcium and thereby contributing to greater bone mass (Bell *et al.*, 1985). Another study that provided adequate dietary calcium found no evidence of a difference in the vitamin D endocrine system (Meier *et al.*, 1991). However, despite lack of differences in dietary calcium and vitamin D intake, it was found that African Americans had significantly lower urinary calcium excretion, and that calcium excretion was inversely related to radial BMD.

4.4. Physical Activity

Physical activity benefits the skeleton throughout all stages of life, and is a lifestyle habit subject to great variation among different groups. Despite varying cultural values and attitudes toward physical activity throughout life, its beneficial effect on bone mass appears ubiquitous. However, multi-cultural studies concerning type of physical activity and accretion of bone density are lacking. It would be especially useful to investigate whether culturally determined activities during adolescence affect lifetime risk for fracture. It could be that habitual activities or work during youth affect adult bone mass and possibly skeletal structure. Physical activity and muscle strength in older adults also affect the risk of falling, another contributor to overall fracture risk.

5. Bone Geometry

5.1. Hip Axis Length

Bone mineral density predicts fracture risk, but there is considerable overlap of BMD in hip fracture cases and controls. Also, there is considerable variation in fracture risk among ethnic groups with similar BMD values. Thus, factors other than bone mass also affect risk for osteoporotic fracture. Analysis of bone densitometry data collected in the SOF suggests that a simple geometric measurement of femoral size, hip axis length (HAL), is related to hip fracture risk (Faulkner *et al.*, 1993). HAL is the distance from the lateral femoral shaft, distal to the greater trochanter, to the inner pelvic brim—on a line that is parallel to the long axis of the femoral neck (Figure 4.3). In the study by Faulkner *et al.* (1993), shorter HAL was associated with a decreased risk of hip fracture. In another study, African Americans and Asian Americans had a significantly shorter HAL when compared to the fracture group (which was predominantly non-Hispanic White) (Cummings *et al.*, 1994). A study comparing Japanese and White Americans demonstrated an association between low fracture risk and short femoral neck (Nakamura *et al.*, 1994). Additionally, the HAL of Mexican American women, another ethnic group with relatively

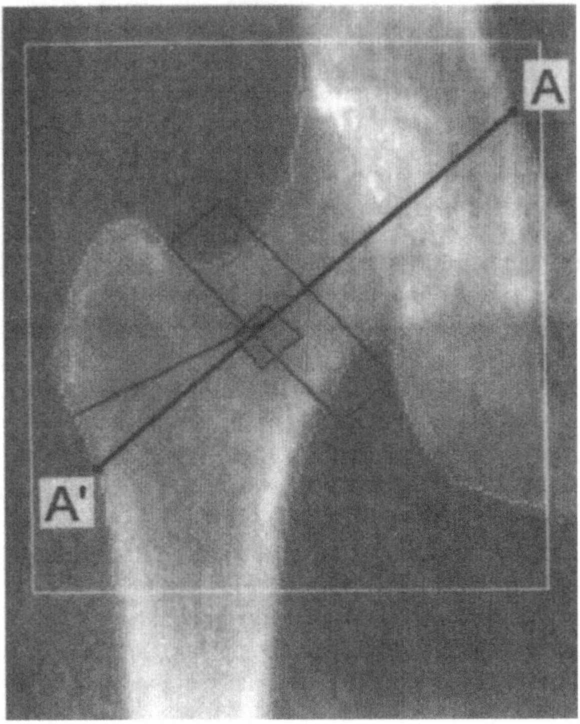

Figure 4.3. Landmarks (A and A′) on the proximal femur that are used for measuring hip axis length (HAL) from a dual-energy x-ray absorptiometry (DEXA) scan. HAL is measured as the distance from A to A′. (Reproduced from *J Bone Miner. Res.* 1994, **9**, 1065–1070 with permission of the American Society for Bone and Mineral Research.)

low risk for hip fracture, averages about the same as for Asian Americans and African Americans (Villa *et al.*, 1995), substantiating the importance of considering bone geometric properties when evaluating fracture risk cross-nationally.

The same cautionary rule applies to assessment of HAL in determining risk for fracture: its application to risk may vary with ethnicity. In a comparison of bone geometric properties as risk factors for hip fracture in European, Chinese, Indian, and Polynesian premenopausal women, Chin and colleagues (1997) found shorter HAL in the Chinese and Indian groups, but longer HAL in European and Polynesian women (Chin *et al.*, 1997). Since Polynesian women enjoy a very low rate of hip fracture, osteoporotic risk factors other than HAL must be considered.

5.2. Cross-Sectional Geometry

The strength of long bones is largely determined by geometric details of their cross-sections. Although both BMD and cross-sectional geometric properties contribute to bone strength, BMD measurements average out structural detail in order to provide an estimate of mineral content per unit area (Nelson *et al.*, 2000). In contrast, cross-sectional geometric measurements are able to provide information about mechanical properties, based on the distribution of bone mineral (Bell *et al.*, 1999). Several studies have suggested that femoral geometric measures change with age, differ in men and women, and vary among different populations (Ruff and Hayes, 1988; Beck *et al.*, 1992; Cummings *et al.*, 1994; Nakamura *et al.*, 1994; Yoshikawa *et al.*, 1994; Mikhail *et al.*, 1996; Peacock *et al.*, 1998; Theobald *et al.*, 1998). In one of these studies, Theobald *et al.* (1998) measured hip bone mass by DEXA, and hip geometric variables on pelvic radiographs, in groups of Nigerian, African American, and White women over the age of 65. They found several significant ethnic differences in the radiographic measurements, independent of BMD.

Hip Structure Analysis, developed by Beck and colleagues for DEXA data, includes assessments of the following variables (Beck *et al.*, 1990): (a) Cross-sectional area: The cortical bone equivalent area of the cross-section of the region of interest (femoral neck or shaft), with all soft tissue voids (trabecular and cellular spaces) eliminated, in cm^2. Cross-sectional area is derived from the integral of the bone mass profile across the narrow region. (b) Cross-sectional moment of inertia (CSMI): A property of the cross-sectional area that represents the magnitude of the greatest bending rigidity of the section, in cm^4. CSMI is derived from the integral of the bone mass profile across the bone together with its center of mass. (c) Section modulus: An index of strength calculated as the CSMI ÷ the distance from the bone edge to the centroid (assumed here to be half the subperiosteal width), in cm^3. These variables, as well as estimates of endocortical diameters (i.e., width of the medullary cavity) and cortical thicknesses (i.e., bone widths), were measured in the femoral neck in a study of African American and White postmenopausal women (Nelson *et al.*, 2000). The results of the Hip Structure Analysis indicated many ethnic differences in BMD, cross-sectional geometry and dimensional variables. The BMD's derived from the narrow cross-sectional region of the neck were significantly greater in African Americans. African American women also had greater measurements for all other variables except endocortical diameter, which was larger in the White women consistent with their thinner cortices.

These results suggest that there are some mechanically important differences in the proximal femur in the African American compared with White women: African American women have longer, narrower femora on average, with smaller medullary cavities than Whites. However, the thicker cortices in African Americans would contribute to both higher BMD values and greater mechanical strength. This architecture would lower bending stresses along the cortical surfaces of the bone during normal physical activities. These observations, along with the greater cross-sectional moments of inertia and section moduli in African Americans, suggest that the spatial distribution of bone is arranged to resist greater loading compared with White women.

In a follow-up study, cross-sectional geometry was assessed in a comparable group of White and Black postmenopausal women living in Johannesburg, South Africa (Nelson *et al.*, 2000). The U.S. groups compared to their South African counterparts (i.e., White and Black) had greater cortical thickness and cross-sectional area despite no significant difference in bone width in the femoral neck. Blacks in both countries had a higher section modulus—an index of bending strength—in the neck, where osteoporotic fractures occur. These results suggest greater hip BMD and bone strength among Blacks in both South Africa and the United States, which would correspond with lower hip fracture risks in these groups.

6. Fracture Incidence

There is a wide variation in the occurrence of osteoporotic hip fractures within and among different ethnic groups. There are also secular trends in hip fracture incidence. In countries where hip fractures are uncommon, fractures due to severe trauma account for a larger proportion of the total number of hip fractures (Melton, 1988).

Studies conducted in ethnically diverse populations using the same methodology for ascertaining hip fractures in all groups are particularly valuable for making inferences about ethnic differences in hip fracture incidence (Stott *et al.*, 1980; Bauer, 1988; Silverman and Madison, 1988; Fisher *et al.*, 1991; Hinton and Smith, 1993; Baron *et al.*, 1994). Most of these studies have been conducted in the United States, and they consistently indicate higher rates among non-Hispanic Whites than among other groups. In a study conducted in Bexar County, Texas, age- and sex-adjusted hip fracture incidence was lowest in African Americans, and highest in non-Hispanic Whites, with intermediate rates for Hispanics (Bauer, 1988). In contrast, Silverman and Madison (1988) found that age- and sex-adjusted incidence of hip fracture in California was lower among Hispanic Whites than among all other groups, including non-Hispanic Whites, African Americans, and Asians. A study comparing hip fracture incidence among native Japanese, Japanese Americans, and non-Hispanic White Americans reported the lowest rates among Japanese Americans and the highest rates among the non-Hispanic Whites (Ross *et al.*, 1991).

Increasing age is an established risk factor for hip fracture in all ethnic groups (Maggi *et al.*, 1991). Although hip fracture incidence increases with age in all ethnic groups, the increase occurs earlier in non-Hispanic White populations than in African American, Asian, and Hispanic populations (Maggi *et al.*, 1991). Studies conducted in non-Hispanic White populations report higher rates of hip fracture among men than women before 50 years of age, whereas after age 50, women have higher rates than men.

7. Summary

There is great variation among populations in bone mass, bone geometry, and fracture incidence. White women have been studied in the greatest detail and it appears that this group has the highest prevalence of and risk for osteoporosis and fractures. It appears that ethnic differences in skeletal health result from complex relationships among bone and body size (which may be largely inherited), morphology, physiological variables, lifestyle factors, migration, and acculturation patterns. Much information may be gleaned from inter-ethnic studies that may help elucidate possible etiologies in the pathogenesis of osteoporosis. Description of study groups should specifically state the basis for identification and classification of the groups being compared.

References

Aloia, J.F., McGowan, D.M., Vaswani, A.N., Ross, P., and Cohn, S.H. (1991). Relationship of menopause to skeletal and muscle mass. *Am. J. Clin. Nutr.* **53**, 1378–1383.

Aloia, J.F., Vaswani, A., Feuerman, M., Mikhail, M., and Ma, R. (2000). Differences in skeletal and muscle mass with aging in black and white women. *Am. J. Physiol. Endocrinol. Metab.* **278**, E1153–1157.

Aspray, T.J., Prentice, A., Cole, T.J., Sawo, Y., Reeve, J., and Francis, R.M. (1996). Low bone mineral content is common but osteoporotic fractures are rare in elderly rural Gambian women. *J. Bone Miner. Res.* **11**(7), 1019–1025.

Baron, J.A., Barrett, J., Malenka, D., Fisher, E., Kniffin, W., Bubolz, T., and Tosteson, T. (1994). Racial differences in fracture risk. *Epidemiol.* **5**, 42–47.

Barondess, D.A., Nelson, D.A., and Schlaen, S.E. (1997). Whole body bone, fat, and lean mass in Black and White men. *J. Bone Miner. Res.* **12**, 967–971.

Bauer, R.L. (1988). Ethnic differences in hip fracture: A reduced incidence in Mexican Americans. *Am. J. Epidemiol.* **127**(1), 145–149.

Beck, T.J., Ruff, C.B., Warden, K.E., Scott, W.W., and Rao, R.U. (1990). Predicting femoral neck strength from bone mineral data: A structural approach. *Invest. Rad.* **25**, 6–18.

Beck, T.J., Ruff, C.B., Scott, W.W., Plato, C.C., Tobin, J.D., and Quan, C.A. (1992). Sex differences in geometry of the femoral neck with aging: A structural analysis of bone mineral data. *Calc. Tiss. Int.* **50**, 24–29.

Bell, N.H., Greene, A., Epstein, S., Oexman, M.J., Shaw, S., and Shary, J. (1985). Evidence for alteration of the vitamin D-endocrine system in Blacks. *J. Clin. Invest.* **76**, 470–473.

Bell, N.H., Shary, J., Stevens, J., Garza, M., Gordon, L., and Edwards, J. (1991). Demonstration that bone mass is greater in black than in white children. *J. Bone Miner. Res.* **6**(7), 719–723.

Bell, K.L., Loveridge, N., Power, J., Garrahan, N., Stanton, M., Lunt, M., Meggitt, B.F., and Reeve, J. (1999). Structure of the femoral neck in hip fracture: Cortical bone loss in the inferoantererior to superoposterior axis. *J. Bone Miner. Res.* **14**, 111–119.

Bhudhikanok, G.S., Wang, M.C., Eckert, K., Matkin, C., Marcus, R., and Bachrach, L.K. (1996). Differences in bone mineral in young Asian and Caucasian Americans may reflect differences in bone size. *J. Bone Miner. Res.* **11**(10), 1545–1556.

Chin, K., Evans, M.C., Cornish, J., Cundy, T., and Reid, I.R. (1997). Differences in hip axis and femoral neck length in premenopausal women of Polynesian, Asian and European origin. *Osteoporos. Int.* **7**(4), 344–347.

Cohn, S.H., Abesamis, C., Zanzi, I., Aloia, J.F., Yasumura, S., and Ellis, K.J. (1977). Body elemental composition: Comparison between black and white adults. *Am. J. Physiol.* **232**, E419–422.

Consensus Development Conference. (1991). Diagnosis; prophylaxis and treatment of osteoporosis. *Amer. J. Med.* **90**, 107–110.

Cummings, S.R., Black, D.M., Nevitt, M.C., Browner, W., Cauley, J., Genant, H.K., Mascioli, S.R., Scott, J.C. *et al.* (1990). Appendicular bone density and age predict hip fracture in women. *JAMA.* **263**, 665–668.

Cummings, S.R., Black, D.M., Nevitt, M.C., Browner, W., Cauley, J., Ensrud, K., Genant, H.K., Palermo, L. *et al.* (1993). Bone density at various sites for prediction of hip fractures. *The Lancet.* **341**, 72–75.

Cummings, S.R., Cauley, J.A., Palermo, L., Ross, P.D., Wasnich, R.D., Black, D., and Faulkner, K.G. (1994). Racial differences in hip axis length might explain racial differences in rates of hip fracture. *Osteoporos. Int.* **4**, 226–229.

Daniels, E.D., Pettifor, J.M., Schnitzler, C.M., Russell, S.W., and Patel, D.N. (1995). Ethnic differences in bone density in female South African nurses. *J. Bone Miner. Res.* **10**(3), 359–367.

DeSimone, D.P., Stevens, J., Edwards, J., Shary, J., Gordon, L., and Bell, N.H. (1989). Influence of body habitus and race on bone mineral density of the midradius, hip, and spine in aging women. *J. Bone Miner. Res.* **4**(6), 827–830.

Dudeja, V., Misra, A., Pandy, R.M., Devina, G., Kumar, G., and Vikram, N.K. (2001). BMI does not accurately predict overweight in Asian Indians in northern India. *Br. J. Nutr.* **86**, 105–112.

Ellis, K.J., and Cohn, S.H. (1975). Correlation between skeletal calcium mass and muscle mass in man. *J. Appl. Physiol.* **38**(3), 455–460.

Faulkner, K.G., Cummings, S.R., Black, D., Palermo, L., Glüer, C.C., and Genant, H.K. (1993). Simple measurement of femoral geometry predicts hip fracture: The Study of Osteoporotic Fractures. *J. Bone Miner. Res.* **8**(10), 1211–1217.

Fisher, E.S., Baron, J.A., Malenka, D.J., Barrett, J.A., Kniffin, W.D., Whaley, F.S., and Bubolz, T.A. (1991). Hip fracture incidence and mortality in New England. *Epidemiol.* **2**, 116–122.

Fujita, T., Okamoto, Y., Tomita, T., Sakagami, Y., Ota, K., and Ohata, M. (1977). Calcium metabolism in aging inhabitants of mountain versus seacoast communities in the Kii peninsula. *J. Am. Geriatr. Soc.* **25**, 254–258.

Gilsanz, V., Roe, T.F., Mora, S., Costin, G., and Goodman, W.G. (1991). Changes in vertebral bone density in black girls and white girls during childhood and puberty. *N. Engl. J. Med.* **325**(23), 1597–1600.

Grisso, J.A., Kelsey, J.L., Strom, B.L., O'Brien, L.A., Maislin, G., LaPann, K., Samelson, L., and Hoffman, S. (1994). Risk factors for hip fracture in black women. *N. Engl. J. Med.* **330**(22), 1555–1559.

Haddock, L., Ortiz, V., Vazquez, M.D., Aguilo, F., Bernard, E., Ayala, A., and Mejias, N. (1996). The lumbar and femoral bone mineral densities in a normal female Puerto Rican population. *P.R. Health Sci. J.* **15**(1), 5–11.

Hagiwara, S., Miki, T., Nishizawa, Y., Ochi, H., Onoyama, Y., and Morii, H. (1989). Quantification of bone mineral content using dual-photon absorptiometry in a normal Japanese population. *J. Bone Miner. Res.* **4**(2), 217–222.

Han, Z.H., Palnitkar, S., Rao, D.S., Nelson, D., and Parfitt, A.M. (1997). Effects of ethnicity and age or menopause on the remodeling and turnover of iliac bone: Implications for mechanisms of bone loss. *J. Bone Miner. Res.* **12**(4), 498–508.

Harper, A.B., Laughlin, W.S., and Mazess, R.B. (1984). Bone mineral content in St Lawrence Island Eskimos. *Hum. Biol.* **56**(1), 63–78.

Heaney, R.P. (1986). Calcium, bone health and osteoporosis. In W. A. Peck (ed.) *Bone and Mineral Research* (vol. 4). Elsevier Science, Amsterdam, New York, Oxford, pp. 255–301.

Heaney, R.P. (1999). Aging and calcium balance. In C. J. Rosen, J. Glowacki, and J. P. Bilezikian (eds) *The Aging Skeleton*. Academic Press, San Diego, pp. 19–26.

Heaney, R.P., and Weaver, C.M. (1992). Plant constituents and food calcium absorbability. *J. Bone Miner. Res.* **7**(Suppl), S136.

Hinton, R.Y., and Smith, G.S. (1993). The association of age, race, and sex with the location of proximal femoral fractures in the elderly. *J. Bone Joint Surg. Am.* **75**(5), 752–759.

Hu, J.F., Zhao, X.H., Jia, J.B., Parpia, B., and Campbell, T.C. (1993). Dietary calcium and bone density among middle-aged and elderly women in China. *Am. J. Clin. Nutr.* **58**(2), 219–227.

Katzman, D.K., Bachrach, L.K., Carter, D.R., and Marcus, R. (1991). Clinical and anthropometric correlates of bone mineral acquisition in healthy adolescent girls. *J. Clin. Endocrinol. Metab.* **73**(6), 1332–1339.

Kleerekoper, M., Nelson, D.A., Flynn, M.J., Pawluszka, A.S., Jacobsen, G., and Peterson, E.L. (1994a). Comparison of radiographic absorptiometry with dual energy x-ray absorptiometry and quantitative computed tomography in normal older white and black women. *J. Bone Miner. Res.* **9**, 1745–1750.

Kleerekoper, M., Nelson, D.A., Peterson, E.L., Flynn, M.J., Pawluszka, A.S., Jacobsen, G., and Wilson, P. (1994b). Reference data for bone mass, calciotropic hormones, and biochemical markers of bone remodeling in older (55–75) postmenopausal white and black women. *J. Bone Miner. Res.* **9**(8), 1267–1276.

Kleerekoper, M., Nelson, D., Peterson, E., Wilson, P., Jacobsen, G., and Longcope, C. (1994c). Body composition and gonadal steroids in older white and black women. *J. Endocrinol. Metab.* **79**, 775–779.

Kumanyika, S. (1987). Obesity in Black women. *Epidemiol. Rev.* **9**, 31–51.

Laraque, D., Arena, L., Karp, J., and Gruskay, D. (1990). Bone mineral content in black pre-schoolers: Normative data using single photon absorptiometry. *Pediatr. Radiol.* **20**(6), 461–463.

Lau, E.M.C., Woo, J., Leung, P.C., Swaminathan, R., and Leung, D. (1992). The effects of calcium supplementation and exercise on bone density in elderly Chinese women. *Osteoporosis Int.* **2**, 168–173.

Lau, E.M., Woo, J., Leung, P.C., and Swaminathan, R. (1993). Low bone mineral density, grip strength and skinfold thickness are important risk factors for hip fracture in Hong Kong Chinese. *Osteoporos. Int.* **3**(2), 66–70.

Lauderdale, D.S., Jacobsen, S.J., Furner, S.E., Levy, P.S., Brody, J.A., and Goldberg, J. (1997). Hip fracture incidence among elderly Asian-American populations. *Am. J. Epidemiol.* **146**(6), 502–509.

Lee, J., Kolonel, L., and Hinds, M. (1981). Relative merits of the weight-corrected-for height indices. *Am. J. Clin. Nutr.* **34**, 2521–2529.

Li, J.Y., Specker, B.L., Ho, M.L., and Tsang, R.C. (1989). Bone mineral content in black and white children 1 to 6 years of age. Early appearance of race and sex differences. *Am. J. Dis. Child.* **143**(11), 1346–1349.

Liel, Y., Edwards, J., Shary, J., Spicer, K.M., Gordon, L., and Bell, N.H. (1988). The effects of race and body habitus on bone mineral density of the radius, hip, and spine in premenopausal women. *J. Clin. Endocrinol. Metab.* **66**(6), 1247–1250.

Looker, A.C., Loria, C.M., Carroll, M.D., McDowell, M.A., and Johnson, C.L. (1993). Calcium intakes of Mexican Americans, Cubans, Puerto Ricans, non-Hispanic whites, and non-Hispanic blacks in the United States. *J. Am. Diet. Assoc.* **93**(11), 1274–1279.

Looker, A.C., Wahner, H.W., Dunn, W.L., Calvo, M.S., Harris, T.B., Heyse, S.P., Johnston, C.C., Jr., and Lindsay, R.L. (1995). Proximal femur bone mineral levels of US adults. *Osteoporos Int.* **5**(5), 389–409.

López, L.M., and Masse, B. (1992). Comparison of body mass indexes and cutoff points for estimating the prevalence of overweight in Hispanic women. *J. Am. Diet. Assoc.* **92**(11), 1343–1347.

Luckey, M.M., Meier, D.E., Mandeli, J.P., DaCosta, M.C., Hubbard, M.L., and Goldsmith, S.J. (1989). Radial and vertebral bone density in white and black women: Evidence for racial differences in premenopausal bone homeostasis. *J. Clin. Endocrinol. Metab.* **69**(4), 762–770.

Maggi, S., Kelsey, J.L., Litvak, J., and Heyse, S.P. (1991). Incidence of hip fractures in the elderly: A cross-national analysis. *Osteoporos. Int.* **1**(4), 232–241.

Marcus, R., Greendale, G., Blunt, B.A., Bush, T.L., Sherman, S., Sherwin, R., Wahner, H., and Wells, B. (1994). Correlates of bone mineral density in the Postmenopausal Estrogen/Progestin Interventions Trial. *J. Bone Miner. Res.* **9**(9), 1467–1476.

Matkovic, V., Kostial, K., Simonovic, I., Buzina, R., Brodarec, A., and Nordin, B.E.C. (1979). Bone status and fracture rates is two regions of Yugoslavia. *Am. J. Clin. Nutr.* **32**, 540–549.

Matsumine, H., Hirato, K., Yanaihara, T., Tamada, T., and Yoshida, M. (1986). Aromatization by skeletal muscle. *J. Clin. Endocrinol. Metab.* **63**(3), 717–720.

Mazess, R.B. (1978). Bone mineral in Vilcabamba, Ecuador. *Am. J. Roentgenol.* **130**, 671–674.

Mazess, R.B., and Mather, W. (1974). Bone mineral content of North Alaskan Eskimos. *Am J. Clin. Nutr.* **27**, 916–925.

McHugh, D., Baumgartner, R.N., Stauber, P.M., Wayne, S., Hicks, V.L., and Heyward, V.H. (1993). Bone mineral in southwest Native American women. *Basic Life Sci.* **60**(87), 87–88.

Meier, D.E., Luckey, M.M., Wallenstein, S., Clemens, T.L., Orwoll, E.S., and Waslien, C.I. (1991). Calcium, vitamin D, and parathyroid hormone status in young white and black women: Association with racial differences in bone mass. *J. Clin. Endocrinol. Metab.* **72**(3), 703–710.

Meier, D.E., Luckey, M.M., Wallenstein, S., Lapinski, R.H., and Catherwood, B. (1992). Racial differences in pre- and postmenopausal bone homeostasis: Association with bone density. *J. Bone Miner. Res.* **7**(10), 1181–1189.

Melton, L.J. (1988). Epidemiology of fractures. In B.L. Riggs, and L.J. Melton (eds) *Osteoporosis: Etiology, Diagnosis and Management*. Raven Press, New York, pp. 111–154.

Mikhail, M.B., Vaswani, A.N., and Aloia, J.F. (1996). Racial differences in femoral dimensions and their relation to hip fracture. *Osteopor. Int.* **6**, 22–24.

Nakamura, T., Turner, C.H., Yoshikawa, T., Slemenda, C.W., Peacock, M., Burr, D.B., Mizuno, Y., Orimo, H. *et al.* (1994). Do variations in hip geometry explain differences in hip fracture risk between Japanese and White Americans? *J. Bone Miner. Res.* **9**(7), 1071–1076.

Najjar, M.F., and Rowland, M. (1987). Anthropometric reference data and prevalence of overweight, United States, 1976–1980. *Vital Health Stat. 11.* **238**, 1–73.

Nelson, D.A. (1996). An anthropological perspective on optimizing calcium consumption for the prevention of osteoporosis. *Osteopor. Int.* **6**, 325–328.

Nelson, D.A., and Barondess, D.A. (1997). Whole body bone, fat and lean mass in children: Comparison of three ethnic groups. *Am. J. Phys. Anthropol.* **103**(2), 157–162.

Nelson, D.A., Kleerekoper, M., and Parfitt, A.M. (1988). Bone mass, skin color and body size among black and white women. *Bone Miner.* **4**, 257–264.

Nelson, D.A., Jacobsen, G., Barondess, D.A., and Parfitt, A.M. (1995). Ethnic differences in regional bone density, hip axis length, and lifestyle variables among healthy Black and White men. *J. Bone Miner. Res.* **10**, 782–787.

Nelson, D.A., Simpson, P.M., Johnson, C.C., Barondess, D.A., and Kleerekoper, M. (1997). The accumulation of whole body skeletal mass in third- and fourth-grade children: Effects of age, gender, ethnicity, and body composition. *Bone* **20**, 73–78.

Nelson, D.A., Barondess, D.A., Hendrix, S.L., and Beck, T.J. (2000). Cross-sectional geometry, bone strength, and bone mass in the proximal femur in black and white postmenopausal women. *J. Bone Miner. Res.* **15**, 1992–1997.

Patel, D.N., Pettifor, J.M., Becker, P.J., Grieve, C., and Leschner, K. (1992). The effect of Ethnic group on appendicular bone mass in children. *J. Bone Miner. Res.* **7**(3), 263–272.

Peacock, M., Liu, G., Carey, M., Ambrosius, W., Turner, C.H., Hui, S., and Johnston, C.C. (1998). Bone mass and structure at the hip in men and women over the age of 60 years. *Osteoporos. Int.* **8**, 231–239.

Perry, H.M., 3rd, Bernard, M., Horowitz, M., Miller, D.K., Fleming, S., Baker, M.Z., Flaherty, J., Purushothaman, R. *et al.* (1998). The effect of aging on bone mineral metabolism and bone mass in Native American women. *J. Am. Geriatr. Soc.* **46**(11), 1418–1422.

Prentice, A., Laskey, M.A., Shaw, J., Cole, T.J., and Fraser, D.R. (1990). Bone mineral content of Gambian and British children aged 0–36 months. *Bone Miner.* **10**, 211–224.

Pruzansky, M.E., Turano, M., Luckey, M., and Senie, R. (1989). Low body weight as a risk factor for hip fracture in both black and white women. *J. Orthop. Res.* **7**(2), 192–197.

Reid, I.R., Mackie, M., and Ibbertson, H.K. (1986). Bone mineral content in Polynesian and white New Zealand women. *Brit. Med. J.* **292**, 1547–1548.

Reid, I.R., Cullen, S., Schooler, B.A., Livingston, N.E., and Evans, M.C. (1990). Calcitropic hormone levels in Polynesians: Evidence against their role in interracial differences in bone mass. *J. Clin. Endocrinol. Metab.* **70**(5), 1452–1456.

Reid, I.R., Plank, L.D., and Evans, M.C. (1992). Fat mass is an important determinant of whole body bone density in premenopausal women but not in men. *J. Clin. Endocrinol. Metab.* **75**(3), 779–782.

Report of a WHO Consultation on Obesity. (1997). Obesity: Preventing and managing the global epidemic. WHO/NUT/NCD/98.1.

Ross, P.D., Norimatsu, H., Davis, J.W., Yano, K., Wasnich, R.D., Fujiwara, S., Hosoda, Y., and Melton, L. (1991). A comparison of hip fracture incidence among native Japanese, Japanese Americans, and American Caucasians. *Am. J. Epidemiol.* **133**(8), 801–809.

Ruff, C.B., and Hayes, W.C. (1988). Sex differences in age-related remodeling of the femur and tibia. *J. Orth. Res.* **6**, 886–896.

Russell-Aulet, M., Wang, J., Thornton, J., Colt, E.W., and Pierson, R.J. (1991). Bone mineral density and mass by total-body dual-photon absorptiometry in normal white and Asian men. *J. Bone Miner. Res.* **6**(10), 1109–1113.

Russell-Aulet, M., Wang, J., Thornton, J.C., Colt, E.W., and Pierson, R.J. (1993). Bone mineral density and mass in a cross-sectional study of white and Asian women. *J. Bone Miner. Res.* **8**(5), 575–582.

Schnitzler, C.M. (1993). Bone quality: A determinant for certain risk factors for bone fragility. *Calcif. Tissue Int.* **53**(Suppl 1), S27–31.

Schnitzler, C.M., Pettifor, J.M., Mesquita, J.M., Bird, M.D., Schnaid, E., and Smyth, A.E. (1990). Histomorphometry of iliac crest bone in 346 normal black and white South African adults. *Bone Miner.* **10**(3), 183–199.

Silverman, S.L., and Madison, R.E. (1988). Decreased incidence of hip fracture in Hispanics, Asians, and blacks: California Hospital Discharge Data. *Am. J. Public Health.* **78**(11), 1482–1483.

Solomon, L. (1979). Bone density in aging Caucasian and African populations. *Lancet.* **2**, 1326–1330.

Stott, S., Gray, D.H., and Stevenson, W. (1980). The incidence of femoral neck fractures in New Zealand. *New Zealand Med. J.* **91**, 6–9.

Theobald, T.M., Cauley, J.A., Gluer, C.C., Bunker, C.H., Ukoli, F.A.M., and Genant, H.K. (1998). Black-White differences in hip geometry. *Osteopor. Int.* **8**, 61–69.

Villa, M.L. (1994). Cultural determinants of skeletal health: The need to consider both race and ethnicity in bone research. *J. Bone Miner. Res.* **9**(9), 1329–1332.

Villa, M.L., Marcus, R., Delay, R.R., and Kelsey, J.L. (1995). Factors contributing to skeletal health of postmenopausal Mexican-American women. *J. Bone Miner. Res.* **10**(8), 1233–1242.

Wang, M.C., Aguirre, M., Bhudhikanok, G.S., Kendall, C.G., Kirsch, S., Marcus, R., and Bachrach, L.K. (1997). Bone mass and hip axis length in healthy Asian, black, Hispanic, and white American youths. *J. Bone Miner. Res.* **12**(11), 1922–1935.

Weinstein, R.S., and Bell, N.H. (1988). Diminished rates of bone formation in normal Black adults. *N. Engl. J. Med.* **319**(26), 1698–1701.

Yano, K., Wasnich, R.D., Vogel, J.M., and Heilbrun, L.K. (1984). Bone mineral measurements among middle-aged and elderly Japanese residents in Hawaii. *Am. J. Epidemiol.* **119**(5), 751–764.

Yano, K., Heilbrun, L.K., Wasnich, R.D., Hankin, J.H., and Vogel, J.M. (1985). The relationship between diet and bone mineral content of multiple skeletal sites in elderly Japanese-American men and women living in Hawaii. *Am. J. Clin. Nutr.* **42**, 877–888.

Yoshikawa, T., Turner, C.H., Peacock, M., Slemenda, C.W., Weaver, C.M., Teegarden, D., Markwardt, P., and Burr, D.B. (1994). Geometric structure of the femoral neck measured using dual-energy x-ray absorptiometry. *J. Bone Miner. Res.* **9**, 1053–1064.

5

Bone Loss, Fracture Histories, and Body Composition Characteristics of Older Males

William A. Stini

1. Background

The National Institutes of Health sponsored a consensus development conference on osteoporosis prevention, diagnosis, and therapy in its Bethesda, Maryland campus in March of 2000 (National Institutes of Health, 2001). This conference was stimulated by the recognition of the fact that osteoporosis has become a major worldwide public health problem. In fact, osteoporosis has already become a major challenge to the health care professions as the number and proportion of the elderly continue to grow. According to the statistics cited at the outset of the conference, 10 million Americans already had osteoporosis at the beginning of the year 2000, and 18 million more had low bone mass that placed them at risk for non-traumatic fractures.

1.1. Definition of Terms

The agreed-upon definition of osteoporosis employed throughout these discussions was "a skeletal disorder characterized by compromised bone strength predisposing to an increased risk of fracture." Bone strength reflects the integration of bone density (grams of mineral per area or volume) and bone quality (determined by architecture, turnover, damage accumulation, and mineralization). When an alteration in any of these factors reduces bone strength, the chance of failure, that is, fracture, during trauma increases. Failure to achieve normal bone density during growth and development may cause a predisposition to osteoporosis late in life even though the rate of bone loss at that time is not excessive. Thus, an area of increasing emphasis is the encouragement of nutritional and activity strategies that maximize peak bone mass early in life. Although the attainment of

William A. Stini • Department of Anthropology, University of Arizona.

Bone Loss and Osteoporosis: An Anthropological Perspective, edited by Sabrina C. Agarwal and Sam D. Stout. Kluwer Academic/Plenum Publishers, New York, 2003.

peak bone mass does not occur at the same time at all sites throughout the body, there is usually no increase in whole-body bone density beyond the age of 30 years.

The operational definition of osteoporosis employed by the World Health Organization (WHO) is a bone density of 2.5 standard deviations below average peak bone density. Since average peak bone density and the age of its attainment are different in males and females, the normative standards used to estimate the level of risk differ as well. Women achieve peak bone density earlier, but at a lower density than that characteristic of men. Moreover, since a period of accelerated bone loss is often associated with the onset of menopause, women are at risk for osteoporotic bone fracture earlier than men are. However, later in life, especially after age 70, the risk of fracture in men increases rapidly. Weight reduction programs that rely upon restriction of energy intake have also been shown to increase bone turnover and to reduce bone density in obese women (Ricci *et al.*, 2001). Malnutrition associated with alcoholism has been found to increase the incidence of osteoporosis in men (Santolaria *et al.*, 2000). Rheumatoid arthritis is associated with reduced bone density (often because of the need for corticosteroid medications) (Sinigaglia *et al.*, 2000). However, osteoarthritis has been found to be associated with greater bone density in the spine in both sexes, presumably as the result of reduced bone turnover (el Miedany *et al.*, 2000).

1.2. Bone Loss in Other Primates

There is a growing body of evidence that the loss of bone density with age is a trait humans share with other primates. In a longitudinal study, Black *et al.* (2001) found that forearm bone density of captive rhesus macaques declined with age and that bone density and lean body mass were positively associated in both sexes. A cross-sectional study of free-ranging macaques living on Cayo Santiago (Cerroni *et al.*, 2000) produced similar results, with females exhibiting attainment of peak bone density at about 9.5 years, and loss of bone density beginning around 17.2 years. Interestingly, male Cayo Santiago macaques not only attained greater peak bone density than females but also achieved it earlier. No loss of bone density was seen in males up to 18.5 years when the observations in this study were discontinued. However, Colman *et al.* (1999) report loss of bone density in older captive male rhesus macaques even in the absence of nutritional or gonadal steroid deficiencies. Changes in sex steroid production appear to play an important role in the acceleration of the rate of bone turnover in non-human primates as well as in humans (Compston, 2001).

1.3. Population Differences

In addition to gender differences in bone density and age-related loss of bone, there are differences between human populations. For instance, the incidence of hip fracture is lower in Japan than in Western countries despite the fact that Japanese have lower bone densities. The difference in fracture risk appears to be attributable to a slower bone loss rate in later life for Japanese (Dennison *et al.*, 1998). Nevertheless, osteoporosis is recognized as a major health problem in Japan (Matsukura *et al.*, 2000; Tsuzuku *et al.*, 2000). Rogucka *et al.* (2000) report that loss of both trabecular and cortical bone in Polish populations occurs by age 60. As the literature on osteoporosis grows, it has become increasingly clear that no population is immune to the damage inflicted by age-related bone loss (see also Chapter 4, this volume for a discussion of ethnic differences in bone loss).

2. Risk Factors

There are certain well-established risk factors for osteoporosis. For women these include a history of atraumatic fracture since age 25, X-ray report of osteopenia, premature menopause before age 45 or a history of amenorrhea of more than 6 months duration, smoking, family history of osteoporosis, and predisposing medical conditions with associated medications, such as corticosteroids. A body mass index (BMI) below 20 kg/m^2 is also indicative of high risk (Frost *et al.*, 2001). Of the factors associated with osteoporosis, BMI, calcium intake, and activity levels can be considered modifiable, that is, at least to some extent under control of the individual (Guthrie *et al.*, 2000a,b; Snelling *et al.*, 2001). Indirect indicators of lean body mass, such as handgrip strength, have also been shown to be positively associated with bone density (Di Monaco *et al.*, 2000).

An epidemiological study of femoral shaft fractures conducted in Finland yielded an incidence of 9.9 fractures per 100,000 person-years, with the highest age and gender specific incidence among young males from 15 to 24 years of age, followed by that for females over age 75 years (Salminen *et al.*, 2000). However, 75% of these fractures were the result of high-energy trauma, 87% of which were attributable to automobile accidents, most of which involved young males. Singer *et al.* (1998), in a study of fracture incidence in Edinburgh, Scotland, calculated that between the ages of 15 and 49 years, males were 2.9 times more likely to sustain a fracture than females, but over age 60, females were 2.3 times as likely to sustain a fracture than males. On the basis of their findings, they identified three peaks of fracture occurrence. The first, just as in the Finnish study, was among young males. The second peak was in the elderly of both sexes, mainly affecting metaphyseal bone such as the proximal femur with a lesser involvement of diaphyseal bone. The third increase in fractures was seen in the wrist, occurring most often in women beyond age 40, at an age some years before menopause for most women. The hip fractures experienced by older women were predominantly nontraumatic. However, the prognosis following hip fracture in older women is far less favorable, with an estimated mortality rate of over 20% worldwide.

The rate of normal bone loss after the attainment of peak bone density is the same for both men and women, about 3%/decade for cortical bone and 7–11%/decade for trabecular bone (O'Flaherty, 2000). In women entering menopause, a period of more-rapid loss is superimposed on the gradual loss already occurring. This menopausal/postmenopausal phase of bone loss may persist for as long as 10 years, and affects both cortical and trabecular bone in roughly equal proportions.

2.1. Factors Influencing Bone Turnover

Bone turnover is subject to seasonal variation (Woitge *et al.*, 1998, 2000), with high levels of serum vitamin D in summer and parathyroid hormone (PTH) in winter. Seasonal fluctuations in serum vitamin D levels have been documented in populations where seasonal differences in day length are relatively slight as well as in areas farther from the equator (El-Hajj *et al.*, 2001; Lips *et al.*, 2001; Nakamura *et al.*, 2001; Patel *et al.*, 2001). Low serum 25-hydroxyvitamin D level has been found to be associated with increased serum alkaline phosphatase and PTH, and lower bone density in the femoral neck (Lips *et al.*, 2001). However, Nakamura *et al.* (2001) found no significant association between serum 25-hydroxyvitamin D and forearm bone density. It should be pointed out that while the femoral neck contains a relatively large proportion of trabecular bone, the diaphysis of the radius used for estimation of forearm bone density is predominantly cortical bone. In their study of the effects of vitamin supplementation on a group of healthy British women, Patel *et al.* (2001) found that while there was significant seasonal variation in serum 25-hydroxyvitamin D, there was no evidence of seasonal variation in serum PTH, calcium absorption, markers of bone turnover, or bone density in the spine, femur, or total body. In a comparison of Black and White, men and women, Bikle *et al.* (1999) found that, compared to Whites, Black subjects maintained lower levels of serum 25-hydroxyvitamin D, but higher levels of 1,25 dihydroxyvitamin D. Calcium excretion was 26% lower in Black men than in White men and 36% lower in Black women than in White women. Serum PTH levels were found to be 29% higher in Black women than in White women while no significant racial difference in PTH levels was found in men.

2.2. Peak Bone Mass

It has long been known that the rate of bone loss in men is lower than in women during the early and middle years of life. In a cross-sectional study conducted in France, Szulc *et al.* (2000) estimated that men attained peak bone density at the lumbar spine and hip between the ages of 25 and 29 years. However, peak bone mass in the distal forearm and for the whole body was not attained until ages 40 and 37 respectively. Both the mineral content and the cross-sectional area of the long bones of the limbs continued to increase up to about age 50. On average, these men lost 13–18% of their peak bone mass by age 80, with the most marked decrease (43%) occurring in the Ward's triangle site of the proximal femur.

2.3. Endocrinological Factors

While the pattern of bone loss in females conforms to expectations based on endocrinological changes occurring with age, male bone loss is less clearly defined. It is quite likely that estrogen plays a significant role in male bone metabolism independent of testosterone (da Silva and Porto, 1997; Maugeri *et al.*, 1998; Ongphiphadhanakul *et al.*, 1998; Oz *et al.*, 2000). One indicator of the importance of estrogen is the fact that male bone mineral density (BMD) is more highly correlated with serum estrogen than with testosterone (Khosla *et al.*, 1999). Fassbender *et al.* (2000) report a significant correlation between estradiol and testosterone levels in male osteoporosis patients. There is considerable evidence that male bones fracture at a higher bone density than those of women, and that the prevalence of vertebral fractures is actually higher in men (Kudlacek *et al.*, 2000). Cody *et al.* (2000) report a different pattern of bone loss associated with fractures of the femoral neck occurring in men from that seen in women. In men, bone density was found to decrease throughout the proximal femur. In women a combination of localized changes including loss of trabecular bone at the fracture site as well as decreased cortical bone at the point of impact was most common. Women lose more height proportionally than men as they age, and the beneficial effects of regular physical exercise in attenuating loss of stature are more pronounced in men than in women (Sagiv *et al.*, 2000). However, women with non-insulin dependent diabetes mellitus (NIDDM) appear to maintain greater bone density than non-diabetic women. No such difference between diabetic and non-diabetic men has been reported (el Miedany *et al.*, 1999). Davies *et al.* (2000) report an interesting negative association between calcium intakes and BMI in women, a relationship that has not to date been reported for males.

In a recently reported Spanish study of healthy elderly men, multiple regression analysis of the relationships of bone density to hormonal and anthropometric variables indicates that body weight, sex hormone binding globulin (SHBG), and intact PTH (iPTH) levels are independent predictors of bone mass. However, most of the BMD was explained by body weight alone. After adjusting for age and BMI, SHBG and insulin-like growth factor 1 (IGF-1) were negatively correlated with bone density (Martinez Diaz-Guerra *et al.*, 2001). There seems to be little doubt that age-related changes in androgen levels have an impact on bone metabolism in males as well as in females. However, the nature of the relationships between estrogenic hormones and testosterone is far from clear. This uncertainty is reflected in the conflicting results reported by investigators concerned with the causes of bone loss in aging men. For instance, contrary to the Khosla *et al.* report cited earlier, that estrogen levels are more highly correlated with bone density than testosterone levels in men, other investigators (D'Amore *et al.*, 2000) report that testosterone levels are the most reliable predictors of bone loss. Rapado *et al.* (1999) found no significant correlation between male sex hormone and decrease in hip BMD, and Boonen *et al.* (1997) found that both serum testosterone and hydroxyvitamin D, and dihydroxyvitamin D were all decreased in hip fracture patients. Combined administration of vitamins D_3 and K_2 has been found effective in increasing the BMD of the lumbar spine in women with osteoporosis (Iwamoto *et al.*, 2000b). Testosterone replacement therapy has been shown to increase bone formation in men diagnosed with idiopathic hypogonadotrophic hypogonadism (IHH), although bone resorption also increases in these patients (Zarate, 2000; DeRosa *et al.*, 2001). However, Medras *et al.* (2001) report that even when long-term testosterone replacement therapy succeeds in normalizing serum androgen levels, elimination of osteopenia does not always occur. The complex interactions between sex hormones, body composition, and behavioral factors (Legroux-Gerot *et al.*, 1999; Winters, 1999), make it extremely difficult to trace direct cause/effect associations between changes in androgen production and bone mineral metabolism.

2.4. Vitamin D and Vitamin D Receptors

The role of the vitamin D receptor (VDR) genotype in predisposition to osteoporosis remains under investigation. Vitamin D, its metabolites and homologues are well-known to have many physiological effects. With respect to the maintenance of bone density, one of the most important and best-understood functions of vitamin D is its regulation of calcium absorption in the small intestine. The most active form of vitamin D in this regulatory function is 1,25 $(OH)_2$ vitamin D_3 (calcitriol). The receptors for this hormone have several known variants, one of which arises from a substitution of a guanine for an adenine at the 3731st position from the 5′ end (Arai *et al.*, 2001). The G-allele exhibits reduced transcriptional activity in promoter region and reduced calcium absorption. Postmenopausal women homozygous for the G-allele were found to have a 12% lower BMD in the lumbar spine than homozygotes for the A-allele. Interactions between alleles at the VDR locus alleles and at the estrogen receptor (ER) locus, which is also polymorphic, are now thought to underlie some of the subtle variation in bone densities found when either VDR or ER genotypes are independently examined (Kim *et al.*, 2001).

Further interactions involving collagen type I alpha 1 (COLIA 1) have been examined by Finnish investigators (Valimaki *et al.*, 2001) who focused on the BB, Bb, and bb VDR genotypes and the SS, Ss, and ss Colia 1 genotypes. Contrary to the findings of Uitterlinden *et al.* (2001) these investigators found no significant relationship between VDR, collagen type, and BMD or hip fracture in their population. However, their results do raise questions concerning genetic and environmental factors that could combine to influence fracture risk at different stages in the life cycle. For instance, in a population of Italian women, Braga *et al.* (2000) found that the products of the COLIA 1 alleles interact with products of alleles at the calcitonin receptor (CTR) locus in a manner that may influence the process of acquiring peak bone mass early in life rather than bone loss later. In view of the complexity of the endocrinological interactions influencing bone growth and maintenance it is not surprising that apparently conflicting results continue to emerge (e.g., Ozisik *et al.*, 2001, who found that VDR genotype has no influence on BMD in Turkish men with IHH) (see also Chapter 9, this volume for further discussion on the role of vitamin D in bone loss).

2.5. Body Composition and Mechanical Factors

As in women, fracture occurrence in men is negatively correlated with BMD, BMI, muscle strength, and level of physical activity (Thorsen *et al.*, 1999; Ismail *et al.*, 2000; Krassas *et al.*, 2001). However, the structural basis for bone density loss in men may differ from that in women (Seeman, 1999). Male periosteal expansion exceeds that of female during growth and development. An important component of certain racial difference in bone density results from similar differences in the early acquisition of bone density. Blacks, both male and female, experience greater periosteal expansion early in life, and therefore have greater bone density than age- and sex-matched Whites. One result of greater periosteal expansion is wider long bones in early adulthood. Structurally, this expansion places cortical bone mineral mass at a greater distance from the neutral axis of the bone in men than in women, and in Blacks than in Whites. Placement of bone mineral mass at a greater distance from the neutral axis of the bone confers a mechanical advantage that enhances the strength of long bones, especially in resistance to torsional stress. One result of this increase in strength is a lowered risk of nontraumatic fracture. Consequently, at peak bone density, both racial and gender differences in bone strength are likely to be attributable to size and not to BMD.

The loss of trabecular bone is similar in both sexes, but women experience greater loss of connectivity, the important relationship between the struts and plates that maintains the structural integrity of the trabeculae. In addition, endocortical resorption is greater in women. Men lose less cortical width for that reason and because of a greater amount of subperiosteal apposition during aging. Men who suffer fractures of the spine have smaller vertebral width (Iwamoto *et al.*, 2000a), and men with hip fractures have a narrower femoral neck. Nonetheless, the average decline in density of the radius experienced by men between the ages of 29 and 76 is about 1% per year (Overton and Basu, 1999). Ultrasound determinations of bone density in the calcaneus have proven effective in predicting fracture risk in men (Pluskiewicz and Drozdzowska, 1999) despite the difference between the structural and functional characteristics of the bones of the forearm and the heel.

3. The Sun City/Tucson Longitudinal Study

The Arizona Bone Density Study was initiated in 1982. The first cohort of subjects was drawn from the Volunteer Association of the Walter O. Boswell Memorial Hospital in Sun City Arizona. These subjects were, by and large, retirees. Most owned their own homes and were financially independent. Almost all were of European ancestry. In order to broaden the demographics of the study, a second cohort was recruited from residents of publicly subsidized retirement housing in Tucson, Arizona. These subjects were, on the average, less affluent than those from Sun City. Also, most of the Tucson subjects had been Arizona residents for a longer period of time, often since birth, and roughly 30% of them were of Hispanic origin as compared to less than 5% in Sun City. A small sample of African American subjects was also recruited in Tucson. From the outset, more women than men were recruited in both the Sun City and Tucson populations. This sampling bias reflected the belief, prevalent at the time, that osteoporosis was a condition primarily affecting women.

3.1. Objectives

The primary objective of the study was to monitor changes in bone density over time. However, other changes were monitored as well. Height and weight were measured on each occasion for all subjects, and bioelectric impedance assessments of body composition were conducted on a sample of 451 (277 men and 174 women), who were enrolled in the wheat bran fiber and piroxicam clinical trials. Alkaline phosphatase levels and concentrations of serum calcium and other minerals were also determined through the analysis of blood samples from these subjects. On each occasion, all subjects were requested to complete questionnaires containing questions about bone fracture histories, medications, stress-inducing experiences, exercise patterns, milk consumption, and use of dietary supplements. On the occasion of their first visit, women were asked to complete an additional questionnaire concerning age at menarche and menopause and reproductive and breast-feeding histories.

3.2. Subjects

From 1982 through 1998 data were collected annually at both Sun City and Tucson (Stini, 2000a,b). Since the average age of the subjects of the first cohort was 70 years, and the loss of subjects for various reasons could be expected, new subjects were added each year. By the end of 1998, the total sample was 5,475 (4,121 women and 1,354 men). One hundred and seventy three subjects (126 women and 47 men) participated for 10 years or more. Over the course of the study, subjects from several rural communities in Pinal County Arizona (Casa Grande, Eloy, and Florence) had been incorporated in the study population, as had subjects enrolled in wheat bran fiber and piroxicam colon cancer prevention clinical trials conducted in Sun City and Tucson.

3.3. Methods

Annual scans of the left radius were conducted using single-beam photon absorptiometry (Lunar Radiation SP-1 and SP-2 Bone Densitometers). While both dual-photon absorptiometry (DPA) and dual-energy X-ray absorptiometry (DEXA) instruments provide more information about clinically sensitive areas such as the lumbar spine and the femoral neck, the objective of comparing serial measurements of cortical bone density was satisfactorily achieved using the single photon devices. The portability of the single photon device was a major consideration in its favor, because in order to reach the target populations of the Arizona study, it was necessary to set up the equipment at a number of sites in several cities and in rural areas. Change in cortical bone density over time can be measured with a high degree of accuracy at the radial site using single-beam photon absorptiometry (SPA). Since cortical bone makes up more than 80% of the total bone mass of the adult, the SPA scanning of this bone as a surrogate for whole-body scanning yields useful results.

Within this limited context, SPA bone scans are a highly reliable method for effecting valid assessments of cortical bone density. When suitable safeguards are taken to assure that all scans are taken at precisely the same site; the method is ideal for the monitoring of bone density change through serial measurements. Thus, when used as a research method for a large sample in a mixed longitudinal study of bone density change, it is a very powerful tool. However, its clinical use as a predictor of fractures at sites where trabecular bone is more abundant cannot be recommended. Since the objectives of the present study did not include estimates of trabecular bone density or changes thereof, the advantages of SPA methodology considerably outweighed its disadvantages. Results of a comparative study involving subjects drawn from the Arizona Bone Density Study, yielded a correlation of 89% between the values for whole-body bone density attained by DEXA measurement and the values for bone density of the distal one third site of the radius attained through SPA measurement (Chen *et al.*, 1997). An additional advantage of the SPA method is that the highly collimated photon stream emitted by its 200 mC ^{125}I source produces a very low radiation dose for the subject, and its low scatter minimizes the risk of radiation to both subjects and investigators.

The measurement of stature to the nearest millimeter was done using a freestanding field anthropometer with the subject shoeless. Weight in kilograms was taken using a portable medical scale. The same anthropometrist took each of these measurements on each scanning occasion throughout the study. BMI was calculated using the equation: BMI = wt (kg)/ ht (m)^2. More than 14,000 records of these measurements as well as bone scan reports, human subjects' consent forms and questionnaires remain on file in The Biological Anthropology Laboratory at the University of Arizona.

3.4. Results

Table 5.1 shows the values for bone density and BMI arranged by 5-year categories for a sample of 4,036 women and 1,264 men for whom complete records are available. The values that appear in this table represent those obtained at each subject's final examination. In some instances, this may be the last of 16 such measurements and in others it is the first

Table 5.1. Final bone densities and body mass index values for Tucson and Sun City women and men

	Bone density (g/cm²)				Body mass index (wt (kg)/ht (m²))	
Age	Women	(n)	Men	(n)	Women	Men
<50	0.6591	(369)	0.7803	(50)	25.79	26.12
50–55	0.6532	(142)	0.7468	(20)	27.36	29.30
55–60	0.6188	(202)	0.7553	(38)	26.97	27.58
60–65	0.5908	(332)	0.7502	(84)	26.17	27.40
65–70	0.5585	(684)	0.7279	(208)	26.16	26.91
70–75	0.5295	(808)	0.7157	(286)	25.79	26.70
75–80	0.4946	(708)	0.7054	(295)	25.34	26.92
80–85	0.4773	(497)	0.6763	(183)	24.94	25.17
85–90	0.4512	(246)	0.6341	(81)	24.31	24.21
90–95	0.4161	(69)	0.5817	(18)	23.58	24.72
95–100	0.3966	(11)	0.4106	(1)	23.26	23.30

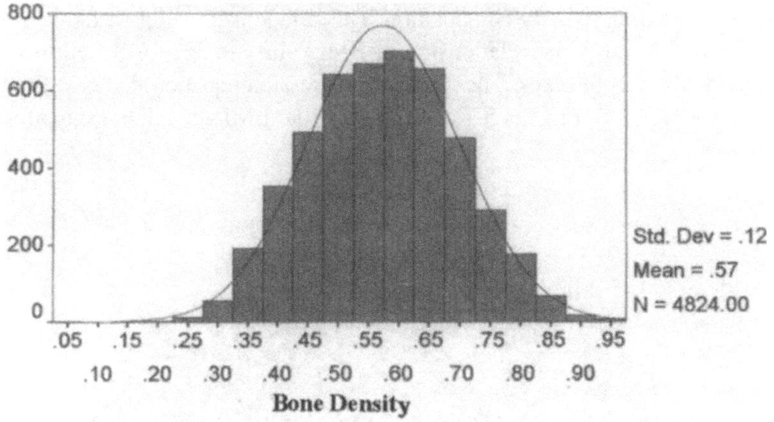

Figure 5.1. The range of values for bone density in the Arizona population (sexes combined). The normal curve is superimposed on the histogram for bone density expressed in g/cm².

and only one. The values shown in this table therefore represent a purely cross-sectional database. Figure 5.1 shows the range of bone density values observed in the Arizona subjects of both sexes.

As the values in Table 5.1 indicate, average cortical bone density declines steadily from age 50 onwards in women. The relatively small sample of men in the 50–55 year age group would appear to experience a sharp decrease in bone density, but it is probable that the apparent acceleration of bone density decrease is an artifact of small sample size in this age group. Succeeding age groups exhibit a rate of decline similar to that seen in the values for women. The decline in bone density in both sexes is sufficient to dispel the widely held notion that bone density decrease is primarily a women's problem. However, the lower average bone densities characteristic of women throughout early adulthood make them susceptible to bone fractures at an earlier age than men.

Figure 5.2 shows the relationship of bone density to age for 5,180 individuals, sexes combined. The "best fit" regression equation for this nonlinear relationship is: $y = a - bx^3$. Figure 5.3 shows the same relationship restricting the analysis to the female sample of 3,942 individuals. Again, the relationship is nonlinear, with the best-fit equation being: $y = a - bx^2$. The relationship of bone density values to age for the male sample of 1,238 individuals (Figure 5.4) is also nonlinear with the same best-fit equation as the combined sex sample. However the value of the intercept (a) is approximately 0.700 for the women while it is about 0.800 for males, reflecting the sex difference in peak bone density. The slopes (b) for all of these curves are negative. Comparison of the slopes for male versus female values clearly shows the steeper rate of decline in bone density experienced by women.

Figure 5.5 shows the range of values for BMI observed in Arizona subjects of both sexes. Although sample size for the male subjects in the <50 age group is small (50), and contains only one individual in the 95–100 age group, BMI values are informative when all age groups are compared. For instance, the highest values for both sexes occur in the 50–55 year age group. The decline in BMI from age 50 to age 95 is quite similar in both sexes. However the observed change in BMI may not accurately reflect the more significant changes occurring in body composition. This relationship will be examined in a later section. Figure 5.6 shows the relationship of BMI values to age for the entire sample of 5,180 individuals of both sexes. The nonlinear regression equation that best fits this relationship is: $y = a - bx^3$. Figures 5.7 and 5.8 show the BMI/age relationships for females

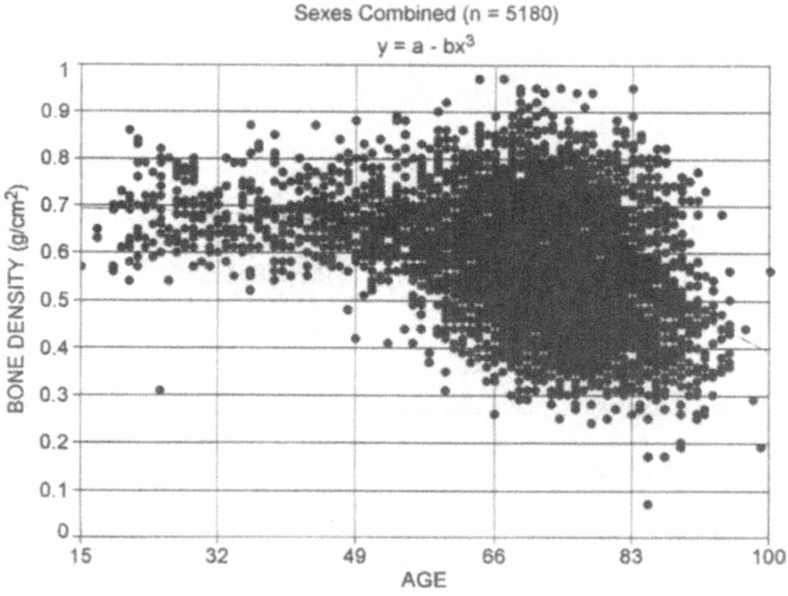

Figure 5.2. Bone density change by age (sexes combined). The abscissa (x-coordinate) has the value 15 at its origin. Reading from left to right along the base of the grid, the succeeding values are 32, 49, 66, 83, and 100. The ordinate (y-coordinate) has its origin at 0. Moving vertically up the grid, the succeeding values are 0.1, 0.2, 0.3, 0.4, 0.5, 0.6, 0.7, 0.8, 0.9, and 1.0.

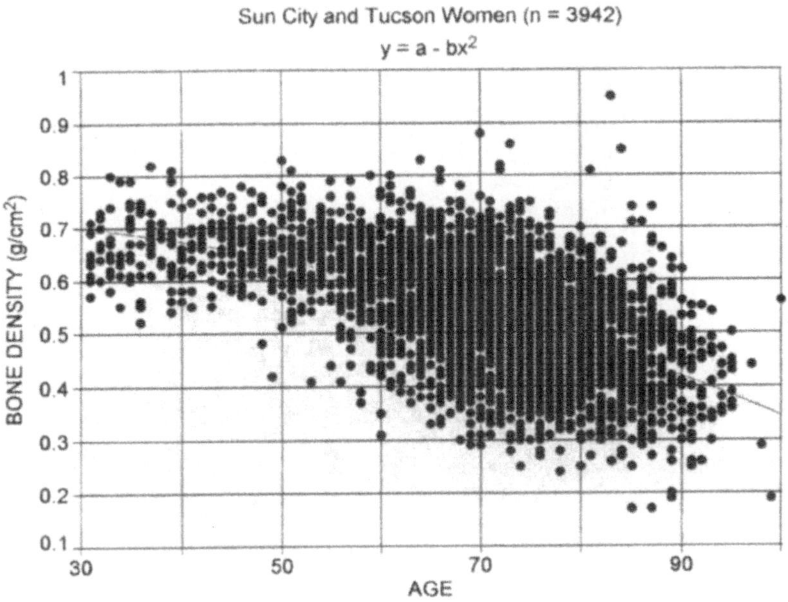

Figure 5.3. Bone density by age (women). The abscissa has the value 30 at its origin, then 50, 70, 90. The ordinate starts at 0.1, then 0.2, 0.3, 0.4, 0.5, 0.6, 0.7, 0.8, 0.9, 1.

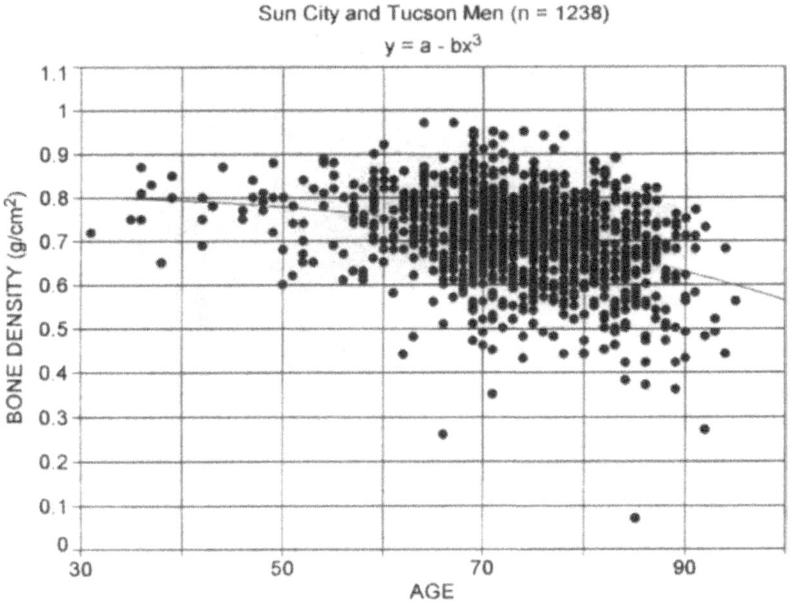

Figure 5.4. Bone density by age (men). The abscissa has the same values as in Figure 5.2. The ordinate has all of the same value plus 1.1 at the top.

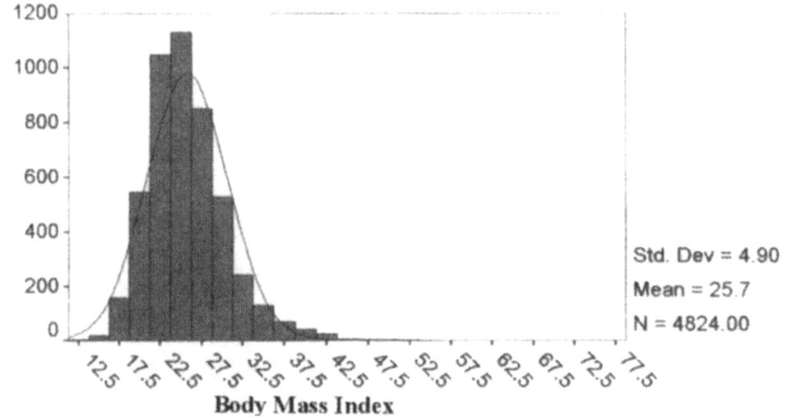

Figure 5.5. The range of values for body mass index (kg/m^2) in the Arizona population of both sexes.

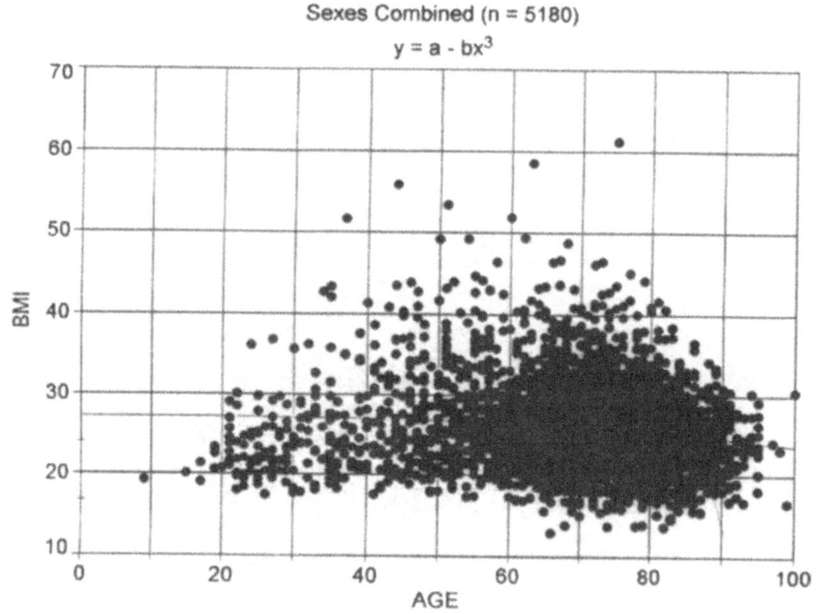

Figure 5.6. BMI and age (sexes combined). The abscissa has the value 0 at its origin, then 20, 40, 60, 80, 100. The ordinate has the value 10 at its origin, then 20, 30, 40, 50, 60, and 70.

and males respectively. As in the case of the bone density values, the slopes of these regressions are all negative.

In Figure 5.9, which represents the nonlinear regression of bone density on BMI, the slope is positive, the best-fit equation being: $y = a - b/x^2$. However, when estimates of percent lean body mass obtained using the bioelectric impedance method were regressed on BMI, the slope was negative (Figure 5.10), while the slope for percent body fat was

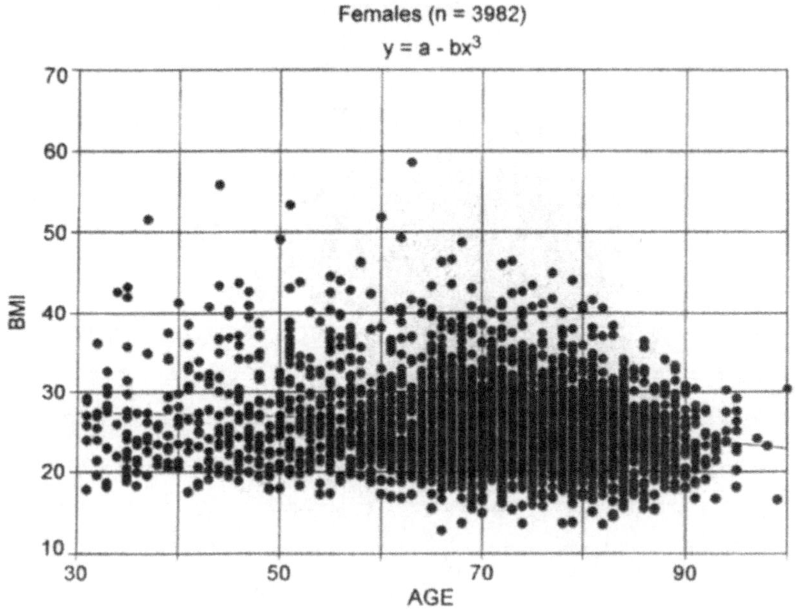

Figure 5.7. BMI and age (females). The abscissa has the value 30 at its origin, then 50, 70, and 90. The ordinate has the value 10 at its origin, then 20, 30, 40, 50, 60, 70.

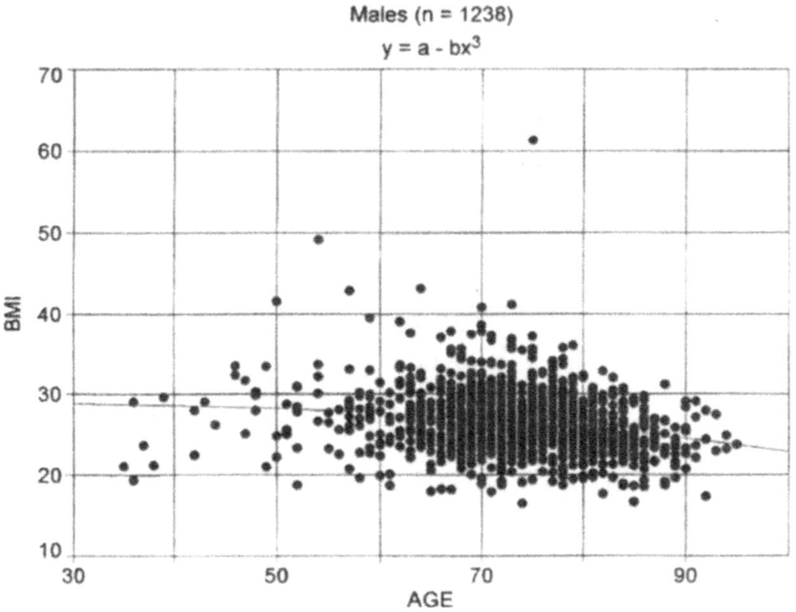

Figure 5.8. BMI and age (males). The abscissa has the value 30 at its origin, then 50, 70, and 90. The ordinate has the value 10 at its origin, then 20, 30, 40, 50, 60, and 70.

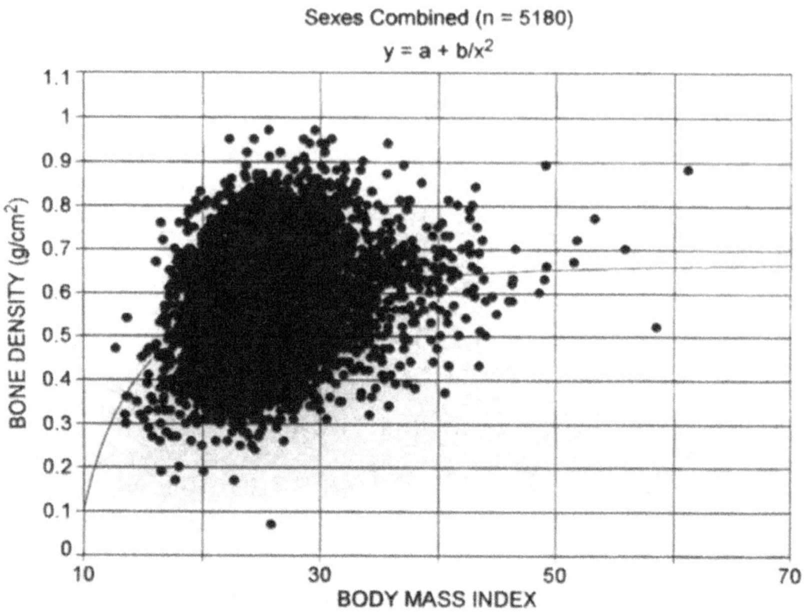

Figure 5.9. Bone density as related to body mass index (sexes combined). The abscissa has the value 10 at its origin, then 30, 50, and 70. The ordinate has the value 0 at its origin, then 0.1, 0.2, 0.3, 0.4, 0.5, 0.6, 0.7, 0.8, 0.9, 1, and 1.1.

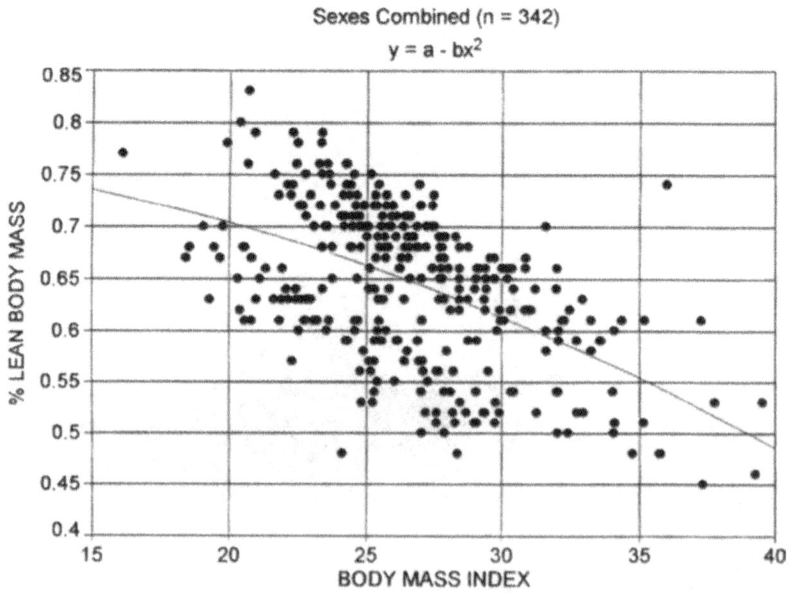

Figure 5.10. Relationship of percent lean body mass to BMI (sexes combined). The abscissa has the value 15 at its origin, then 20, 25, 30, 35, and 40. The ordinate has the value 0.4 at its origin, then 0.45, 0.5, 0.55, 0.6, 0.65, 0.7, 0.75, 0.8, and 0.85.

positive (Figure 5.11). These relationships reflect the degree to which the proportions of lean as opposed to adipose tissue affect BMI values.

Bone density values obtained through single SPA are expressed as grams of bone mineral per square centimeter of area. However, these values can be used to estimate the three-dimensional configuration of the radial diaphysis and, by applying certain assumptions, the cross-sectional areas of the cortex and medullary cavity can be estimated. The method used in making these estimates is described in detail elsewhere (Stini *et al.*, 1992). Normal remodeling of the diaphysis of long bones such as the radius usually involves resorption at the endosteal surface and appositional growth at the subperiosteal surface. With increasing age, the deposit of new bone at the subperiosteal surface declines while resorption at the endosteal surface continues. The result is a thinning of the cortex. In its earlier stages, the increased cross sectional area of the diaphysis may confer an advantage in withstanding torsional stress. However, thinning of the cortex eventually leads to increased vulnerability to fractures produced by buckling of the cortex. Therefore, estimation of changes in the ratio of cortical area to total cross-sectional area (PCA) of the radius provides a useful means of estimating the risk of fracture in the radius. Table 5.2 shows the average initial and final values for PCA for women and men.

As can be seen from the values for PCA in Table 5.2, women enter the postmenopausal period with PCA values as high or higher than those of men. However, they are already experiencing a decline in cortical area in the 50–55 year age interval, while men show little change until the 65–70 year interval. Because of the differences in age of onset and rate of decrease in PCA, initial values for men in the 80–85 year age group are

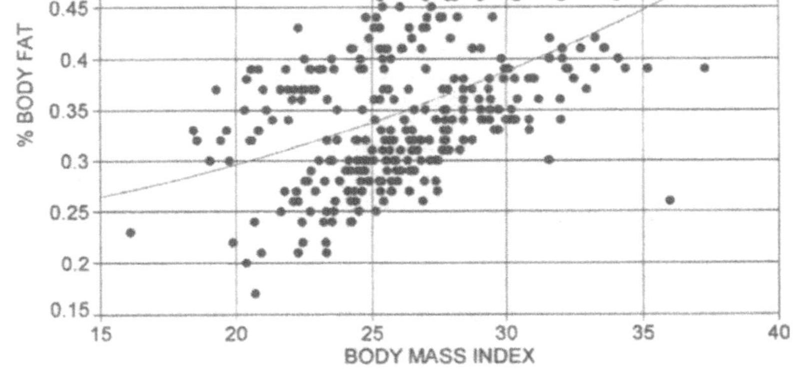

Figure 5.11. Relationship of percent body fat to BMI (sexes combined): The abscissa has the value 15 at its origin, then 20, 25, 30, 35, and 40. The ordinate has the value 0.15 at its origin, then 0.2, 0.25, 0.3, 0.35, 0.4, 0.45, 0.5, 0.55, and 0.6.

Table 5.2. Initial and final percent cortical area, sexes compared

Age	Women		Men	
	Initial PCA	Final PCA	Initial PCA	Final PCA
50–55	64.6	63.5	61.0	61.0
55–60	59.5	58.6	59.3	59.1
60–65	58.0	57.4	59.1	59.1
65–70	54.5	53.3	58.0	57.3
70–75	52.4	50.5	57.9	56.6
75–80	49.0	47.0	57.4	55.7
80–85	48.7	45.5	54.8	52.8
85–90	46.0	43.1	54.3	49.8
90–95	42.6	39.1	50.4	45.9

Table 5.3. PCA values in three age groups and by BMI category

	Female	Male
Age group 60–70		
Average BMI	26.1	26.7
Average PCA	54.6 (n = 928)	57.9 (n = 212)
PCA (BMI >28)	56.9 (n = 288)	58.7 (n = 62)
PCA (BMI <20)	50.4 (n = 60)	54.5 (n = 5)
Age group 70–80		
Average BMI	25.6	26.8
Average PCA	48.9 (n = 1423)	56.2 (n = 418)
PCA (BMI >28)	51.2 (n = 348)	56.7 (n = 147)
PCA (BMI <20)	45.8 (n = 115)	52.9 (n= 12)
Age group 80–90		
Average BMI	24.8	24.8
Average PCA	44.7 (n = 732)	51.9 (n = 250)
PCA (BMI >28)	47.8 (n = 144)	53.6 (n = 36)
PCA (BMI <20)	41.4 (n = 86)	45.1 (n = 15)

higher than those for women in the 65–70 year age group. The rate of loss in the later years of life, however, is very similar in both sexes.

As the regression line shown in Figure 5.9 shows, there is a positive correlation between BMI and cortical bone density. The relationships between BMI and PCA at various ages are shown in Table 5.3. In Table 5.3, BMI values conventionally used to assign the designations "obese" (BMI >28.0), and "excessively lean" (BMI <20.0) were applied to average values in the 10-year age categories: 60–70, 70–80, and 80–90, to assess the relationship between extreme BMI values and PCA. Along with the aforementioned decline in PCA with age, the PCA values for subjects of both sexes with high BMI values are seen to be substantially higher than for those with low BMI values.

When the values for PCA, bone mineral content, and bone density for subjects drawn from the low BMI ($n = 370$) and high BMI ($n = 1228$) categories are compared the differences for all three of these indicators of bone fracture risk are highly significant ($p < 0.0001$). This is true of all age categories whether calculated by sex or with sexes combined. Analysis of variance to test the relationship of PCA to BMI at all ages yields an F value of 91.9 ($p < 0.0001$) sexes combined. Separate analyses of variance for the male and the female samples yield F values of 15.5 and 65.9 respectively, both also significant at the $p < 0.0001$ level.

Normative bone density values, developed from a number of studies conducted in various geographic areas of the United States, are consistently higher than the averages for each age group for both sexes in the Arizona study. When the mean percent of the national normative values for Arizona subjects is compared to their mean BMI values, a t-test yields a 2-tailed significance < 0.0001, similar to the level of significance for the comparison of means for BMI and percent of peak bone density.

All subjects filled out questionnaires that contained questions about fracture histories. Although, there was often some doubt about the bone fractured, the response level to this question was high, and the locations indicated usually made it possible to assign the fracture to such broad categories as "hip," "thigh," "leg," "arm," "rib," and so on. Fractures associated with automobile accidents were excluded from analysis. Of the 3,939 records containing usable fracture histories, 1,066 individuals (878 women and 188 men), reported at least one fracture. The relationship between bone density and fracture histories was equivocal for the male subjects before the age of 80 but was highly significant in the 80–90 year age group. However, as can be seen in Table 5.4, there is an increasingly clear relationship in the female subjects with increased age.

Analysis of variance of bone density values within and between the fracture history categories yields F values of 0.389 (n.s.) for the 50–60 age group; $F = 9.828$ ($p = 0.003$) for the 60–70 age group; $F = 16.14$ ($p < 0.0001$) for the 70–80 age group; and $F = 12.2$ ($p < 0.0001$) for the 80–90 age group. These values reflect the age of occurrence of first and subsequent fractures that the subjects reported. The average age of occurrence of the first fracture for women was 64.4 years. The average age at which men experienced their first fracture was 62.7 years. Of the 301 individuals (268 women and 33 men) reporting a second fracture, the average age of occurrence was 70 years for women and 67.8 years for men. A third fracture was reported by 102 women, with an average age of occurrence of 72.2 years. Only three men reported a third fracture, the average age being 68.3 years.

Table 5.4. Bone densities of women with different fracture histories

	No fractures		1 fracture		>1 fracture		
Age group	*n*	BMD	*n*	BMD	*n*	BMD	Percent*
50–60	192	0.6366	17	0.6393	3	0.6217	9.4
60–70	435	0.5732	152	0.5509	37	0.5233	30.2
70–80	635	0.5203	340	0.4998	102	0.4809	41.0
80–90	291	0.4823	244	0.4454	102	0.4335	54.3

*Percent of women in each age group reporting 1 or more fractures.

4. Discussion

The major objectives of the Arizona Bone Density Study were: (a) to record actual changes in bone density over time; (b) to identify other changes in body composition occurring as a part of the aging process; and (c) to compare the loss of bone density experienced by the most-vulnerable component of the Arizona population, women, with that reported in other populations.

4.1. Observed Bone Loss

The rate of bone loss observed in both sexes in the Arizona population was greater than that derived from normative values used for diagnostic purposes. This is true whether the comparison is with the cross-sectional mean values shown in Table 5.1, or with averaged longitudinal values. In order to make the last-mentioned comparison, only individuals who were scanned five times during the 5-year period represented by their age group were included. Thus, the decline in bone density recorded in women in the 50–55 year age group who had been scanned at ages 50, 51, 52, 53, and 54 was calculated by subtracting the bone density value observed at age 54 from that observed at age 50. While reducing the sample size substantially this procedure made it possible to compare averages derived from individual experience with averages derived from a local population and a national one. In some age groups, the longitudinal data are inadequate to permit meaningful statistical comparisons, but most age groups are sufficiently well represented to provide indicators of similarity and differences. The results of this comparison are shown in Table 5.5, where sample sizes for the cross-sectional and longitudinal components of the Arizona population are entered in parentheses.

As can be seen by comparison of the values in Table 5.5, the rate of density decrease for Arizona subjects is more rapid than national normative values would predict at most ages. Bone density values are also lower for both sexes and all age groups. Following the convention that values above 90% of peak bone density can be considered normal, Arizona average values remain within the normal category until the 55–60 age group, by the 65–70 age

Table 5.5. Rates of bone density loss derived from normative, cross-sectional, and longitudinal values

	Women			Men		
Ages	Standard	Cross-Sectional	Longitudinal	Standard	Cross-Sectional	Longitudinal
50–55	0.0106	0.0059 (142)	0.0594 (7)	0.0335	0.0335 (20)	0.0420 (1)
55–60	0.0405	0.0344 (202)	0.0366 (16)	0.0305	0.0000 (38)	0.0790 (2)
60–65	0.0250	0.0280 (332)	0.0366 (15)	0.0199	0.0051 (84)	0.0310 (1)
65–70	0.0378	0.0323 (684)	0.0445 (68)	0.0145	0.0223 (208)	0.0352 (13)
70–75	0.0297	0.0290 (808)	0.0363 (147)	0.0435	0.0122 (286)	0.0296 (32)
75–80	0.0292	0.0349 (708)	0.0427 (163)	0.0065	0.0103 (295)	0.0431 (50)
80–85	0.0384	0.0173 (497)	0.0544 (165)	0.0048	0.0291 (183)	0.0384 (58)
85–90	0.0287	0.0261 (246)	0.0532 (77)	0.0648	0.0422 (81)	0.0838 (29)
90–95	0.0181	0.0351 (69)	0.0576 (25)	0.0331	0.0524 (18)	0.1226 (5)

group, average values have declined to less than 80% of peak density, and by 75–80 are below 70% of peak density, a level usually considered diagnostic of osteoporosis. Average values for men do not fall below the 90% level until the 65–70 year age group, and below the 80% level after age 85. However, the longitudinal data indicate that male bone loss actually exceed female in a number of age categories. Because of their greater peak bone density, men are less vulnerable to osteoporosis than women, but are clearly not immune to bone loss.

4.2. Changes in Body Composition

The widely used estimate of body composition, BMI is one obvious measure of change that merits careful attention. However, BMI values can be misleading. For instance, young individuals with high lean body mass (LBM)/ total body mass (TBM) ratios will exhibit higher BMI values than those with normal amounts of total body fat (TBF). This is because the LBM compartment of TBM is of higher density. In fact the Seri equations used to calculate TBF and LBM by comparison of a conventional measure of weight with one taken with the subject immersed in water are based on the specific gravity values for TBF and LBM. As can be seen from the regression lines in Figures 5.8 and 5.9, in the age groups represented in the Arizona population, increasing BMI is negatively correlated with increased LBM, and positively correlated with TBF. These results are consistent with those reported by Kehayias *et al.* (1997) in their analysis of total body potassium (Table 5.6). These investigators estimate a decline of total body potassium (TBK) of 7.2 mgK/kg body weight/year in women, and 9.2 mgK/kg/year in men. The steady decline in TBK is closely related to a decline in intracellular fluid (ICF) mass and therefore cell number. Cell number is directly related to basal metabolic rate (BMR). Therefore, the decline in TBK is a measure of the decline in required energy intake associated with increasing age. An average daily energy intake of 1,910 kcal was reported for the 1,303 individuals of both sexes (average age 66.2 years) who completed the Wheat Bran Fiber Colon Cancer Prevention Study.

Another way of estimating energy requirements is to calculate body surface area (SA) using height and weight values. This is the most commonly used method of estimating BMR. When the male and female values for SA are compared for a total of 3,858

Table 5.6. Age changes in body mass index and total body potassium in women and men (From Kehayias *et al.*, 1997)

	Women				Men			
Age	BMI	TBK (g)	TBK/Ht	TBK/Wt	BMI	TBK (g)	TBK/Ht	TBK/Wt
20–29	22.8	101.4	0.62	1.67	24.8	164.5	0.92	2.06
30–39	23.6	98.7	0.60	1.59	25.0	145.6	0.83	1.90
40–49	25.3	96.4	0.58	1.41	27.6	148.3	0.84	1.72
50–59	27.5	95.8	0.59	1.35	28.4	146.1	0.83	1.68
60–69	24.3	85.2	0.53	1.36	25.3	128.2	0.74	1.70
70–79	26.6	79.8	0.51	1.24	25.6	120.2	0.69	1.56
80–89	23.6	72.3	0.46	1.26	26.3	106.8	0.64	1.46

women and 1,166 men, the female average SA is 1.71 m^2 and the male average is 1.95 m^2. Since the same values, height and weight, are used to derive both BMI and SA it is expected that BMI and SA would be highly correlated, as indeed they are ($r = 0.838$ for women and 0.781 for men). Also expected would be a decline in SA with age. SA is negatively correlated with age in both sexes (−0.166 for women and −0.249 for men). All of these correlations are significant at the 0.01 level (2-tailed test). Perhaps more interesting is the high positive correlation between percent body fat and SA, and negative correlations between percent lean tissue and SA ($r = 0.761$ for women and $r = 0.644$ for men), derived from bioelectric impedance values for 128 women and 214 men participating in the Wheat Bran Fiber Study.

The 2-compartment method of estimating body composition by hydrostatic weighing had long been considered the "gold standard" of body composition analysis. However, the components of the lean tissue compartment are more variable with respect to mass and density than are those of the adipose compartment. This is especially true of the portion of LBM represented by bone, which is much denser than skeletal muscle but has lower energy requirements. Thus, the impact of declining bone density will be more significant from the perspective of LBM than from that of BMR. The nonlinear relationship between bone density and BMI can clearly be seen in Figure 5.9, where the best-fit regression equation is $y = a + b/x^2$. The decline in bone density with age as seen in Figures 5.2–5.4, is clearly more precipitous than the decline in BMI with age as seen in Figures 5.6–5.8.

The implications of this disparity raise questions about the appropriateness of using BMI values to estimate energy requirements in older populations although the decline in TBK with age indicates a steady decline in BMR. It should come as no surprise that weight control is often a problem during late middle age, when the proportion of fat to lean tissue is rising, in consequence of decreases in both skeletal muscle mass and bone density. Even maintenance of a constant body weight can mask substantial accumulation of fat when the increase is offset by loss of both high density bone mineral and metabolically active skeletal muscle. By the same token, the early stages of bone density decline often go undiagnosed, since there are no obvious indications of bone density decrease in the absence of *in vivo* monitoring using sophisticated instrumentation.

Jones *et al.* (2001), report that urinary potassium is positively associated with both dietary potassium intake and BMD independently of BMI in calcium-replete children. The focus of this study was on the relationship of potassium intake and the attainment of peak bone mass. A subsample of the Arizona bone density project population was sampled longitudinally for serum mineral values, including potassium. The values ranged between 2.8 and 5.0, with a mean of 4.18. Figure 5.12 shows the distribution and values for serum potassium. Analysis of variance of quartile values for potassium as related to BMC at the distal one third site of the radius yielded an F value of 5.15 for 3 and 342 d.f. (significant at the 0.002 level). The F value for BMD and serum potassium was 4.252 (significant at the 0.006 level). No effect of sex or BMI was found. The organic component has been shown to contain the majority of the sodium and potassium in bone, and it has been suggested (Bushinsky *et al.*, 2000) that it is the organic material in bone and not the mineral itself that is responsible for the buffering of hydrogen ions during metabolic acidosis. On the basis of serum values of both calcium and copper observed in the Arizona study (Figures 5.13 and 5.14), it would appear that greater attention to variation in these values could yield diagnostic benefits.

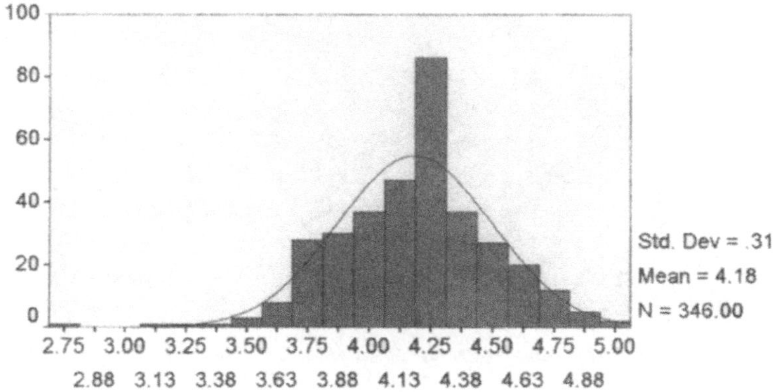

Figure 5.12. Serum potassium values for a subsample of 346 Arizona subjects of both sexes.

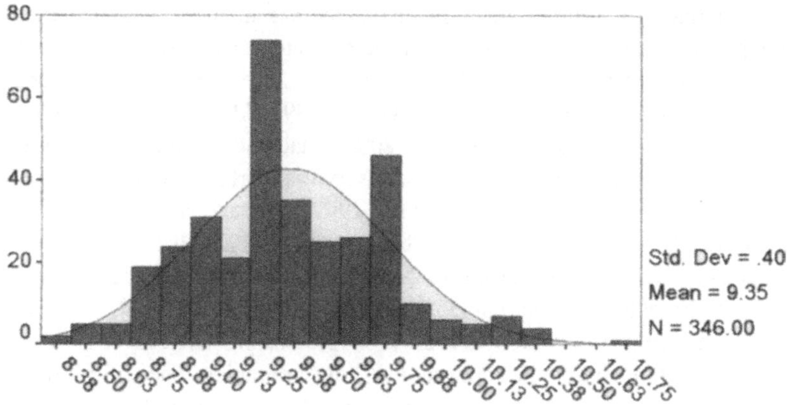

Figure 5.13. Serum calcium values for a subsample of 346 Arizona subjects of both sexes.

4.3. Nutrition, Bone Density, and Prostate Cancer

The bone density of African Americans is, on the average, greater than that of individuals of European or Asian ancestry. African American men also have a higher incidence of prostate cancer than men of European or Asian origin. This difference in prostate cancer incidence does not appear to be explained by dietary or lifestyle factors (Platz *et al.*, 2000). For the general population, beneficial effects of such compounds as isoflavones, lycopenes, selenium, vitamin A, and vitamin D, as well as deleterious effects of calcium and fatty acids have been reported (Chan *et al.*, 1998a,b, 2000; Blumenfeld *et al.*, 2000; Damber, 2000). Although dairy products are unquestionably a rich source of calcium, there is considerable evidence that they are associated with increased risk of prostate cancer (Chan *et al.*, 1998a,b). The relationship between calcium intake and prostate cancer is thought to derive from the effects of calcium and phosphate intake on vitamin D levels (Giovannucci, 1998; Kapur, 2000).

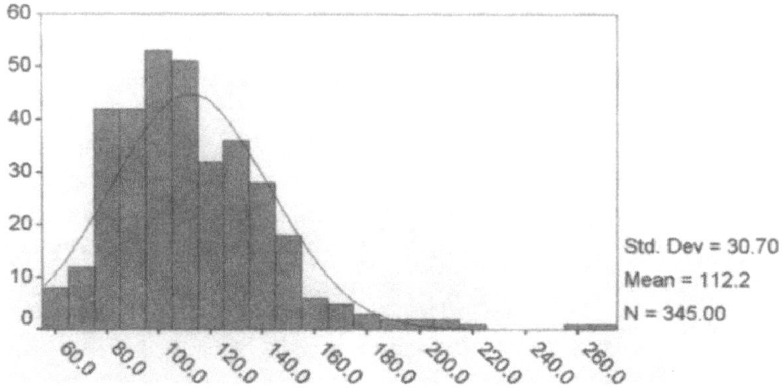

Figure 5.14. Serum copper values for a subsample of 346 Arizona subjects of both sexes.

Epidemiological studies have shown that there is an inverse association between sunlight exposure and the risk for cancers of the prostate, breast, and colon (McCarty, 2000). Both 1,25$(OH)_2$ Vitamin D and 25(OH) Vitamin D have been found to reduce the risk of prostate cancer (Miller, 1998–99; Nomura *et al.*, 1998; Ahonen *et al.*, 2000; Barreto *et al.*, 2000; Brawley and Parnes, 2000; Holick, 2000; Zhao and Feldman, 2001). Vitamin receptor polymorphisms have also been shown to serve as markers for prostate cancer susceptibility (Yu *et al.*, 1998; Correa-Cerro *et al.*, 1999). Prostate cancer cells contain specific receptors for 1,25$(OH)_2$ vitamin D_3 (Chen *et al.*, 1998a,b). It has also been found that when prostate cancers metastasize to bone, endocrine changes caused by cancer cells affect both phosphate and vitamin D metabolism (Satani *et al.*, 1997).

The mechanism by which vitamin D suppresses prostate cancer involves inhibition of cell proliferation and the promotion of cell differentiation. The anti-proliferation effect of 1,25$(OH)_2$ vitamin D_3 has also been in breast cancer cells (Campbell *et al.*, 2000). In some types of prostate cancer cells, inhibition is androgen dependent while in others it is androgen independent (Zhao *et al.*, 2000). Important aspects of the mechanism include inhibition of overall invasion, cell adhesion, and migration to the basement membrane matrix protein laminin through modulation of certain cell surface adhesion molecules (Sung and Feldman, 2000). Developmental biologists have demonstrated the importance of calcium-dependent adhesion in the establishment and maintenance of segmental organization early in embryonic development (McCarthy *et al.*, 2001). In view of the several lines of evidence cited here, routine recommendations of increased calcium intake to prevent osteoporosis (Bendich *et al.*, 1999), must be seriously questioned, particularly when made to men.

5. Summary and Conclusions

There has long been a tendency to view bone density loss as a problem for women. However, as information concerning bone density status of men accumulates, it has become increasingly clear that osteoporosis in males is a problem of significant concern.

During the course of a 16-year mixed-longitudinal study of bone density change in an Arizona population, the rate of bone loss of males and females has been monitored on an annual basis, along with measurement of stature, weight, and questionnaire responses on food intakes, exercise patterns, and health status. Included in the latter category was an annual update of bone fracture histories. When male and female statistics on bone fracture rates for 2,947 women and 815 men were compared, it was found that the rate of fracture occurrence beyond age 50 was slightly higher (0.41) for men than for women (0.37) after correction for such traumatic causes of injury as automobile accidents. This result was surprising in view of the fact that the PCA of the radius at the distal one third site in men averaged 55.3 as compared with a value of 50.2 for women. Preliminary data also indicate that the consequences of bone fracture in the ages beyond 75 are more serious for men than for women in terms of long-term morbidity and mortality.

Several investigators have observed that the risk of osteoporosis in men is more closely associated with estrogen than with testosterone levels, and that the process of bone remodeling in men differs from that in women. In the Arizona population, it has been observed that loss of LBM is more rapid in men than in women after age 80.

As an increasing number of men survive into their 80s and 90s, the problem of age-associated bone loss among men may emerge as a public health concern as serious as that already recognized in women although the mechanisms underlying the process are different. The function of vitamin D in human physiology goes well beyond the maintenance of bone (Stini, 2000c). It is possible that calcium intakes high enough to reduce vitamin D synthesis may increase the risk of prostate cancer.

References

Ahonen, M.H., Tenkanen, L., Teppo, L., Hakama, M., and Tuohimaa, P. (2000). Prostate cancer risk and prediagnostic serum 25-hydroxyvitamin D levels (Finland). *Cancer Causes Control* **11**(9), 847–852.

Arai, H., Miyamoto, K.I., Yoshida, M., Yamamoto, H., Taketani, Y., Morita, K., Kubota, M., Yoshida *et al.* (2001). The polymorphism in the caudal-related homeodomain protein Cdx-2 binding element in the human vitamin D receptor gene. *J. Bone Miner. Res.* **16**(7), 1256–1264.

Barreto, A.M., Schwartz, G.G., Woodruff, R., and Cramer, S.D. (2000). 25-Hydroxyvitamin D3, the prohormone of 1,25-dihydroxyvitamin D3, inhibits the proliferation of primary prostatic epithelial cells. *Cancer Epidemiol. Biomarkers Prev.* **9**(3), 265–270.

Bendich, A., Leader, S., and Muhuri, P. (1999). Supplemental calcium for the prevention of hip fracture: potential health-economic benefits. *Clin. Ther.* **21**(6), 1058–1072.

Bikle, D.D., Ettinger, B., Sisney, S., Tekawa, I.S., and Tolan, K. (1999). Differences in calcium metabolism between black and white men and women. *Miner. Electrolyte Metab.* **25**(3), 178–184.

Black, A., Tilmont, E.M., Handy, A.M., Scott, W.W., Shapses, S.A., Ingram, D.K., Roth, G.S., and Lane, M.A. (2001). A nonhuman primate model of age-related bone loss: A longitudinal study in male and premenopausal female rhesus monkeys. *Bone* **28**(3), 295–302.

Blumenfeld, A.J., Fleshner, N., Casselman, B., and Trachtenberg, J. (2000). Nutritional aspects of prostate cancer: A review. *Can. J. Urol.* **7**(1), 927–935.

Boonen, S., Vanderschueren, D., Cheng, X.G., Verbeke, G., Dequeker, J., Geusens, P., Broos, P., and Bouillon, R. (1997). Age-related (type II) femoral neck osteoporosis in men: Biochemical evidence for both hypovitaminosis D- and androgen deficiency-induced bone resorption. *J. Bone Miner. Res.* **12**(12), 2119–2126.

Braga, V., Mottes, M., Mirandola, S., Lisi, V., Malerba, G., Sartori, L., Bianchi, G., Gatti, D. *et al.* (2000). Association of CTR and COLIA1 alleles with BMD values in peri- and postmenopausal women. *Calcif. Tissue Int.* **67**(5), 361–366.

Brawley, O.W., and Parnes, H. (2000). Prostate cancer prevention trials in the USA. *Eur. J. Cancer* **36**(10), 1312–1315.

Bushinsky, D.A., Gavrilov, K.L., Chabala, J.M., and Levi-Setti, R. (2000). Contribution of organic material to the ion composition of bone. *J. Bone Miner. Res.* **15**(10), 2026–2032.

Campbell, M.J., Gombart, A.F., Kwok, S.H., Park, S., and Koeffler, H.P. (2000). The anti-proliferative effects of 1alpha,25$(OH)_2$D3 on breast and prostate cancer cells are associated with induction of BRCA1 gene expression. *Oncogene* **19**(44), 5091–5097.

Cerroni, A.M., Tomlinson, G.A., Turnquist, J.E., and Grynpasa, M.D. (2000). Bone mineral density, osteopenia, and osteoporosis in the rhesus macaques of Cayo Santiago. *Am. J. Phys. Anthropol.* **113**(3), 389–410.

Chan, J.M., Giovannucci, E., Andersson, S.O., Yuen, J., Adami, H.O., and Wolk, A. (1998a). Dairy products,calcium, phosphorus, vitamin D, and risk of prostate cancer (Sweden). *Cancer Causes Control* **9**(6), 541–543.

Chan, J.M., Giovannucci, E., Andersson, S.O., Yuen, J., Adami, H.O., and Wolk, A. (1998b). Dairy products, calcium, phosphorus, vitamin D, and risk of prostate cancer. *Cancer Causes Control.* **9**(6), 559–566.

Chan, J.M., Pietinen, P., Virtanen, M., Malina, N., Tangrea, J., Albanes, D., and Vitamo, J. (2000). Diet and prostate cancer in a cohort of smokers, with a specific focus on calcium and phosphorus (Finland). *Cancer Causes Control* **11**(9), 859–867.

Chen, Z., Lohman, T.G., Stini, W.A., Ritenbaugh, S., and Aiken, M. (1997). Fat or lean tissue mass: Which one is the major determinant of bone mineral mass in healthy post-menopausal women? *J. Bone Miner. Res.* **12**, 144–151.

Chen, T.C., Schwartz, G.G., Burnstein, K.L., Lokeshwar, B.L., and Holick, M.F. (2000). The *in vitro* evaluation of 25-hydroxyvitamin D3 and 19-nor-1 alpha,25-dihydroxyvitamin D2 as therapeutic agents for prostate cancer. *Clin. Cancer Res.* **6**(3), 901–908.

Cody, D.D., Divine, G.W., Nahigian, K., and Kleerekoper, M. (2000). Bone density distribution and gender dominate femoral neck fracture risk predictors. *Skeletal Radiol.* **29**(3), 151–161.

Colman, R.J., Lane, M.A., Binkley, N., Wegner, F.H., and Kemnitz, J.W. (1999). Skeletal effects of aging in male rhesus macaques. *Bone* **24**(1), 17–23.

Compston, J.E. (2001). Sex steroids and bone. *Physiol. Rev.* **81**(1), 419–447.

Correa-Cerro, L., Berthon, P., Haussler, J., Bochum, S., Drelon, E., Mangin, P., Fournier, G., Paiss, T. *et al.* (1999). Vitamin D receptor polymorphisms as markers in prostate cancer. *Hum. Genet.* **105**(3), 281–287.

Damber, J.E. (2000). Diet probably plays an important role in the development of prostatic cancer. *Lakartidningen* **97**(32–33), 3475–3480.

D'Amore, M., Bottalico, C., D'Amore, S., Di Chio, A., and Scagliusi, P. (2000). Sex hormones and male osteoporosis. A physiologic prospective for prevention and therapy. *Minerva Med.* **91**(11–12), 283–289.

Da Silva, J.A., and Porto, A. (1997). Sex hormone and osteoporosis: A physiological prospective for prevention and therapy. *Acta. Med. Port.* **10**(10), 689–695.

Davies, K.M., Heaney, R.P., Recker, R.R., Lappe, J.M., Barger-Lux, M.J., Rafferty, K., and Hinders, S. (2000). Calcium intake and body weight. *J. Clin. Endocrinol. Metab.* **85**(12), 4635–4638.

Dennison, E., Yoshimura, N., Hashimoto, T., and Cooper, C. (1998). Bone loss in Great Britain and Japan: A comparative longitudinal study. *Bone* **23**(4), 379–382.

DeRosa, M., Paesano, L., Nuzzo, V., Zarrilli, S., Del Puente, A., Oriente, P., and Lupoli, G. (2001). Bone mineral density and bone markers in hypogonadotropic and hypergonadotropic hypogonadal men after prolonged testosterone treatment. *J. Endocrinol. Invest.* **24**(4), 246–252.

Di Monaco, M., Di Monaco, R., Manca, M., and Cavanna, A. (2000). Handgrip strength is an independent predictor of distal radius bone mineral density in postmenopausal women. *Clin. Rheumatol.* **19**(6), 473–476.

El-Hajj Fuleihan, G., Nabulsi, M., Choucair, M., Salamoun, M., Hajj Shahine, C., Kizirian, A., and Tannous, R. (2001). Hypovitaminosis D in healthy children. *Pediatrics* **107**(4), E53.

el Miedany, Y.M., el Gaafary, S., and el Baddini, M.A. (1999). Osteoporosis in older adults with non-insulin-dependent diabetes mellitus: Is it sex related? *Clin. Exp. Rheumatol.* **17**(5), 561–567.

el Miedany, Y.M., Mehanna, A.N., and El Baddini, M.A. (2000). Altered bone mineral metabolism in patients with osteoarthritis. *Joint Bone Spine* **67**(6), 521–527.

Fassbender, W.J., Balli, M., Gortz, B., Hinrichs, B., Kaiser, H.E., and Tracks, H.S. (2000). Sex steroids, biochemical markers, bone mineral density and histomorphometry in male osteoporosis patients. *In Vivo* **14**(5), 611–618.

Frost, M.L., Blake, G.M., and Fogelman, I. (2001). Quantitative ultrasound and bone mineral density are equally strongly associated with risk factors for osteoporosis. *J. Bone Miner. Res.* **16**(2), 406–416.

Giovannucci, E. (1998). Dietary influences of 1,25$(OH)_2$ vitamin D in relation to prostate cancer: A hypothesis. *Cancer Causes Control* **9**(6), 567–582.

Guthrie, J.R., Dennerstein, L., and Wark, J.D. (2000a). Risk factors for osteoporosis: A review. *Medscape Women's Health* **5**(4), E1.

Guthrie, J.R., Ebeling, P.R., Dennerstein, L., and Wark, J.D. (2000b). Risk factors for osteoporosis: Prevalence, change, and association with bone density. *Medscape Women's Health* **5**(5), E2.

Holick, M.F. (2000). Calcium and vitamin D. Diagnostics and therapeutics. *Clin. Lab Med.* **20**(3), 569–590.

Ismail, A.A., O'Neill, T.W., Cooper, C., and Silman, A.J. (2000). Risk factors for vertebral deformities in men: Relationship to number of vertebral deformities. European Vertebral Osteoporosis Study Group. *J. Bone Miner. Res.* **15**(2), 278–283.

Iwamoto, J., Takeda, T., Ichimura, S., Tsukimura, Y., and Toyama, Y. (2000a). Age-related changes in cortical bone in men: Metacarpal bone mass measurement study. *J. Orthop. Sci.* **5**(1), 4–9.

Iwamoto, J., Takeda, T., and Ichimura, S. (2000b). Effect of combined administration of vitamin D3 and vitamin K2 on bone mineral density of the lumbar spine in postmenopausal women with osteoporosis. *J. Orthop. Sci.* **5**(6), 546–551.

Jones, G., Riley, M.D., and Whiting, S. (2001). Association between urinary potassium, urinary sodium, current diet, and bone density in prepubertal children. *Am. J. Clin. Nutr.* **73**(4), 839–844.

Kapur, S. (2000). A medical hypothesis: Phosphorus balance and prostate cancer. *Cancer Invest.* **18**(7), 664–649.

Kehayias, J.J., Fiatarone, M.A., Hong, Z., and Roubenoff, R. (1997). Total body potassium and body fat: Relevance to aging. *Am. J. Clin. Nutr.* **66**, 904–910.

Khosla, S., Melton, L.J. 3rd, and Riggs, B.L. (1999). Osteoporosis: Gender differences and similarities. *Lupus* **8**(5), 393–396.

Kim, J.G., Lim, K.S., Kim, E.K., Choi, Y.M., and Lee, J.Y. (2001). Association of vitamin D receptor and estrogen receptor gene polymorphisms with bone mass in postmenopausal Korean women. *Menopause* **8**(3), 222–228.

Krassas, G.E., Papadopoulou, F.G., Doukidis, D., Konstantinidis, T.H., and Kalothetou, K. (2001). Age-related changes in bone density among healthy Greek males. *J. Endocrinol. Invest.* **24**(5), 326–333.

Kudlacek, S., Schneider, B., Resch, H., Freudenthaler, O., and Willvonseder, R. (2000). Gender differences in fracture risk and bone mineral density. *Maturitas* **36**(3), 173–180.

Legroux-Gerot, I., Blanckaert, F., Solau-Gervais, E., Negahban, M., Duquesnoy, B., Delcambre, B., and Cortet, B. (1999). Causes of osteoporosis in males. A review of 160 cases. *Rev. Rhum. Engl. Ed.* **66**(7–9), 404–409.

Lips, P., Duong, T., Oleksik, A., Black, D., Cummings, S., Cox, D., and Nickelsen, T. (2001). A global study of vitamin D status and parathyroid function in postmenopausal women with osteoporosis: Baseline data from the multiple outcomes of raloxifene evaluation clinical trial. *J. Clin. Endocrinol. Metab.* **86**(3), 1212–1221.

Martinez Diaz-Guerra, G., Hawkins, F., Rapado, A., Ruiz Diaz, M.A., and Diaz-Curiel, M. (2001). Hormonal and anthropometric predictors of bone mass in healthy elderly men: Major effect of sex hormone binding globulin, parathyroid hormone and body weight. *Osteoporosis Int.* **12**(3), 178–184.

Matsukura, T., Kagamimori, S., Yamagami, T., Nishino, H., Iki, M., Kajita, E., Kagawa, Y., Yoneshima, H. *et al.* (2000). Reference data of forearm bone mineral density in healthy Japanese male and female subjects in the second decade based on calendar age and puberty onset: Japanese Population Based Osteoporosis (JPOS) study. *Osteoporosis Int.* **11**(10), 858–865.

Maugeri, D., Panebianco, P., Barbagallo, P., Malaguarnera, M., Curasi, M.P., Russo, M.S., Santangelo, A. Speciale, S. *et al.* (1998). Estrogens and euosteogenesis in men. *Eur. Rev. Med. Pharmacol. Sci.* **2**(5–6), 189–192.

McCarthy, M., Na, E., Neyt, C., Langston, A., and Fishell, G. (2001). Calcium-dependent adhesion is necessary for the maintenance of prosomeres. *Dev. Biol.* **233**(1), 80–94.

McCarty, M.F. (2000). Parathyroid hormone may be a cancer promoter—an explanation for the decrease in cancer risk associated with ultraviolet light, calcium, and vitamin D. *Med. Hypotheses.* **54**(3), 475–482.

Medras, M., Jankowska, E.A., and Rogucka, E. (2001). Effects of long-term testosterone substitutive therapy on bone mineral content in men with hypergonadotrophic hypogonadism. *Andrologia.* **33**(1), 47–52.

Miller, G.J. (1998). Vitamin D and prostate cancer: Biologic interactions and clinical potentials. *Cancer Metastasis Rev.* **99**(4), 353–360.

Nakamura, K., Nashimoto, M., and Yamamoto, M. (2001). Are the serum 25-hydroxyvitamin D concentrations in winter associated with forearm bone mineral density in healthy elderly Japanese women? *Int. J. Vitam. Nutr. Res.* **71**(1), 25–29.

National Institutes of Health (2001). NIH Consensus Development Panel on Osteoporosis Prevention, Diagnosis, and Therapy, March 27–29, 2000: Highlights of the conference. *South Med. J.* **94**(6), 569–573.

Nomura, A.M., Stemmermann, G.N., Lee, J., Kolonel, L.N., Chen, T.C., Turner, A., and Holick, M.F. (1998). Serum vitamin D metabolite levels and the subsequent development of prostate cancer (Hawaii, United States). *Cancer Causes Control.* **9**(4), 541–543.

O'Flaherty, E.J. (2000). Modeling normal aging bone loss, with consideration of bone loss in osteoporosis. *Toxicol. Sci.* **55**(1), 171–188.

Ongphiphadhanakul, B., Rajatanavin, R., Chanprasertyothin, S., Piaseu, N., and Chailurkit, L. (1998). Serum oestradiol and oestrogen-receptor gene polymorphism are associated with bone mineral density independently of serum testosterone in normal males. *Clin. Endocrinol. (Oxf).* **49**(6), 803–809.

Overton, T.R., and Basu, T.K. (1999). Longitudinal changes in radial bone density in older men. *Eur. J. Clin. Nutr.* **53**(3), 211–215.

Oz, O.K., Zerwekh, J.E., Fisher, C., Graves, K., Nanu, L., Millsaps, R., and Simpson, E.R. (2000). Bone has a sexually dimorphic response to aromatase deficiency. *J. Bone Miner. Res.* **15**(3), 507–514.

Ozisik, G., Mergen, H., Ozata, M., Uyanik, C., Caglayan, S., Turan, M., Bolu, E., Ilgin, S. *et al.* (2001). Vitamin d-receptor gene polymorphisms and vertebral bone density in men with idiopathic hypogonadotrophic hypogonadism. *Med. Sci. Monit.* **7**(2), 233–237.

Patel, R. Collins, D. Bullock, S. Swaminathan, R. Blake, G.M., and Fogelman, I. (2001). The effect of season and vitamin D supplementation on bone mineral density in healthy women: A double-masked crossover study. *Osteoporosis Int.* **12**(4), 319–325.

Platz, E.A., Rimm, E.B., Willett, W.C., Kantoff, P.W., and Giovannucci, E. (2000). Racial variation in prostate cancer incidence and in hormonal system markers among male health professionals. *J. Natl. Cancer Inst.* **92**(24), 2009–2017.

Pluskiewicz, W., and Drozdzowska, B. (1999). Ultrasound measurements at the calcaneus in men: Differences between healthy and fractured persons and the influence of age and anthropometric features on ultrasound parameters. *Osteoporosis Int.* **10**(1), 47–51.

Rapado, A., Hawkins, F., Sobrinho, L., Diaz-Curiel, M., Galvao-Tellas, A., Arver, S., Melo Gomes, J., Mazer, N. *et al.* (1999). Bone mineral density and androgen levels in elderly males. *Calcif. Tissue Int.* **65**(6), 417–421.

Ricci, T.A., Heymsfield, S.B., Pierson, R.N., Stahl, T., Chowdhury, H.A., and Shapses, S.A. (2001). Moderate energy restriction increases bone resorption in obese postmenopausal women. *Am. J. Clin. Nutr.* **73**(2), 347–352.

Rogucka, E., Bielicki, T., Welon, Z., Medras, M., and Susanne, C. (2000). Variation in bone mineral density in adults in Poland: Age and sex differences. *Ann. Hum. Biol.* **27**(2), 139–148.

Sagiv, M., Vogelaere, P.P., Soudry, M., and Ehrsam, R. (2000). Role of physical activity training in attenuation of height loss through aging. *Gerontology* **46**(5), 266–270.

Salminen, S.T., Pihlajamaki, H.K., Avikainen, V.J., and Bostman, O.M. (2000). Population based epidemiologic and morphologic study of femoral shaft fractures. *Clin. Orthop.* **372**, 241–249.

Santolaria, F., Gonzalez-Reimers, E., Perez-Manzano, J.L., Milena, A., Gomez-Rodriguez, M.A., Gonzalez-Diaz, A., dela Vega, M.J., and Martinez-Riera, A. (2000). Osteopenia assessed by body composition analysis is related to malnutrition in alcoholic patients. *Alcohol* **22**(3), 147–157.

Satani, H., Yamakawa, K., Kawamura, J., Mori, O., Saito, K., Kato, H., Tochigi, H., Sakurai, M. *et al.* (1997). Bone metabolism and phosphorus metabolism in patients with prostate cancer: Paracrine and endocrine effects produced by prostate neoplasm. *Hinyokika Kiyo* **43**(12), 849–854.

Seeman, E. (1999). The structural basis of bone fragility in men. *Bone* **25**(1),143–147.

Singer, B.R., McLauchlan, G.L., Robinson, C.M., and Christie, J. (1998). Epidemiology of fractures in 15,000 adults: The influence of age and gender. *J. Bone Joint. Surg. Br.* **80**(2), 243–248.

Sinigaglia, L., Nervetti, A., Mela, Q., Bianchi, G., Del Puente, A., Di Munno, O., Frediani, B., Cantatore, F. *et al.* (2000). A multicenter cross sectional study on bone mineral density in rheumatoid arthritis. Italian Study Group on Bone Mass in Rheumatoid Arthritis. *J. Rheumatol.* **27**(11), 2582–2589.

Snelling, A.M., Crespo, C.J., Schaeffer, M., Smith, S., and Walbourn, L. (2001). Modifiable and nonmodifiable factors associated with osteoporosis in postmenopausal women: Results from the Third National Health and Nutrition Examination Survey, 1988–1994. *J. Womens Health Gend Based Med.* **1**, 57–65.

Stini, W.A. (2000a). Bone Loss, Body Mass Index, and Fracture Histories in an Arizona Elderly Population. In R. Watson (ed.) *Handbook of Nutrition and the Aged (3rd edn.)* Washington, CRC Press pp. 115–135.

Stini, W.A. (2000b). Nutrition and Aging. In A. Siniarska and N. Wolanski (eds) *Ecology of Aging. J. Human Ecology* (Special Issue) 8, pp. 63–91.

Stini, W.A. (2000c). Calcium metabolism and evolutionary opportunism. In M. Scultz, K. Christianson, H. Greil, W. Henke, A. Kemkes-Grottenthaler, C. Niemitz, H. Rothe, W. Schieefenhovel, H.D. Schmidt, I. Schroder, H. Schutkowski, M. Teschler-Nicola, and V. Wittwer-Backofen (eds) *Schnittslelle Mensch – Umwelt in Vergangenheit, Gegenwart und Zukunft*. Gottingen, Cuvillier Verlag pp. 215–222.

Stini, W.A., Stein, P. and Chen, Z. (1992). Bone remodeling in old age: longitudinal monitoring in Arizona. *American Journal of Human Biology* **4**, 47–55.

Stini, W.A., Chen, Z., and Stein, P. (1994). Aging, bone loss and body mass index in Arizona retirees. *Am. J. Hum. Biol.* **6**(1), 43–50.

Sung, V., and Feldman, D. (2000). 1,25-Dihydroxyvitamin D3 decreases human prostate cancer cell adhesion and migration. *Mol. Cell Endocrinol.* **164**(1–2), 133–143.

Szulc, P., Marchand, F., Duboeuf, F., and Delmas, P.D. (2000). Cross-sectional assessment of age-related bone loss in men: The MINOS study. *Bone* **26**(2), 123–129.

Thorsen, K., Nordstrom, P., Lorentzon, R., and Dahlen, G.H. (1999). The relation between bone mineral density, insulin-like growth factor, I. lipoprotein (a), body composition, and muscle strength in adolescent males. *J. Clin. Endocrinol. Metab.* **84**(9), 3025–3029.

Tsuzuku, S., Niino, N., Ando, F., and Shimokata, H. (2000). Bone mineral density obtained by peripheral quantitative computed tomography (pQCT) in middle-aged and elderly Japanese. *J. Epidemiol.* **10**(1 Suppl), S39–45.

Uitterlinden, A.G., Weel, A.E., Burger, H., Fang, Y., van Duijn, C.M., Hofman, A., van Leeuwen, J.P., and Pols, H.A. (2001). Interaction between the vitamin D receptor gene and collagen type I alpha1 gene in susceptibility for fracture. *J. Bone Miner. Res.* **16**(2), 379–385.

Valamaki, S., Tahtela, R., Kainulainen, K., Laitinen, K., Loyttyniemi, E., Sulkava, R., Valimaki, M., and Kontula, K. (2001). Relation of collagen type 1 alpha 1 (COLIA 1) and vitamin D receptor genotypes to bone mass, turnover, and fractures in early postmenopausal women and to hip fractures in elderly people. *Eur. J. Intern. Med.* **12**(1), 48–56.

Winters, S.J. (1999). Current status of testosterone replacement therapy in men. *Arch. Fam. Med.* **8**(3), 257–263.

Woitge, H.W., Scheidt-Nave, C., Kissling, C., Leidig-Bruckner, G., Meyer, K., Grauer, A., Scharla, S.H., Ziegler, R. *et al.* (1998). Seasonal variation of biochemical indexes of bone turnover: Results of a population-based study. *J. Clin. Endocrinol. Metab.* **83**(1), 68–75.

Woitge, H.W., Knothe, A., Witte, K., Schmidt-Gayk, H., Ziegler, R., Lemmer, B., and Seibel, M.J. (2000). Circaannual rhythmes and interactions of vitamin D metabolites, Parathyroid hormone, and biochemical markers of skeletal homeostasis: A prospective study. *J. Bone Miner. Res.* **15**(12), 2443–2450.

Yu, D.M., Tokuda, N., Naito, S., Yoshikawa, M., Takahashi, K., Uozumi, J., and Kumazawa, J. (1998). Antiproliferative effect of calcitriol on human prostatic cancer cell lines: Unrelated to the expression of major histocompatability complex antigens or intercellular adhesion molecule-1. (ICAM-1). *Int. J. Urol.* **5**(6), 595–600.

Zarate, A., Basurto, L., and Fanghanel, G. (2000). Osteoporosis in males is a frequently overlooked risk. *Gac. Med. Mex.* **136**(1), 83–86.

Zhao, X., and Feldman, D. (2001). The role of vitamin D in prostate cancer. *Steroids* **66**(3–5), 293–300.

Zhao, X.Y., Peehl, D.M., Navone, N.M., and Feldman, D. (2000). 1 alpha,25-dihydroxyvitamin D3 inhibits prostate cancer cell growth by androgen-dependent and androgen-independent mechanisms. *Endocrinology* **141**(7), 2548–2556.

6

The Histomorphometry of the Subadult Rib: Age-Associated Changes in Bone Mass and the Creation of Peak Bone Mass

Margaret Streeter and Sam D. Stout

1. Introduction

Increased bone fragility and other problems associated with age-associated bone loss are primarily manifested in the later years of life, and much of the research on this important health problem has focused upon the skeletal systems of adults. There is considerable evidence, however, that the accumulation of bone mass that occurs during the growth period in subadults plays an important role in determining achieved peak bone mass, and in turn the risk of osteopenia, bone fragility, and osteoporosis in later life. Whereas considerable attention has been paid to age-associated bone loss in older adults, few studies have addressed bone mass during the first two decades of life (Gilsanz *et al.*, 1988). In addition, while loss of cancellous bone with age is particularly well documented, histomorphometric data on the loss of cortical bone with age is less well studied (Compston, 1999). This is particularly significant, since the process of bone loss is not homogeneous and trabecular bone and cortical bone are independently "modulated" (Burckhardt and Cichel, 1989).

This chapter will present the results of a study of age-associated changes in the histomorphometry of a modern sample of subadult ribs. It examines the pattern of change in cross-sectional area, as well as several static histomorphometric indicators of bone remodeling.

1.1. Intracortical Bone Remodeling in the Subadult Rib

The cortical bone morphology of the subadult rib reflects the processes of growth, modeling, and remodeling. During growth, the rib cage expands to adult proportions.

Margaret Streeter • Department of Anthropology, University of Missouri.

Sam D. Stout • Department of Anthropology, The Ohio State University.

Bone Loss and Osteoporosis: An Anthropological Perspective, edited by Sabrina C. Agarwal and Sam D. Stout. Kluwer Academic/Plenum Publishers, New York, 2003.

In ribs of the very young bone remodeling plays a minor role, while growth and modeling work together to determine their shape. This is achieved by periosteal apposition and modeling drifts that coordinate resorption and formation to expand and move the cortex away from the pleural cavity out toward the cutaneous surface. Unlike remodeling, where resorption and formation occur in a tethered sequence, these processes are independent in bone modeling (for a more detailed discussion of the processes of bone remodeling and modeling see also Chapters 1 and 2, this volume). Because of the relatively rapid and extensive turnover and replacement of cortical bone that occurs with growth and modeling, the age-related pattern of intracortical histomorphology of subadult bones is complex.

Histomorphometric methods that have been developed to estimate age at death (Robling and Stout, 2000) and bone remodeling rates (Stout and Lueck, 1995) are not applicable to subadult bones because of the very young mean tissue ages resulting from the extensive growth and modeling drifts. These methods are based upon the relatively gradual and continued accumulation of the basic structural units of bone remodeling (osteons) that occurs in adult cortical bone. The age from which osteons observed in an adult bone have accumulated depends upon the effective age of birth for the adult compacta, rather than physical birth. For the midshaft of the rib, the effective age of birth for adult compacta has been estimated to be approximately 12.5 years (Wu *et al.*, 1970). Epker *et al.* (1965) report that the number of Haversian canals per mm^2 is initially relatively high ($13/mm^2$) for children in the first decade of life. During the next decade, the number of these structures decreases to an average of $7/mm^2$. The number of haversian canals then increases gradually for the remaining decades of life.

Studies to date have included relatively small samples of subadults (≤ 20) and have lumped cases by broad age groups (decades) that tends to obscure changes and patterns that occur in relation to developmental stages of growth or other patterns that are not revealed by using arbitrary 10 year age groups. Germane to this issue are the results of a longitudinal study of the density and volume of bone in the axial and the appendicular skeletons of 40 healthy children using computed tomography (Loro *et al.*, 2000). Bone density and volume measurements exhibited distinct patterns relative to the Tanner stages of sexual development. In order to establish age-associated changes and variability of intracortical histomorphometry in the immature skeleton, and how they relate to major stages of growth and development, further research is needed that focuses upon subadult samples.

1.2. Peak Bone Mass and Age-Associated Bone Loss

There are several important studies that have examined how cross-sectional area measurements of the rib change with age (Sedlin and Frost, 1963; Sedlin, 1964; Epker *et al.*, 1965). In their study of variations in cortical cross-section area of ribs, Sedlin *et al.* (1963) report that the mean cross-sectional area for the cortex of ribs increases from infancy until skeletal maturity, after which it begins to decline with advancing age. In a subsequent study, it was established that both the total area and area occupied by the marrow cavity also increase from birth to adulthood, but the relative amount of the total cross-sectional area of a rib that is composed of cortical bone declines steadily after infancy (Sedlin, 1964). This proportional loss of cortical bone results from a greater rate of expansion of the marrow cavity relative to periosteal expansion.

Peak bone mass is a major factor determining the risk of bone fragility in later life (Rubin *et al.*, 1999). It is generally reported that peak bone mass is achieved sometime during the fourth and fifth decades of life (Kleerekoper and Avioli, 1998), although recent studies report that it occurs earlier during the second decade of life (Audran, 1992; Kanis, 1994; Teegarden *et al.*, 1995). The amount of bone that is gained during adolescence is a major contributor to peak bone mass (Loro *et al.*, 2000), and much of the increase in bone density in subadults results from an increase in cortical area (Burckhardt and Cichel, 1989). The higher the peak bone density, the less likely an individual is to eventually develop osteoporosis. Therefore, the amount of bone accrued during postnatal and pubertal growth is an important determining factor in the development of osteoporosis (Richman *et al.*, 2001). A clear understanding of the normal patterns and variations in the gain and loss of bone in subadults, therefore, is important to our understanding of the mechanisms leading to adult age-associated bone loss and conditions of osteopenia.

1.3. Factors Determining Peak Bone Mass

There are many factors that determine peak bone mass. Genetics may play a role in determining an individual's potential peak bone mass (Heaney and Matkovic, 1995; Deng *et al.*, 1999). Studies have shown that 60–70% of variance in peak bone density is determined genetically (Richman *et al.*, 2001). The heritability of bone mass extends to prepubertal children, is gender- and site-specific, and under different genetic control than growth (Jones and Nguyen, 2000). Seeman (1999) notes, however, that these estimates are based upon heritability studies that reflect the proportional contributions of genetics and environment to the phenotype and, therefore, do not measure absolute "genetic variation."

As might be expected, given the heritability of bone mass, race has been reported to be a major factor determining peak bone mass (Key and Bell, 1999). (See also Chapter 4, this volume, and its critique of the use of "race" and "ethnicity" in the biomedical literature.)

Nutrition, especially during growth and development, is an important variable determining achieved peak bone mass (Lloyd and Cusatis, 1999; New *et al.*, 2000). In addition to calcium intake, other possible dietary factors include protein, caffeine, phosphorous, and other minerals (Slemenda and Johnson, 1990). (For a discussion of the importance and evolution of vitamin D nutrition and bone see also Chapter 9, this volume.)

Hormones are important in the development, maintenance, and loss of bone mass. Their role is particularly significant for the development of bone mass in both the growing and aged skeleton (RussellAulet *et al.*, 1998; Warren, 1999; Bouillon and Prodonova, 2000). Hormones may also be responsible for the existence of gender differences in bone mass and risk of osteoporosis (LeBoff and Glowacki, 1999; Sowers, 2000). (See also Chapter 5, this volume.)

Biomechanics, especially physical activity, is increasingly viewed as an important determinant of peak bone mass (van der Meulen and Carter, 1999). In a study designed to investigate whether ethnicity, anthropometrics, and lifestyle are important factors in intraskeletal differences in bone mass of young adult women, Davis *et al.* (1999) report that geographical–regional differences in bone mass can be at least partially explained by differences in anthropometrics and lifestyle during skeletal maturation. More specifically, a longitudinal study of bone mass and level of physical activity during adolescence and the young adult period found a significant positive correlation between degree of physical fitness and the bone mineral density (BMD) observed at the end of skeletal growth in both males and females (Kemper *et al.*, 2000). In this study, neuromotor fitness, but not cardiopulmonary fitness, was found to be related to adult BMD, and no significant correlations were found for the wrist, a bone site that is less involved in physical activity and fitness. Similarly, Lloyd *et al.* (2000) report that adult females who exercised on a regular basis as teenagers, exhibit greater peak hipbone mass compared to their sedentary peers. This study also did not find a significant correlation between adult bone mass and teenage calcium intake. Frost and Schönau (2000) point out the potential value of load bearing exercise in children and adolescents for bone strength, and to minimize osteopenia and bone fragility in adult life. (For a discussion of biomechanics and age-related bone loss see Chapter 2, this volume.)

2. A Study of Subadult Rib Histomorphometry

The following presents the results of a study of age-associated changes in the histomorphometry of subadult ribs. All ribs were taken at autopsy from individuals that died of traumatic deaths and judged to be metabolically normal. Bone samples were taken from the middle third of the 5th, 6th, or 7th rib. The sample consists of 48 males and 19 females ranging in age from 2 to 20 years with a mean age of 15.2 ± 0.58 years. Mean ages for males and females are not significantly different and exhibit similar distributions (Figure 6.1). Table 6.1 summarizes the results of this analysis.

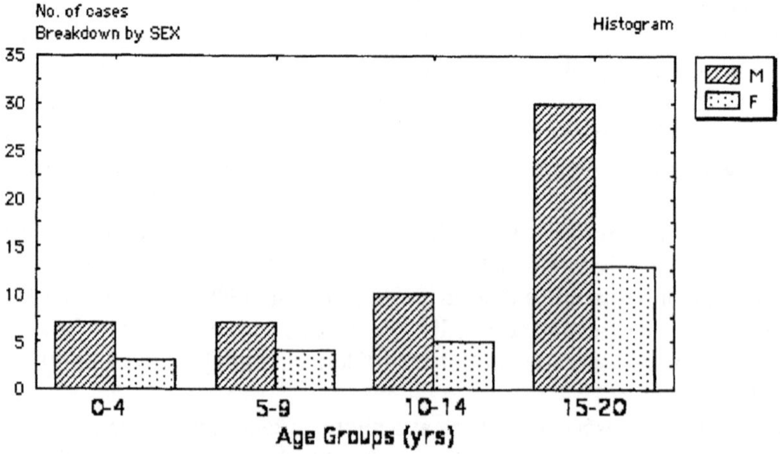

Figure 6.1. Age distribution for the subadult rib sample.

Table 6.1. Descriptive Statistics by Sex

	Male ($N = 48$)	Female ($N = 19$)	Combined ($N = 67$)
Age (yrs):	15.3 ± 0.67	14.9 ± 1.21	15.2 ± 0.58
%CA:	44.2 ± 1.66	48.3 ± 2.83	45.4 ± 1.44
TA (mm^2)*:	61.8 ± 3.13	48.1 ± 4.47	57.9 ± 2.69
MA (mm^2)*:	36.1 ± 2.51	25.5 ± 2.36	33.1 ± 2.07
CA (mm^2):	25.7 ± 1.12	22.5 ± 2.36	24.8 ± 1.05
OPD (#/mm^2):	9.3 ± 0.74 ($N = 41$)	7.7 ± 1.20 ($N = 13$)	8.8 ± 0.65 ($N = 54$)
ONAr (mm^2):	0.039 ± 0.0018 ($N = 39$)	0.38 ± 0.0031 ($N = 12$)	0.038 ± 0.0016 ($N = 51$)

*Males and females significantly different ($p < 0.05$).

2.1. Cross-Sectional Areas and Bone Mass

Similar to the findings of earlier studies (Sedlin, 1964; Takahashi and Frost, 1965) and consistent with what we know about skeletal growth, ribs exhibit continuous growth until the age of approximately 20 years, after which there is little change in their absolute size (Figure 2a). While total cross-sectional area, which is the area of bone contained within the periosteal border of a rib, for males is significantly greater than for females ($p < 0.05$), a significant sex difference exists only when ages over 15 years are considered. These findings are consistent with those of Takahashi and Frost (1965) who reported no sex-related difference in the total cross-sectional area of ribs of children under the age of 15 years. Whereas the total cross-sectional area of female ribs peaks by the middle of the second decade of life, male ribs continue to grow into the third decade (Figures 6.2b, 6.2c). The greater average size (total cross-sectional area) of male ribs, therefore, appears to be the result of their longer duration of appositional growth.

Both the mean area of the marrow cavity (MA) and cortical area (CA) are greater in males than females (Table 1), but the difference is significant only for MA ($p < 0.05$). Similar to total area, the area of the marrow cavity determined for the combined sexes asymptotes during the early third decade of life (Figures 6.2a), and when the sexes are considered separately, expansion of the marrow cavity of females asymptotes earlier, during the later half of the second decade, and the MA even begins to decrease (Figures 6.2b, 6.2c). These findings are consistent with existence of endosteal expansion related to puberty in females discussed by Martin in this volume. CA also increases in subadults, but its increase is less dramatic than for that of either total subperiosteal or MA and appears to asymptote at about the same age in both sexes (Figures 6.2a–6.2c).

When CA is divided by total subperiosteal area (%CA), it is found that this normalized measure of CA decreases steadily from infancy on (Figure 2a). This is consistent with the findings of others (Sedlin, 1964). Contrary to findings for adults, and even though they have smaller absolute measures of cortical bone (i.e., TA and CA), subadult females exhibit greater, but not statistically significant ($p = 0.207$), relative CA than males (Table 1 and Figures 6.2b, 6.2c). The sex difference in the relative amount of cortical bone (%CA) is most notable after adolescence (≥ 15 years). This difference appears to be due to an

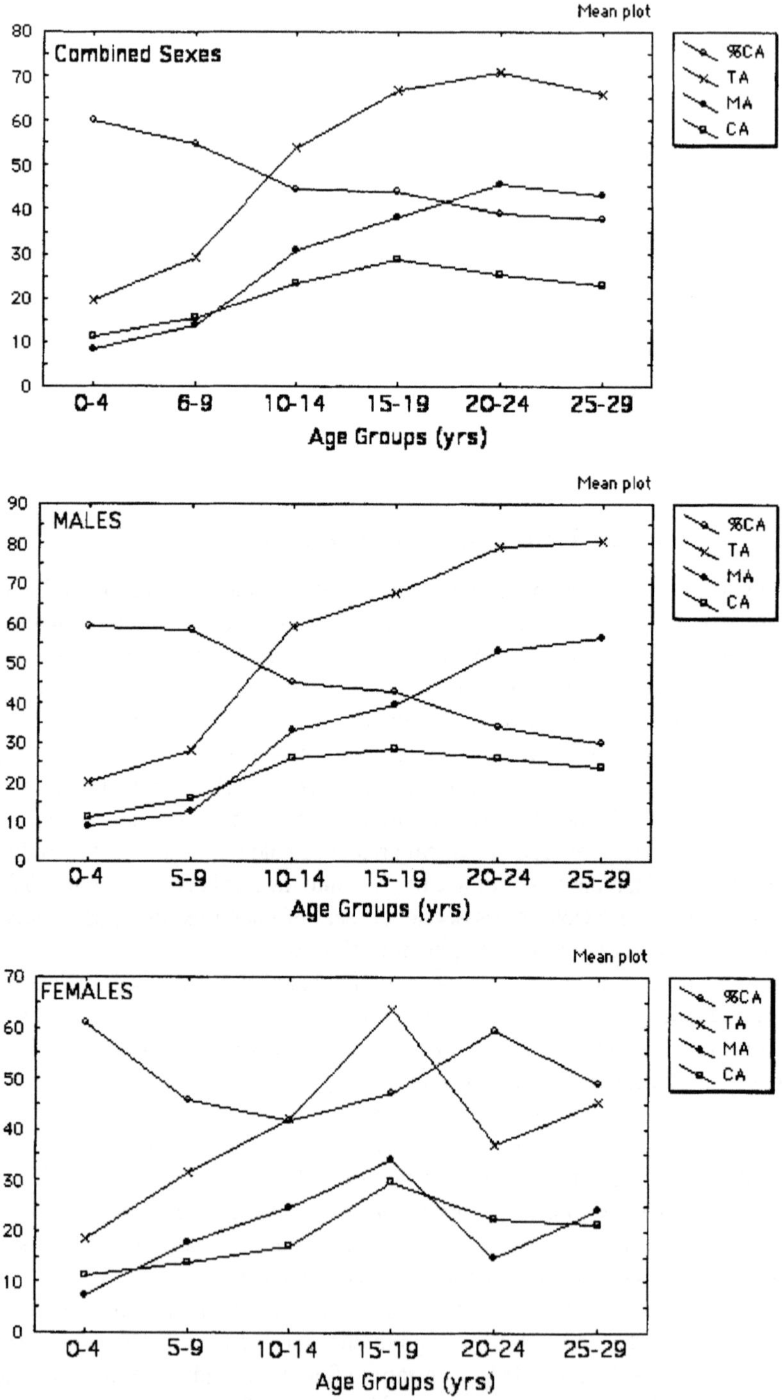

Figure 6.2. (a) Mean plot for subadult total subperiosteal cross-sectional area (TA), cortical area (CA), area of marrow, and relative cortical area (%CA). Means for the adult age categories 20–24 and 25–29 are added to include the young adult age range over which peak bone mass is reported to occur. (b) Same as (a), but for males only. (c) Same as (a), but for females only.

earlier peak and less dramatic expansion of the marrow cavity in females than males. These sex differences in %CA also parallel the patterns for the relationship between whole body bone mineral content and lean body mass described by Martin in this volume.

2.2. Intracortical Remodeling: Osteon Population Density and Osteon Size

Since bone remodeling occurs continuously from birth to death and osteons are produced by bone remodeling, the number of osteons in a cross-section of bone increases with age. The pattern of age-associated changes in the numbers of osteons for several elements of the adult skeleton, such as the femur, tibia, rib, and clavicle, are well established. This relationship between age and numbers of osteons is the basis for most of the histological methods that are used to estimate age commonly employed in bioarchaeology and forensic anthropology. The applicability of these methods to subadult skeletal remains, however, is yet to be demonstrated. (For a review of histological age estimation methods the reader should consult Robling and Stout [2000].) Age-associated change in the number of osteons in cross-sections of subadult bones is poorly understood.

The results of this study confirm that the number of osteons increases with age, but that the increase in osteon population density (OPD) is apparent only for ages above approximately 14 years (Figure 6.3a). The apparent stasis or even decrease in OPD probably results from the combined effects of increase in size and the rapid bone turnover due to growth and modeling during the first one and a half decades of life. The resulting relatively young mean tissue ages suggests that osteon-based age estimation methods may not be practical for ages younger than about 15 years. It is interesting that these findings are consistent with the estimated age for the birth of adult compacta of 12.5 years for the rib (Wu *et al.*, 1970).

Similar to reports for adult ribs (Stout and Paine, 1992), there is no difference in OPD between male and female subadults. While OPD tended to be higher in males than females (Table 6.1), the difference is not statistically significant ($p > 0.2$). This lack of difference between the sexes holds when comparisons are made between specific age groups as well. When the numbers of intact and fragmentary osteons per square millimeter are considered separately, it is revealed that the number of fragmentary osteons makes a relatively small contribution to OPD and begins to increase significantly only after the age of approximately 14 years (Figure 6.3b).

The average amount of bone contained within the cement lines of osteons (ONAr), which is a measure of the amount of bone formed by each remodeling unit (BMU) does not change with age ($p > 0.5$), and there is not a significant difference in osteon size between the sexes ($p > 0.4$).

3. Summary and Conclusions

Results for OPD indicate that this observable indicator of cortical bone remodeling does not exhibit the relatively simple linear pattern of increase in OPD with age observed in the adult rib. The combined effects of bone growth and modeling create a pattern of relatively low and unchanging OPDs in subadults below about 15 years of age even though bone remodeling rates are significantly higher during this age period (Frost, 1969). As a

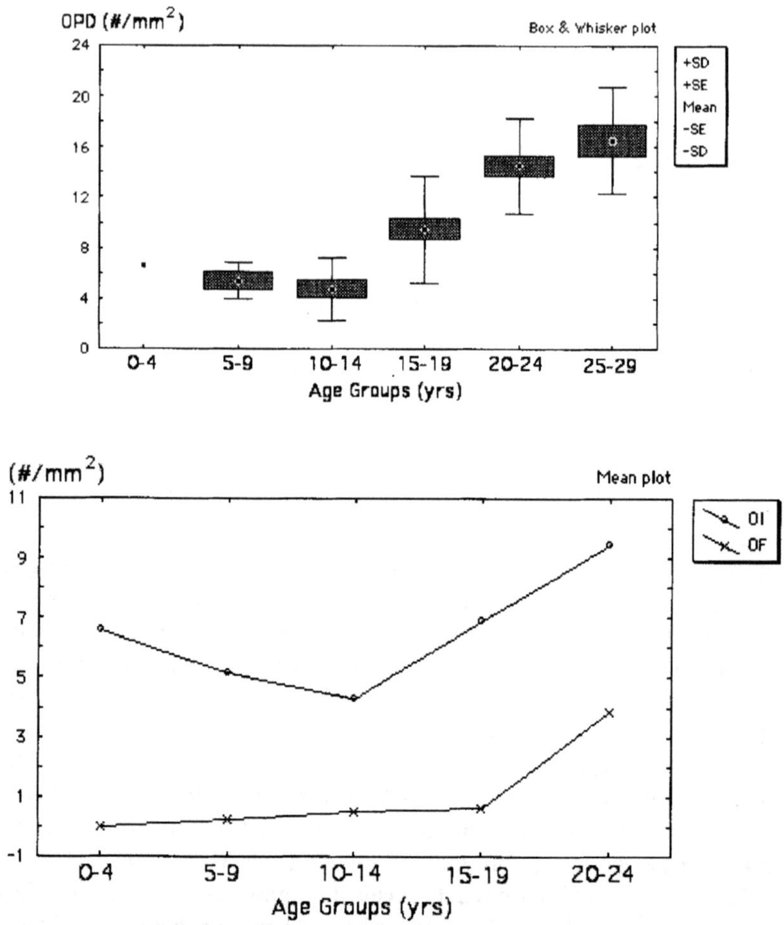

Figure 6.3. (a) Box and whisker plot for osteon population density (OPD) in subadults. The adult age categories 20–24 and 25–29 are included to better illustrate the transition from subadult to adult rates of change. (b) Mean plot of intact osteons (OI) and fragmentary osteons (OF) illustrating their relative contributions to OPD.

result, mean tissue age is significantly lower than chronological age during most of the subadult years.

This study builds upon earlier histomorphological studies of age-associated changes in bone mass (Sedlin *et al.*, 1963; Epker *et al.*, 1965; Takahashi and Frost, 1966) and remodeling (Pirok *et al.*, 1966; Frost, 1969). It expands our understanding of the patterns of histomorphological changes in the subadult rib and how these relate to the development of peak bone mass. Although these results pertain specifically to the rib, it is noteworthy that these histomorphological results for the rib are similar to those reported for the mid-shaft of the 5th metacarpal by Garn (1972) using radiography. Both periosteal (TA) and endosteal expansion (MA) are relatively slow during childhood, accelerate during adolescence, and plateau with adulthood (Figures 6.2a–6.2c).

The amount of bone mass an individual possesses when they enter adult life is an important factor determining their risk of osteopenia, bone fragility, and osteoporosis in

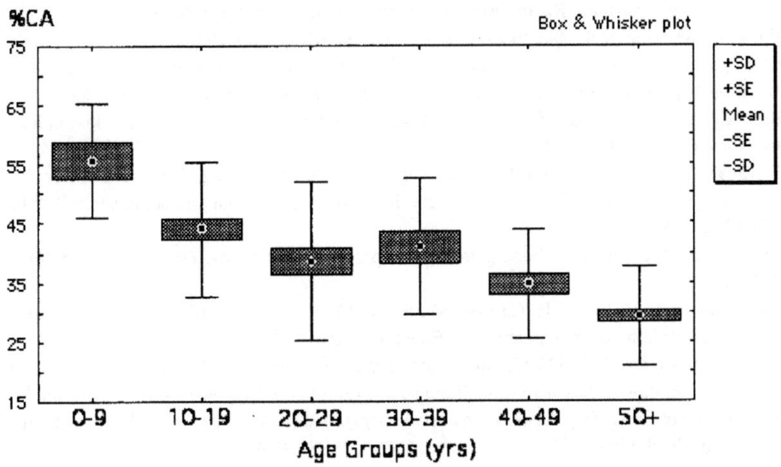

Figure 6.4. Box and whisker plot of the means for relative cortical area (%CA) for a combined sample of subadult and adult ribs.

later life. Although absolute measures of bone mass, such as total subperiosteal area and CA increase in subadults, this increase reflects changes rib size. When CA is normalized to size (%CA), it is observed that the relative amount of cortical bone contained in the cross-section of a rib actually decreases from its maximum in early childhood to a smaller value that will be carried into adulthood (Figure 6.4).

Factors that affect the relative amounts and rates of periosteal apposition and expansion of the marrow cavity in the subadult rib determine the peak bone mass that exists at the end of bone growth and modeling. Figure 6.4 illustrates the range of variation in the relative amount of cortical bone (%CA) that occurs for ribs at various ages. Factors that account for this variation affect adult peak bone mass and need to be identified and analyzed. The results of this study also suggest that the higher degree of osteopenia and susceptibility of older adult females to osteoporosis may not necessarily be due to their achieving a smaller peak bone mass as subadults. Significant factors that are responsible for observed differences in adult bone mass between males and females must exert their influence on the adult skeleton. It is hoped that this chapter will stimulate greater interest and further research in age-associated changes in bone mass in the subadult skeleton. Given reported population differences in the risk of osteoporosis, further research that includes samples derived from populations that differ geographically, culturally, and temporally is needed.

References

Audran, M.J. (1992). Epidemiology, etiology, and diagnosis of osteoporosis. *Curr. Opin. Rheumat.* **4**, 394–401.

Bouillon, R., and Prodonova, A. (2000). Growth hormone deficiency and peak bone mass. *JPEM* **13**(6), 1327–1336.

Burckhardt, P., and Cichel, C. (1989). The peak bone mass concept. *Clin. Rheumatol.* **8**, 16–21.

Compston, J. (1999). Histomorphometric manifestations of age-related bone loss. In C.J. Rosen, J. Glowacki and J.P. Bilezikian (eds.) *The Aging Skeleton* Academic Press, NY, pp. 251–261.

Davis, J., Novotny, R., Wasnich, R., and Ross, P. (1999). Ethnic, anthropometric, and lifestyle associations with regional variations in peak bone mass. *Calcif. Tissue Int.* **65**(2), 100–105.

Deng, H., Stegman, M., Davies, K., Conway, T., and Recker, R. (1999). Genetic determination of variation and covariation of peak bone mass at the hip and spine. *J. Clin. Densitometry* **2**(3), 251–263.

Epker, B.N., Kelin, M., and Frost, H.M. (1965). Magnitude and location of cortical bone loss in human rib with aging. *Clin. Orthop.* **41**, 198–203.

Frost, H. (1969). Tetracycline based histological analysis of bone remodeling. *Calcif. Tissue Res.* **3**, 211–237.

Frost, H.M., and Schönau, E. (2000). The "Muscle-Bone Unit" in children and adolescents: A 2000 overview. *JPEM* **13**, 571–590.

Garn, S.M. (1972). The course of bone gain and the phases of bone loss. *Orthop. Clin. of North Am.* **3**(3), 503–519.

Gilsanz, V., Gibbens, D.T., Roe, T.F., Carlson, M., Senac, M.O., Boechat, M.I., Huang, H., Schultz, E.E. *et al.* (1988). Vertebral bone density in children: Effect of parity. *Radiology* **166**, 847–850.

Heaney, R.P., and Matkovic, V. (1995). Inadequate peak bone mass. In B.L. Riggs and L.J. Melton (eds.) *Osteoporosis: Etiology, Diagnosis, and Management* (2nd edn.). Lippincott-Raven, Philadelphia.

Jones, G., and Nguyen, T. (2000). Associations between maternal peak bone mass and bone mass in prepubertal male and female children. *J. Bone Miner. Res.* **15**(10), 1998–2004.

Kanis, J.A. (1994). *Osteoporosis*. Blackwell Science, Oxford.

Kemper, H., Twisk, J., van Mechelen, W., Post, G., Roos, J., and Lips, P. (2000). A fifteen-year longitudinal study in young adults on the relation of physical activity and fitness with the development of the bone mass: The Amsterdam growth and health longitudinal study. *Bone* **27**(6), 847–853.

Key, L.L., and Bell, N.H. (1999). Racial determinants of peak bone mass. In C.J. Rosen, J. Glowacki and J.P. Bilezikian (eds.) *The Aging Skeleton* Academic Press, NY, pp. 127–141.

Kleerekoper, M., and Avioli, L.V. (1998). Osteoporosis pathogenesis and therapy. In L.V. Avioli and S.M. Krane (eds.) *Metabolic Bone Disease and Clinicallly Related Disorders* (3rd edn.) academic Press, NY, pp. 387–409.

LeBoff, M.S., and Glowacki, J. (1999). Sex steroids, bone, and aging. In C.J. Rosen, J. Glowacki and J.P. Bilezikian (eds.) *The Aging Skeleton* Academic Press, NY, pp. 159–174.

Lloyd, T., and Cusatis, D.C. (1999). Nutritional determinants of peak bone mass. In C.J. Rosen, J. Glowacki and J.P. Bilezikian (eds.), *The Aging Skeleton* Academic Press, NY, pp. 95–114.

Lloyd, T., Taylor, D., Lin, H., Matthews, A., Eggli, D., and Legro, R. (2000). Oral contraceptive use by teenage women does not affect peak bone mass: A longitudinal study. *Fertil. Steril.* **74**(4), 734–738.

Loro, M., Sayre, J., Roe, T., Goran, M., Kaufman, F., and Gilsanz, V. (2000). Early identification of children predisposed to low peak bone mass and osteoporosis later in life. *J. Clin. Endocrinol. Metab.* **85**(10), 3908–3918.

New, S.A., Pearson, C.E., Gowing, A.M., and Keay, N.J. (2000). Influence of dietary intake on peak bone mass attainment in elite female ballet dancers and healthy age-matched controls: Baseline results from a three-year longitudinal study. *Proc. Nutr. Soc.* **59**, A26.

Pirok, D.J., Ramser, J.R., Takahashi, H., Villanueva, A.R., and Frost, M.D. (1966). Normal histological, tetracycline and dynamic parameters in human, mineralized bone sections. *Henry Ford Hosp. Med. Bull.* **14**, 195–218.

Richman, C., Kutilek, S., Miyakoshi, N., Srivastava, A.K., Beamer, W.G., Donahue, L.R., Rosen, C.J., Wergedal, J.E. *et al.* (2001). Postnatal and pubertal skeletal changes contribute predominantly to the differences in peak bone density between C3H/HeJ and C57BL/6J mice. *J. Bone Miner. Res.* **16**(2), 386–397.

Robling, A.R., and Stout, S.D. (2000). Methods of determining age at death using bone microstructure. In M.A. Katzenberg and S.R. Saunders (eds.) *Biological Anthropology of the Human Skeleton* Wiley-Liss, NY, pp. 187–205.

Rubin, L., Hawker, G., Peltekova, V., Fielding, L., Ridout, R., and Cole, D. (1999). Determinants of peak bone mass: Clinical and genetic analyses in a young female Canadian cohort. *J. Bone Miner. Res.* **14**(4), 633–643.

RussellAulet, M., Shapiro, B., Jaffe, C.A., Gross, M.D., and Markan, A.L. (1998). Peak bone mass in young healthy men is correlated with the magnitude of endogenous growth hormone secretion. *J. Clin. Endocrinol. Metab.* **83**(10), 3463–3468.

Sedlin, E.D., and Frost, H.M. (1963). Variations in rate of human osteon formation. *Can. J. Biochem. Physiol.* **41**, 19–22.

Sedlin, E.D., Frost, H.M., and Villanueva, B.S. (1963). Variations in cross-section area of rib cortex with age. *J. Gerontol.* **18**(1), 9–13.

Sedlin, N.A. (1964). The ratio of cortical area to total cross-section area in rib diaphysis: A quantitative index of osteoporosis. *Clin. Orthop.* **36**, 161–168.

Seeman, E. (1999). Genetic determinants of the population variance in bone mineral density. In C.J. Rosen, J. Glowacki and J.P. Bilezikian (eds.) *The Aging Skeleton* Academic Press, NY, pp. 77–94.

Slemenda, C.W., and Johnson, C.C. (1990). Osteoporotic fractures. In D.J. Simmons (ed.) *Nutrition and Bone Development* Oxford University Press, NY, pp. 131–147.

Sowers, M. (2000). Lower peak bone mass and its decline. *Best Practice and Research Clin. Endocrinol. Metab.* **14**(2), 317–329.

Stout, S., and Lueck, R. (1995). Bone remodeling rates and skeletal maturation in three archaeological skeletal populations. *Am. J. Phys. Anthropol.* **98**, 161–171.

Stout, S.D., and Paine, R.R. (1992). Histological age estimation using rib and clavicle. *Am. J. Phys. Anthropol.* **87**, 111–115.

Takahashi, H., and Frost, H.M. (1965). Correlation between body habitus and cross-sectional area of ribs. *J. Physiol. Pharmacol.* **43**, 773–781.

Takahashi, H., and Frost, H.M. (1966). Age and sex related changes in the amount of cortex in normal human ribs. *Acta Orthop. Scand.* **37**, 122–130.

Teegarden, D., Proulx, W.R., Martin, B.R., Zhao, J. McCabe, G.P., Lyle, R.M., Peacock, M., Slemenda, C. *et al.* (1995). Peak bone mass in young women. *J. Bone Miner. Res.* **10**, 711–715.

van der Meulen, M.C.H., and Carter, D. (1999). Mechanical determinants of peak bone mass. In C.J. Rosen, J. Glowacki and J.P. Bilezikian (eds.) *The Aging Skeleton* Academic Press, NY, pp. 105–125.

Warren, M.P. (1999). Hormonal influences on the establishment of peak bone mass. In C.J. Rosen, J. Glowacki and J.P. Bilezikian (eds.) *The Aging Skeleton* Academic Press, NY, pp. 115–125.

Wu, K., Schubeck, K., Frost, H., and Villanueva, A. (1970). Haversian bone formation rates determined by a new method in a mastadon and in human diabetes mellitus and osteoporosis. *Calcif. Tissue Res.* **6**, 204–219.

Part III

Evolutionary Perspectives

7

An Evolutionary and Biocultural Approach to Understanding the Effects of Reproductive Factors on the Female Skeleton

Sabrina C. Agarwal and Patricia Stuart-Macadam

1. Introduction

Osteoporosis is a systemic skeletal disease characterized by a reduction in bone mass and a deterioration of the microstructure of bone tissue, with a consequent increase in bone fragility and susceptibility to fracture. The precise mechanisms and etiology of the disease are incompletely understood. Age-related bone loss is found in both sexes, but is accelerated in females with the onset of menopause. Bone loss in postmenopausal years averages anywhere between 1–5% per year, increasing the risk of a 50-year old white woman sustaining a fracture at any skeletal site to 30–40% (Melton, 1995). Further, secular trends in Europe and North America indicate that the incidence of fragility fracture has doubled over the last three decades, creating a serious social and financial burden (Melton, 1995).

However, a woman's risk of developing osteoporosis is greatly mediated by factors that are independent of the menopause-induced drop in estrogen levels, such as genetics, nutrition, and physical activity. Pregnancy and lactation can also play potentially important roles in female bone maintenance. Substantial transfer of calcium from the mother to the fetus or infant occurs during pregnancy and lactation. Mineralization of the fetal skeleton has been estimated to require approximately 30 g of calcium from maternal sources (Nguyen *et al.*, 1995; Kojima *et al.*, 2002). This fetal or infant need for calcium can be met through three possible compensatory maternal mechanisms: increased intestinal absorption of calcium, renal calcium conservation, or from the maternal skeleton (Kent *et al.*, 1990; Sowers, 1996). It is unclear under what circumstances and to what extent the maternal skeleton may be compromised to fulfill this requirement. Further, both

---

Sabrina C. Agarwal • Department of Anthropology, University of Toronto.

Patricia Stuart-Macadam • Aurora Homepathics, Adelaide, Australia.

Bone Loss and Osteoporosis: An Anthropological Perspective, edited by Sabrina C. Agarwal and Sam D. Stout. Kluwer Academic/Plenum Publishers, New York, 2003.

lactation and lactation-related amenorrhea have been suggested to contribute to maternal bone loss. However, studies that have investigated bone mass during pregnancy and postpartum have been inconsistent, often reporting no change in bone mineral density (BMD), site-specific bone loss, or a combination of loss and gain. Studies of parity have been equally unclear.

Here we review the studies examining the association between parity and bone loss and the effects of pregnancy and lactation on the maternal skeleton. These studies have implemented various types of study design, methods, and sample sizes and have examined different bone sites. We provide insight into the role of reproductive factors in bone maintenance that has been obtained with the use of animal models. Finally, we examine the data on the effects of pregnancy and lactation on the maternal skeleton from an evolutionary perspective, and look at the possible role of pregnancy and lactation on bone fragility in historical populations.

2. Pregnancy

Studies of bone turnover have clearly indicated pregnancy to be a biologically active period (Martinez *et al.*, 1985; Cole *et al.*, 1987; Rodin *et al.*, 1989; Seki *et al.*, 1991; Cross *et al.*, 1995; Black *et al.*, 2000; Naylor *et al.*, 2000). Pregnancy was initially regarded as a state of secondary hyperparathyroidism, however several studies have reported no elevation in Parathyroid harmone (PTH) levels during pregnancy (Cross *et al.*, 1995; Sowers, 1996; Naylor *et al.*, 2000). Improved calcium absorption during pregnancy is thought to be related to increased levels of total 1,25-dihydroxyvitamin D, however, several other possible pathways for increased calcium absorption, such as estrogen and prolactin, have also been suggested (Cross *et al.*, 1995; Sowers, 1996). Recently insulin-like growth factor I (IGF-I) has been suggested to be partly responsible for the elevation in bone turnover during pregnancy (Naylor *et al.*, 2000).

Despite the still unknown mechanism controlling bone turnover during pregnancy, the majority of studies generally agree that early pregnancy shows increased bone resorption, followed by bone formation in the late third trimester of pregnancy (Black *et al.*, 2000). Observed changes in bone density during pregnancy tend to support these biochemical findings. While a few case studies of pregnancy-associated osteoporosis have been reported (Yamamoto *et al.*, 1994; Phillips *et al.*, 2000), osteoporotic fracture in pregnancy is rare. A number of longitudinal and cross-sectional studies have attempted to examine in greater detail the change in BMD during pregnancy. An early study by Lamke *et al.* (1977) reported trabecular bone loss in the forearm of pregnant women. A longitudinal study of BMD in six pregnant women also found decreased bone density in the radial shaft as well as the femoral neck, although no change in density was found in the weight-bearing tibial site (Drinkwater and Chesnut, 1991). Further longitudinal studies have shown similar losses of BMD to occur at several skeletal sites. For example, in a large 2-year prospective study of 59 pregnant women, Kolthoff *et al.* (1998) found BMD to vary depending on skeletal site with the most pronounced loss in the spine (5.2% in 3 months after delivery). A more recent study by More *et al.* (2001) reported similar results, finding a significant difference between baseline and delivery BMD in both the spine and the radius. Black *et al.* (2000) further substantiated the observation of early pregnancy losses in bone density with corresponding changes in biochemical markers of bone turnover.

Turnover was found to be uncoupled during the first two trimesters with increased bone resorption followed by an increase in bone formation in the third trimester. While longitudinal studies have traditionally relied upon non-invasive methods such as X-ray or absorptiometry to assess BMD during pregnancy, several recent studies have also examined the effects of pregnancy on aspects that relate more directly to bone quality. For example, two recent longitudinal studies using ultrasound found both speed of sound (SOS) and broadband ultrasound attenuation (BUA) (indicators related to bone density) to be significantly lower by the third trimester (Gambacciani *et al.*, 1995; Yamaga *et al.*, 1996). A unique cross-sectional study by Shahtaheri *et al.* (1999b) of trabecular microarchitecture in the iliac crest during early and late pregnancy found standard bone structural variables, such as bone volume and trabecular thickness, to decrease significantly during early pregnancy. However, Shahtaheri *et al.* (1999b) also note that bone structure was restored in late pregnancy primarily due to an increase in the trabecular number.

Cross-sectional studies of BMD have reported similar findings. For example in a comparison of 73 postpartum women with 55 age-matched controls, Karlsson *et al.* (2001) found lumbar spine BMD and total body BMD to be significantly lower in the postpartum group. However, the researchers did not find any difference in BMD between women with multiple pregnancies (range 4–7) as compared to women with fewer pregnancies (range 0–2). This finding highlights the question of whether pregnancy associated decreases in BMD translates into pregnancy as a risk factor for later bone fragility. Black *et al.* (2000) suggest that while the early loss of BMD during pregnancy may be problematic in cases where pregnancy ends in miscarriage in the early trimester, in pregnant women requiring drug steroid therapy, or in women with preexisting bone loss, is it unlikely to have any long-term consequences. Increased bone loss and risk may also exist in the case of still-growing young adolescent mothers (Sowers *et al.*, 2000). However, the overwhelming majority of studies have demonstrated that while decreases in BMD do occur during pregnancy, these losses are usually spontaneously compensated for during lactation and with the return of menses (Lamke *et al.*, 1977; Drinkwater and Chesnut, 1991; Kolthoff *et al.*, 1998; Holmberg-Marttila *et al.*, 1999; Black *et al.*, 2000; Karlsson *et al.*, 2001; More *et al.*, 2001). Similarly, the study by Shahtaheri *et al.* (1999b) suggests that the compensation and restoration of bone in late pregnancy may occur at the microstructural level. These indications of compensation may further explain the lack of apparent long-term bone loss in the epidemiological studies of parity.

3. Parity

While there have been a number of epidemiological and retrospective studies on parity, these studies have not provided an entirely clear picture of the relationship with bone mass and fragility. Several studies have shown no association between BMD and parity. For example, Melton *et al.* (1993) found no association with BMD and parity even after adjusting for age and examining several skeletal sites. Hreshchyshyn *et al.* (1988) found no significant difference in lumbar BMD between nulliparous and multiparous women, but did find a decrease in femoral BMD with increasing parity. Similarly, cross-sectional studies by Hu *et al.* (1994) and Kojima *et al.* (2002) found no association between parity and BMD in both pre- and post-menopausal women. In contrast, in studies of early postmenopausal women Grainge *et al.* (2001) and Murphy *et al.* (1994) have both reported an increase in BMD at the femoral neck and total radius with increasing parity. Fox *et al.* (1993) specifically found a 1.4% increase in the distal radius BMD with each additional birth in a large study of postmenopausal women. Sowers *et al.* (1992) found nulliparity to be associated with lower levels of BMD, and Forsmo *et al.* (2001) have reported nulliparous women to have lower BMD as compared to parous women, although they found no linear relationship between parity and BMD. The effect of multiparity on bone mass has also been investigated. A study by Bererhi *et al.* (1996) of Omani women found no significant association between number of children and BMD in the lumbar spine despite the fact that Omani mothers had a large number of child births (0–14 childbirths with mean surviving children of 5.1) and practiced extended lactation. Henderson *et al.* (2000) recently conducted a similar but more detailed study. The authors examined BMD of the spine, femoral neck, and radius in a small sample of grand multiparous Finish American women (each with at least 6 children), and found no significant difference between the multiparous and nulliparous women in the population. These studies are interesting as they suggest that BMD is unaffected by repeated and closely spaced pregnancies with extended lactation.

Increased estrogen levels during pregnancy and subsequent renal and intestinal absorption of calcium may also explain the positive effect of parity on BMD (Fox *et al.*, 1993; Kojima *et al.*, 2002). Grainge *et al.* (2001) suggest that reduced levels of PTH during pregnancy may also explain the association between BMD and parity. However, retrospective studies on parity are often limited by recall bias whereby women are asked to recall past reproductive events (Fox *et al.*, 1993; Grainge *et al.*, 2001). Also, while researchers studying parity have generally used absorptiometry to measure BMD, they investigated differing skeletal sites and skeletal tissue (both trabecular and cortical) making attempts at comparison difficult. Sowers (1996) also notes that confounding findings of the relationship between parity and BMD may also be related to differences in the ability to conceive and maintain a viable fetus. There may be a similar problem with the use of nulliparous women as controls, as they may have insufficient hormonal environments, preventing conception or compromising their bone mineralization, making them inappropriate in comparisons with parous women (Sowers, 1996).

It is also suggested that parity is related to risk of fracture. Hoffman *et al.* (1993) found live birth to be associated with reduced odds of hip fracture and Mallmin *et al.* (1994) found nulliparous women to have an increased risk of forearm fracture. The explanation for the observed association between parity and reduced risk of fracture may be related to increased weight-bearing activity after pregnancy and weight gain during and after pregnancy in parous women (Hoffman *et al.*, 1993; Sowers, 1996; Kojima *et al.*, 2002).

4. Lactation

During lactation there is potentially continued demand for calcium from the maternal skeleton dependant on the duration of breast-feeding (Sowers, 1996). Further, increased calcium absorption has not largely been observed during lactation (Kent *et al.*, 1990; Specker *et al.*, 1991; Sowers, 1996). Studies on BMD and lactation, although seemingly contradictory, appear to be dependent upon the duration of the study (Sowers, 1996).

Several studies have shown no association between lactational history and BMD (Johnell and Nillson, 1984; Feldblum *et al.*, 1992), while a study by Lissner *et al.* (1991) reports a negative association between the number of months of recalled lactation and bone mineral content. However, as with studies on BMD and parity, these association studies are limited by their reliance on the use of recall information of past lactation practices.

Longitudinal studies that have examined bone mass during lactation have consistently demonstrated that bone loss can occur with lactation (Lamke *et al.*, 1977; Chan *et al.*, 1982; Hayslip *et al.*, 1989; Drinkwater and Chesnut, 1991; Kent *et al.*, 1993; Sowers *et al.*, 1993,1995; Affinito *et al.*, 1996; Lopez *et al.*, 1996; Sowers, 1996). Several of these studies have shown lactational bone loss to be site-specific primarily affecting cancellous bone (Hayslip *et al.*, 1989; Kent *et al.*, 1990; Drinkwater and Chesnut, 1991; Kent *et al.*, 1993). Further, there is convincing evidence from longitudinal studies that despite initial loss with extended lactation, recovery can occur during weaning and post-weaning (Kent *et al.*, 1990; Sowers *et al.*, 1993, 1995; Kalkwarf and Specker, 1995; Affinito *et al.*, 1996; Lopez *et al.*, 1996; Sowers, 1996; Kolthoff *et al.*, 1998; More *et al.*, 2001). However, although Chan *et al.* (1982) examined loss in young women with low calcium intake, it has been noted that few studies have examined bone loss under conditions of low dietary intakes of calcium or vitamin D deficiency, or with various aged subjects (Sowers, 1996). A study of Saudi females suggests that BMD may be significantly lower in Saudi females who have a high rate of pregnancies and long duration of breast-feeding in combination with prevalent vitamin D deficiency (Ghannam *et al.*, 1999). While it is generally hypothesized that extended lactation may pose a particular risk to maternal bone density, this has not been substantiated in longitudinal studies of extended lactation, even in the presence of short recovery periods in the case of multiple pregnancies (Sowers *et al.*, 1993; Henderson *et al.*, 2000).

The epidemiological study by Hreshchyshun *et al.* (1988) found that, if all females who had breast-fed were compared with those who had not, there was no significant difference in BMD, but if only parous females were considered then females who breast-fed had a higher lumbar spine BMD than those who did not. The data showed that there was a 1.5% increase in bone mineral density per breast-fed child. Feldblum *et al.* (1992) found that females who had breast-fed had an estimated 41 mg/cm^2 higher lumbar BMD after controlling for parity, body mass index, physical activity, and menopausal status. Studies have also suggested a positive effect of lactation on fracture risk. For example, Cumming and Klineberg (1993) found that parous females who had not breast-fed had twice the risk of hip fracture as nulliparous females. An increased average duration of breast-feeding per child was associated with a greater reduction in risk of hip fracture. Kreiger *et al.* (1982) found a 40% reduction in risk of hip fracture for each 12 months of breast-feeding during a female's lifetime. Alderman *et al.* (1986) found a similar magnitude of risk reduction among females who had breast-fed for longer than 12 months overall. Studies by Aloia *et al.* (1983) and Kelsey *et al.* (1992) have shown that breast-feeding protects against fractures of the vertebrae.

The pattern of significant bone loss during lactation and subsequent recovery with weaning is also supported by the measurement of biochemical markers during lactation (Cole *et al.*, 1987; Kent *et al.*, 1990; Cross *et al.*, 1995; Sowers *et al.*, 1995; Affinito *et al.*, 1996; Lopez *et al.*, 1996). These studies also indicate a return to baseline values and a period of increased bone formation postweaning and with the reestablishment of menses consistent with the recovery of bone mass (Kent *et al.*, 1990; Cross *et al.*, 1995; Sowers *et al.*, 1995; Lopez *et al.*, 1996). Examination of calciotropic hormone levels during lactation does not seem to provide an explanation for the observed loss and recovery observed during lactation. Authors have reported either a decrease in PTH levels with duration of lactation (Specker *et al.*, 1991; Cross *et al.*, 1995) or no change in PTH levels during lactation (Kent *et al.*, 1990; Kent *et al.*, 1993) with levels increasing post-weaning. Similarly, researchers have found no change in levels of 1,25-dihydroxyvitamin D or in levels of vitamin D metabolites (Specker *et al.*, 1991; Kent *et al.*, 1993). As mentioned earlier with pregnancy, Cross *et al.* (1995) have suggested that hormonal changes in levels of estrogen and prolactin could play a role in calcium homeostasis during lactation; other researchers have suggested a possible role for parathyroid hormone related-protein (PTHrP) during lactation (Kent *et al.*, 1993; Sowers, 1996).

5. Animal Models

A number of animal models have also been utilized to better understand the loss of bone mineral and bone turnover during pregnancy and lactation. Studies of bone mineral and lactation in the rat have shown an increase in bone formation and bone mass with pregnancy in the maternal skeleton, followed by increased turnover and loss of bone mineral during lactation (Miller *et al.*, 1986; Hagaman *et al.*, 1990; Bowman and Miller, 1999; Shahtaheri *et al.*, 1999a; Zeni *et al.*, 1999). In a study of cancellous bone microstructure in uniparous and multiparous rats, Shahtaheri *et al.* (1999a) found that while the first pregnancy cycle showed dramatic bone formation (a 40% increase in the lumbar spine cancellous bone volume as compared to age-matched virgin controls), a rapid succession of pregnancy cycles with lactation resulted in a loss of cancellous bone and connectivity in low-weight bearing sites. The authors did note that lactating multiparous animals might have had the benefit of recovery and perhaps a compensatory period before subsequent pregnancy (Shahtaheri *et al.*, 1999a). The post-lactational period in the rat has been described as "anabolic," demonstrating an accelerated rate of bone gain and recovery with adequate dietary conditions (Hagaman *et al.*, 1990; Bowman and Miller, 1999). A similar pattern of bone accumulation during pregnancy followed by decreased bone mineral content and increased bone remodeling and turnover during lactation has also been reported in dog models (Miller *et al.*, 1989; Fukuda and Iida, 1993). Few longitudinal studies on the effects of pregnancy and lactation have been made utilizing large animals. Studies with nonhuman primates are particularly valuable in understanding the effects of pregnancy and lactation in humans. A histomorphometric study of iliac crest bone in cynomolgus monkeys by Lees and Jerome (1998) found no change in bone formation rates with pregnancy, but a significant increase during lactation. Increased levels of the bone markers alkaline phosphatase and bone gla-protein supported the observation of increased turnover during lactation (Lees and Jerome, 1998). While no effect on bone mineral content was found to occur during pregnancy, large decreases were observed during peak lactation (Lees and Jerome, 1998). However, Lees and Jerome (1998) suggest that observed subsequent gains by 10 months postpartum and increased trabecular thickness at 9 months postpartum, indicate that at least cancellous bone is capable of recovery from lactational losses. The authors further found estrogen levels to change greatly during pregnancy and lactation, and suggest that low postpartum estradiol concentrations may explain the observed changes in bone turnover (Lees and Jerome, 1998). In another recent study of pregnancy and lactation in young macaques by Ott *et al.* (1999) an increase in total bone density was found during early pregnancy, with no changes observed during late pregnancy and parturition. Vertebral bone density did show a decrease during pregnancy and 6 months of lactation, however, both bone density measurements were found to recover 3 months after weaning (Ott *et al.*, 1999). Histomorphometric measurements demonstrated an increase in bone formation parameters between pregnancy and weaning (Ott *et al.*, 1999). Osteocalcin levels showed a decrease during mid-pregnancy with a dramatic increase during lactation, while in the opposite direction, 1,25-dihydroxyvitamin D levels significantly decreased after lactation (Ott *et al.*, 1999). The authors interpreted the results to support the hypothesis of reduced mid-pregnancy bone formation with increased cancellous resorption, followed by lactational loss of bone with subsequent increased formation post-weaning (Ott *et al.*, 1999). Both studies of nonhuman primates concur with studies of human females that lactation is a period of increased bone turnover, resulting in bone loss that, with increased post-weaning bone formation, can facilitate recovery (Lees and Jerome, 1998; Ott *et al.*, 1999). Further, these studies do not indicate any permanent structural changes in the maternal skeleton that would compromise skeletal integrity, and both have demonstrated an increase in trabecular bone thickness with pregnancy and lactation that may in fact hint at compensatory mechanisms for improved bone quality (Lees and Jerome, 1998; Ott *et al.*, 1999).

6. Evolutionary and Historical Evidence

When considering BMD and female reproductive factors it is valuable to take the data out of the strictly modern clinical studies into the context of a larger evolutionary perspective. It is only by looking at the whole picture that we may gain an understanding of the patterns and factors involved. To gain this broader perspective, reproductive patterns of our closest living relatives, the apes, women in non-industrialized societies, and women from historical populations will be examined.

Large-bodied nonhuman primates such as gorillas and chimpanzees, our genetically closest primate relatives, usually experience their first birth soon after menarche, late weaning age with a lactation period duration of 3–4 years with frequent nursing, and typically about 5 offspring (Dettwyler, 1995). Based on comparative primate data on specifically lactation and weaning, Dettwyler (1995) further suggests that the natural age of weaning for humans, without the cultural modification of lactation behavior, could likely fall between 2.5 and as long as 7.0 years of age. It is likely that for much of our evolutionary history women would have followed a reproductive pattern similar to this, with an average of 5 children and 4 years of breast-feeding per child. Certainly non-industrialized female life cycles are typically characterized by late menarche, frequent pregnancies, prolonged lactation, and early menopause (Sperling and Beyene, 1997).

Reproductive patterns have changed substantially only within the last century, resulting in a dramatic shift in the hormonal milieu of modern Western females. Sperling and Beyene (1997) illustrate this point in their comparison of estimated reproductive histories in non-industrialized and post-industralized Western populations. They suggest non-industrialized females usually experience late menarche, first birth soon after, 3–4 years lactation, an average family size of about 5, and early menopause; resulting in a total number of menstrual cycles of approximately 4 years, or 48 cycles (Eaton *et al.*, 1994; Sperling and Beyene, 1997; Weaver, 1998). These estimates suggest a long period of lactational amenorrhea (3 years upwards). An estimate of the number of menstrual cycles under natural fertility based on longitudinal data on the Dogon women of Mali by Strassmann (1997), suggests the median lifetime number of menses to be about 109 cycles. In comparison, post-industrialized Western females experience early menarche, little or no breast-feeding, an average family size of 2.5, and late menopause, resulting in a total number of menstrual cycles of about 35 years, or 420 cycles (Eaton *et al.*, 1994; Sperling and Beyene, 1997; Weaver, 1998). Even compared to the empirical data estimates of Strassman (1997), this suggests a significantly greater number of cycles in the lifetime of the Western post-industrialized woman. This raises the question of whether there are consequences for the female skeleton as a result of this dramatic hormonal shift.

We may be able to get some clues by looking at skeletons from the past. The study of female skeletons in past populations gives us a unique opportunity to examine bone in populations with very different reproductive patterns, patterns that are more consistent with those found throughout the majority of human evolution. This can provide insight into the long-term effects of reproductive factors on bone maintenance. Several researchers studying bone loss in archeological skeletons have discussed the possible role of pregnancy and lactation. For example, investigators have suggested that pregnancy and lactation stress combined with nutritional deficiency could have resulted in early age bone loss in Nubian archeological populations (Armelagos *et al.*, 1972; Martin and Armelagos, 1979, 1985; Martin, 1981; Martin *et al.*, 1984, 1985). Similarly, Poulsen *et al.* (2001) suggest that significant decreases in BMD in Danish medieval female skeletons of young age could be the result of pregnancy and lactation stress. The authors in fact suggest that the physiological demands associated with pregnancy and breast-feeding may have increased mortality in young medieval women, although no evidence is given of the circumstances in which reproduction would have been so detrimental (Poulsen *et al.*, 2001). In contrast, Vogel *et al.* (1990) suggest that parity may have played a role in better trabecular connectivity as compared to modern populations in female skeletons from European historical populations. A recent study by Agarwal (2001) and Agarwal *et al.* (2003) of vertebral trabecular architecture in the Medieval British skeletal population, Wharram Percy, provides an example of how reproductive factors may have influenced bone maintenance and fragility in the post-reproductive years. The study of 55 individuals divided into three broad age categories, found significant age-related change in trabecular bone structure to occur primarily by middle age (with significant differences between the youngest and two older age groups in the population), but neither sex showed continuing change in trabecular structure between middle and old age (Agarwal *et al.*, 2003). Further, while males showed a similar pattern of age-related change in parameters related to bone connectivity, females showed no statistical differences between the age groups in bone connectivity at all (Agarwal *et al.*, 2003). These patterns of trabecular bone loss and fragility contrast with those generally found in modern populations that typically report continuing loss of bone structure and connectivity between middle and old age, and suggest greater loss in females. It is possible that reproductive factors such as high parity and extended periods of lactation could have played a key role in female bone maintenance in this historic population. Although no direct evidence of pregnancy and lactation practices are available for the archaeological population in this study, parity would likely have been higher in the rural medieval population, as compared to modern populations. Extended lactation was also practiced in medieval times. Rural medieval peasants, such as those in the study population, would likely have had to nurse their own children (Gies and Gies, 1990). The health benefits of breast-feeding for both the mother and child (Gies and Gies, 1990) and the possible contraceptive function of breast-feeding were also known by the medieval period, perhaps accounting for later weaning ages in the medieval period (Fildes, 1995). Agarwal (2001) and Agarwal *et al.* (2003) suggest that the patterns of age-related change in trabecular architecture in the female skeletons in this study may be related to the unique hormonal environment created by these reproductive practices. Increased parity and extended lactation would also have resulted in lower steroid exposure in the historic females, in comparison to modern Western females who give birth to fewer children and practice little or no breast-feeding (Sperling and Beyene, 1997; Pollard, 1999). Further, age of menarche is known to show a secular change, specifically decreasing in recent modern populations (Treloar, 1974; Sperling and Beyene, 1997), and although age at menopause has been regarded as generally stable through human evolution (Pavelka and Fedigan, 1991), there is evidence that many populations show earlier onset of menopause in comparison to industrialized Western populations (Eaton *et al.*, 1994; Sperling and Beyene, 1997). Although it is uncertain where the reproductive patterns in the archaeological population of Wharram Percy would fall in relation to the menstrual cycle estimates discussed earlier, it is clear that the hormonal milieu would have been different in these historical females. The less dramatic change in vertebral trabecular bone after menopause observed in this archaeological population may simply reflect the lower levels of steroid exposure in these historical females (Agarwal *et al.*, 2003). Weaver (1998) suggests that the pattern of bone loss in modern females may be related to the sudden down regulation of bone forming osteoblast cells that are elevated with the chronically high levels of estrogen. At the same time, reproductive patterns may additionally explain the observation in archaeological studies of poor bone density and trabecular bone architecture in young historical females. We may simply be observing skeletons of premenopausal women of reproductive age who were pregnant or breast-feeding at the time of death. Their maternal skeletons may not have had the sufficient time to recover from the demands of pregnancy or the start of lactation, which it is capable of doing. While interpreting the patterns of bone loss in the past is speculative, it is known that reproductive patterns were undoubtedly different historically. It is not surprising that the patterns of bone loss in the historical females differ from modern Western patterns. These observations of bone loss and fragility in historical females may shed light on our current understanding of bone maintenance in modern Western women.

7. Discussion

Although reproductive factors have long been hypothesized as risk factors for the maternal skeleton, from an evolutionary perspective it would be maladaptive if the female skeleton were incapable of efficient bone maintenance under the normal conditions of pregnancy and lactation. After all, pregnancy and lactation are not pathological states, but aspects of normal female physiological functioning. However, many modern clinical studies and most anthropological studies on past human populations have focused on the detrimental effects of pregnancy and lactation on the maternal skeleton. Often there has been an assumption that the "stress" and "demands" of pregnancy and lactation produce a "drain" on the maternal skeleton. It is true that these reproductive states are characterized by increased metabolic activity involving bone metabolism but this reflects a dynamic, flexible, and adaptive response to changing requirements. There has not been an appreciation of the plasticity and adaptability of bone metabolism during these states, when calcium availability can be increased by two important compensatory maternal mechanisms, renal calcium conservation and increased intestinal absorption of calcium, in addition to bone turnover of the maternal skeleton.

Pregnancy and lactation are associated with numerous physiological adaptations mediated by an extremely complex interplay of hormones. These reproductive states trigger a hormonal cascade effect that produces both short- and long-term changes in female physiology, metabolism, and health. During pregnancy estrogen levels rise, as well as prolactin and oxytocin levels. During lactation estrogen levels fall while prolactin and oxytocin levels remain high (Leake *et al.*, 1983; Widstrom *et al.*, 1984; Silber *et al.*, 1991). As Peaker (1976) says: "The secretion of milk...markedly affects the whole maternal organism." Cardiovascular changes occur including high blood flow to the mammary glands, alimentary tract, and liver, as well as higher cardiac output, particularly to the mammary glands, gastrointestinal tract, and skin (Leake *et al.*, 1983). Lactating women have been shown to have higher levels of serum parathyroid hormone, 1,25-dihydroxyvitamin D_3, and phosphorous, and these differences may persist even after weaning; urinary calcium excretion decreases rapidly in early lactation, and declines further as lactation continues (Feldblum *et al.*, 1992). There is an increase in the gastrointestinal endocrine system during lactation and hormones such as gastrin, cholecystokinin (CCK), insulin, glucagon, and somatostatin are affected (Silber *et al.*, 1991). These hormones enhance digestion and stimulate anabolic metabolism by promoting insulin release. The main hormones of pregnancy and lactation, estrogen, prolactin, and oxytocin, have incredibly complex relationships with other hormones and factors and are involved in a number of metabolic functions.

It is obvious that, because of quite different reproductive patterns, the hormonal milieu during much of the life of most modern Western women would be quite different from the hormonal milieu of our ancestors or a woman from a non-industrialized society following traditional reproductive patterns. However, because of the exceedingly slow pace of evolution, the biology of women and their children would still be adapted to these ancient patterns of reproduction, patterns that have been followed for more than 99% of our time on earth. These reproductive patterns are associated with an evolutionary "health package" mediated by hormonal, metabolic, and physiological factors that support the health of women and their children. For example, the health benefits of breast-feeding for infants and children are well known and include a reduction in jaundice, gastrointestinal disease, eczema, malocclusion, juvenile diabetes, SIDS, childhood cancers, respiratory disease, ear infections, and other diseases (Stuart-Macadam, 1995). The health benefits of lactation for women are less well known, but include a reduction in postpartum bleeding and uterine hemorrhage, placental retention, postnatal depression, perhaps enhanced maternal behavior, and a reduced risk of reproductive cancers including ovarian, breast, and possibly endometrial cancer. The benefits of breast-feeding on breast cancer risk increase with increasing duration of breast-feeding (Stuart-Macadam and Dettwyler, 1995).

It is very possible that bone health is one aspect of this evolutionary "health package." Modern clinical studies assessing the relationship between BMD and reproductive factors have been contradictory; some showing a detrimental effect, some showing no effect, and some showing a protective effect. The problem is that there have been weaknesses in most of these studies, with small sample sizes, different sample sites, and deficiencies in addressing specific issues relating to lactation, such as duration, timing, and intensity. There have only been a handful of studies that have sampled women who come close to practicing the reproductive patterns of our ancestors. There does seem to be agreement that there is often loss of bone density (primarily cancellous) during pregnancy and lactation, but that this is reversed with weaning. Some studies show that parity and breast-feeding are associated with higher BMD and fewer osteoporotic fractures later in life (Kreiger *et al.*, 1982; Aloia *et al.*, 1983; Alderman *et al.*, 1986; Hreshchyshyn *et al.*, 1988; Feldblum *et al.*, 1992; Kelsey *et al.*, 1992; Cumming and Klineberg, 1993). In fact, there are hints that there may be a "dose dependent" relationship between parity, lactation, and bone health in the sense that with greater parity and longer duration of breast-feeding the greater the protective effect on bone density and fracture incidence later in life (Kreiger *et al.*, 1982; Alderman *et al.*, 1986; Hreshchyshyn *et al.*, 1988).

Studies on nonhuman primates support these findings and show that lactation is a period of increased bone turnover with bone loss that is recovered after weaning. They have also suggested an increase in trabecular bone thickness with pregnancy and lactation that suggest a compensatory mechanism for improved bone quality. The studies on females from historical populations that have considered the influence of reproductive factors are few and contradictory. Further, these are not directly comparable, as some examine bone quantity by measuring BMD (Armelagos *et al.*, 1972; Martin *et al.*, 1984; Martin *et al.*, 1985; Poulsen *et al.*, 2001), while only two examine bone quality parameters (Vogel *et al.*, 1990; Agarwal *et al.*, 2003).

Since modern clinical studies and primate data indicate that it is quite normal to have a temporary reduction in bone mass during the reproductive years it is not surprising that researchers should find a reduction in BMD in young reproductive-age historical females. In an archaeological sample, this means that females who die during the reproductive life phase would likely show reduced BMD. However, it may be totally unrelated to diet, cause of death, or bone health, and have everything to do with the fact that they were pregnant, recently pregnant, or lactating at the time of death. It is important to appreciate that while pregnancy and lactation are metabolically active states, bone loss during pregnancy and weaning does not necessarily translate into lower BMD in later life. On the contrary, the data from modern clinical studies and nonhuman primates show that the trend of reduction in bone mass is normally reversed after birth and during weaning and even hint that these reproductive factors may actually be protective against low BMD and osteoporotic fracture later in life.

8. Conclusions

To understand the relationship between bone density and female reproductive factors it is important to take a broad evolutionary perspective, and to view bone health and maintenance within the larger context of the changing female life cycle. A synthesis of data from modern clinical studies, animal models, and historical populations indicates that bone loss does occur in women of reproductive age during pregnancy and lactation. However, this bone loss appears to primarily affect cancellous tissue and is reversed during and after weaning. Interestingly, some studies show that parity and lactation are actually protective factors against low BMD and osteoporotic fracture later in life. There are hints that there could be a "dose-dependent" effect in the sense that greater parity and longer lactation provide even more protection.

Reproductive patterns of Western women have changed dramatically in the last century, and associated with this is a very different hormonal experience for the modern woman as compared with our ancestors and many women in non-industrial societies. Studies of female BMD and bone quality from the past are vitally important as they give us the opportunity to consider the effect of reproductive patterns that existed and were maintained throughout most of human evolution. These studies not only shed light on bone maintenance in historical populations, but may also provide clues as to the modern Western phenomenon of increasing bone loss and fragility fracture incidence in older women.

References

Affinito, P., Tommaselli, G.A., di Carlo, C., Guida, F., and Nappi, C. (1996). Changes in bone mineral density and calcium metabolism in breastfeeding women: A one year follow-up study. *J. Clin. Endocrinol. Metab.* **81**, 2314–2318.

Agarwal, S.C. (2001). The effects of pregnancy and lactation on the maternal skeleton: A historical perspective. *Am. J. Phy. Anthropol.* **32**, 30.

Agarwal, S.C., Dumitrui, M., Tomilnson, G.A., and Grynpas, M.D. Medieval trabecular architecture: The influence of age sex, and lifestyle. *Am. J. Phys. Anthropol.* 2003. in press.

Alderman, B.W., Weiss, N.S., Daling, J.R., Ure, C.L., and Ballard, J.H. (1986). Reproductive history and post-menopausal risk of hip and forearm fracture. *Am. J. Epidemiol.* **124**, 262–267.

Aloia, J.F., Vaswani, A.N., Yeh, J.K., Ross, P., Ellis, K., and Cohn, S.H. (1983). Determinants of bone mass in postmenopausal women. *Arch. Intern. Med.* **143**, 1700–1704.

Armelagos, G.J., Mielke, J.H., Owen, K.H., Van Gerven, K.H., Dewey, J.R., and Mahler, P.E. (1972). Bone growth and development in prehistoric populations from Sudanese Nubia. *J. Hum. Evol.* **1**, 89–119.

Bererhi, H., Kolhoff, N., Constable, A., and Nielsen, S.P. (1996). Multiparity and bone mass. *Br. J. Obstet. Gynaecol.* **103**, 818–821.

Black, A.J., Topping, J., Durham, B., Farquharson, R.G., and Fraser, W.D. (2000). A detailed assessment of alterations in bone turnover, calcium homeostasis, and bone density in normal pregnancy. *J. Bone Miner. Res.* **15**, 557–563.

Bowman, B.M., and Miller, S.C. (1999). Skeletal mass, chemistry, and growth during and after multiple reproductive cycles in the rat. *Bone* **25**, 553–559.

Chan, G.M., Slater, P., Ronald, N., Roberts, C.C., Thomas, M.R., Folland, D., and Jackson, R. (1982). Bone mineral status of lactating mothers of different ages. *Am. J. Obstet. Gynecol.* **144**, 438–441.

Cohen, M.N. (1994). The osteological paradox reconsidered. *Curr. Anthropol.* **35**, 629–631.

Cole, D.E., Gundberg, C.M., Stirk, L.J., Atkinson, S.A., Hankey, D.A., Ayer, L.M., and Baldwin, L.S. (1987). Changing osteocalcin concentrations during pregnancy and lactation: Implications for maternal mineral metabolism. *J. Clin. Endo. Metab.* **65**, 290–294.

Cross, N.A., Hillman, L.S., Allen, S.H., Krause, G.F., and Vieira, N.E. (1995). Calcium homeostasis and bone metabolism during pregnancy, lactation, and postweaning: A longitudinal study. *Am. J. Clin. Nutr.* **61**, 514–523.

Cumming, R.G., and Klineberg, R.J. (1993). Breastfeeding and other reproductive factors and the risk of hip fractures in elderly women. *Int. J. Epidemiol.* **22**, 684–691.

Dettwyler, K.A. (1995). A time to wean: The hominid blueprint for the natural age of weaning in modern human populations. In P. Stuart-Macadam and K.A. Dettwyler (eds) *Breastfeeding: Biolcultural Perspectives.* Aldine de Gruyter, New York, pp. 39–74.

Drinkwater, B.L. and Chesnut, C.Hd. (1991). Bone density changes during pregnancy and lactation in active women: A longitudinal study. *Bone Miner.* **14**, 153–160.

Eaton, S.B., Pike, M.C., Short, R.V., Lee, N.C., Trussell, J., Hatcher, R.A., Wood, J.W., Worthman, C.M. *et al.* (1994). Women's reproductive cancers in evolutionary context. *Q. Rev. Biol.* **69**, 353–367.

Feldblum, P.J., Zhang, J., Rich, L.E., Fortney, J.A., and Talmage, R.V. (1992). Lactation history and bone mineral density among perimenopausal women. *Epidemiology* **3**, 327–531.

Fildes, V. (1995). The culture and biology of breastfeeding: An historical review of Western Europe. In P. Stuart-Macadam and K.A. Dettwyler (eds) *Breastfeeding: Biolcultural Perspectives.* Aldine de Gruyter, New York, pp. 101–126.

Forsmo, S., Schei, B., Langhammer, A., and Forsen, L. (2001). How do reproductive and lifestyle factors influence bone density in distal and ultradistal radius of early postmenopausal women? The Nord-Trondelag Health Survey, Norway. *Osteoporos Int.* **12**, 222–229.

Fox, K.M., Magaziner, J., Sherwin, R., Scott, J.C., Plato, C.C., Nevitt, M., and Cummings, S. (1993). Reproductive correlates of bone mass in elderly women. Study of Osteoporotic Fractures Research Group. *J. Bone Miner. Res.* **8**, 901–908.

Fukuda, S., and Iida, H. (1993). Histomorphometric changes in iliac trabecular bone during pregnancy and lactation in beagle dogs. *J. Vet Med. Sci.* **55**, 565–569.

Gambacciani, M., Spinetti, A., Gallo, R., Cappagli, B., Teti, G.C., and Facchini, V. (1995). Ultrasonographic bone characteristics during normal pregnancy: Longitudinal and cross-sectional evaluation. *Am. J. Obstet. Gynecol.* **173**, 890–893.

Ghannam, N.N., Hammami, M.M., Bakheet, S.M., and Khan, B.A. (1999). Bone mineral density of the spine and femur in healthy Saudi females: Relation to vitamin D status, pregnancy, and lactation. *Calcif. Tissue Int.* **65**, 23–28.

Gies, F., and Gies, G. (1990). Life in a medieval village. Harper Row, London.

Grainge, M.J., Coupland, C.A., Cliffe, S.J., Chilvers, C.E., and Hosking, D.J. (2001). Reproductive, menstrual and menopausal factors: Which are associated with bone mineral density in early postmenopausal women? *Osteoporos. Int.* **12**, 777–787.

Hagaman, J.R., Ambrose, W.W., and Hirsch, P.F. (1990). A scanning electron microscopic and photon absorptiometric study of the development, prolongation, and pattern of recovery from lactation-induced osteopenia in rats. *J. Bone Miner. Res.* **5**, 123–132.

Hayslip, C.C., Klein, T.A., Wray, H.L., and Duncan, W.E. (1989). The effects of lactation on bone mineral content in healthy postpartum women. *Obstet. Gynecol.* **73**, 588–592.

Henderson, P.H., 3rd, Sowers, M., Kutzko, K.E., and Jannausch, M.L. (2000). Bone mineral density in grand multiparous women with extended lactation. *Am. J. Obstet. Gynecol.* **182**, 1371–1377.

Hoffman, S., Grisso, J.A., Kelsey, J.L., Gammon, M.D., and O'Brien, L.A. (1993). Parity, lactation and hip fracture. *Osteoporos. Int.* **3**, 171–176.

Holmberg-Marttila, D., Sievanen, H., and Tuimala, R. (1999). Changes in bone mineral density during pregnancy and postpartum: Prospective data on five women. *Osteoporos. Int.* **10**, 41–46.

Hreshchyshyn, M.M., Hopkins, A., and Zylstra, S. (1988). Associations of parity, breastfeeding, and birth control pills with lumbar spine and femoral neck bone densities. *Am. J. Obstet. Gynecol.* **159**, 318–322.

Hu, J.F., Zhao, X.H., Chen, J.S., Fitzpatrick, J., Parpia, B., and Campbell, T.C. (1994). Bone density and lifestyle characteristics in premenopausal and postmenopausal Chinese women. *Osteoporos. Int.* **4**, 288–297.

Johnell, O., and Nillson, B. (1984). Lifestyle and bone mineral mass in perimenopausal women. *Calcif. Tissue Int.* **36**, 354–356.

Kalkwarf, H.J., and Specker, B.L. (1995). Bone mineral loss during lactation and recovery after weaning. *Obstet. Gynecol.* **86**, 26–32.

Karlsson, C., Obrant, K.J., and Karlsson, M. (2001). Pregnancy and lactation confer reversible bone loss in humans. *Osteoporos. Int.* **12**, 828–834.

Kelsey, J.L., Browner, W.S., Seeley, D.G., Nevitt, M.C., and Cummings, S.R. (1992). Risk factors for fractures of the distal forearm and proximal humerus. The Study of Osteoporotic Fractures Research Group. *Am. J. Epidemiol.* **135**, 477–489.

Kent, G.N., Price, R.I., Gutteridge, D.H., Allen, J.R., Rosman, K.J., Smith, M., Bhagat, C.I., Wilson, S.G., and Retallack, R.W. (1993). Effect of pregnancy and lactation on maternal bone mass and calcium metabolism. *Osteoporos. Int.* **3** (Suppl 1), 44–47.

Kent, G.N., Price, R.I., Gutteridge, D.H., Smith, M., Allen, J.R., Bhagat, C.I., Barnes, M.P., Hickling, C.J. *et al.* (1990). Human lactation: Forearm trabecular bone loss, increased bone turnover, and renal conservation of calcium and inorganic phosphate with recovery of bone mass following weaning. *J. Bone Miner. Res.* **5**, 361–369.

Kojima, N., Douchi, T., Kosha, S., and Nagata, Y. (2002). Cross-sectional study of the effects of parturition and lactation on bone mineral density later in life. *Maturitas* **41**, 203–209.

Kolthoff, N., Eiken, P., Kristensen, B., and Nielsen, S.P. (1998). Bone mineral changes during pregnancy and lactation: A longitudinal cohort study. *Clin. Sci.* (Lond) **94**, 405–412.

Kreiger, N., Kelsey, J.L., Holford, T.R., and O'Connor, T. (1982). An epidemiologic study of hip fracture in postmenopausal women. *Am. J. Epidemiol.* **116**, 141–148.

Lamke, B., Brundin, J., and Moberg, P. (1977). Changes of bone mineral content during pregnancy and lactation. *Acta. Obstet. Gynecol. Scand.* **56**, 217–219.

Leake, R.D., Waters, C.B., Rubin, R.T., Buster, J.E., and Fisher, D.A. (1983). Oxytocin and prolactin responses in long-term breast-feeding. *Obstet. Gynecol.* **62**, 565–568.

Lees, C.J., and Jerome, C.P. (1998). Effects of pregnancy and lactation on bone in cynomolgus macaques: Histomorphometric analysis of iliac biopsies. *Bone* **22**, 545–549.

Lissner, L., Bengtsson, C., and Hansson, T. (1991). Bone mineral content in relation to lactation history in pre- and postmenopausal women. *Calcif. Tissue Int.* **48**, 319–325.

Lopez, J.M., Gonzalez, G., Reyes, V., Campino, C., and Diaz, S. (1996). Bone turnover and density in healthy women during breastfeeding and after weaning. *Osteoporos. Int.* **6**, 153–159.

Mallmin, H., Ljunghall, S., Persson, I., and Bergstrom, R. (1994). Risk factors for fractures of the distal forearm: A population-based case-control study. *Osteoporos. Int.* **4**, 298–304.

Martin, D.L. (1981). Microstructural examination: Possibilities for skeletal analysis. In D.L. Martin and M.P. Bumstead (eds) *Biocultural Adaptation: Comprehensive Approaches to Skeletal Analysis*. University of Massachusetts, Amherst, pp. 96–107.

Martin, D.L., and Armelagos, G.J. (1979). Morphometrics of compact bone: An example from Sudanese Nubia. *Am. J. Phys. Anthropol.* **51**, 571–578.

Martin, D.L., and Armelagos, G.J. (1985). Skeletal remodelling and mineralization as indicators of health: An example from prehistoric Sudanese Nubia. *J. Hum. Evol.* **14**, 527–537.

Martin, D.L., Armelagos, G.J., Goodman, A.H., and Van Gerven, D.P. (1984). The effects of socioeconomic change in prehistoric africa: Sudanese Nubia as a case study. In M.N. Cohen and G.J. Armelagos (eds) Paleopathology at the origins of agriculture. Academic Press, New York, pp. 193–214.

Martin, D.L., Goodman, A.H., and Armelagos, G.J. (1985). Skeletal pathologies as indicators of quality and quantity of diet. In R.I. Gilbert and J.H. Mielke (eds) *The Analysis of Prehistoric Diets*. Academic Press, New York, pp. 227–279.

Martinez, M.E., de Pedro, C., Catalan, P., Salinas, M., Balaguer, G., and Ordas, J. (1985). Levels of osteocalcin in normal pregnancy. *Am. J. Obstet. Gynecol.* **153**, 708–709.

Melton, L. (1995). How many women have osteoporosis now? *J. Bone Miner. Res.* **10**, 175–177.

Melton, L.J., Bryant, S.C., Wahner, H.W., O'Fallon, W.M., Malkasian, G.D., Judd, H.L., and Riggs, B.L. (1993). Influence of breastfeeding and other reproductive factors on bone mass later in life. *Osteoporosis Int.* **3**, 76–83.

Miller, M.A., Omura, T.H., and Miller, S.C. (1989). Increased cancellous bone remodeling during lactation in beagles. *Bone* **10**, 279–285.

Miller, S.C., Shupe, J.G., Redd, E.H., Miller, M.A., and Ohura, T.H.B. (1986). Changes in bone mineral and bone formation rates during pregnancy and lactation in rats. *Bone* **7**, 283–287.

More, C., Bettembuk, P., Bhattoa, H.P., and Balogh, A. (2001). The effects of pregnancy and lactation on bone mineral density. *Osteoporos Int.* **12**, 732–737.

Murphy, S., Khaw, K.T., May, H., and Compston, J.E. (1994). Parity and bone mineral density in middle-aged women. *Osteoporos Int.* **4**, 162–166.

Naylor, K.E., Iqbal, P., Fledelius, C., Fraser, R.B., and Eastell, R. (2000). The effect of pregnancy on bone density and bone turnover. *J. Bone Miner. Res.* **15**, 129–137.

Nguyen, T.V., Jones, G., Sambrook, P.N., White, C.P., Kelly, P.J., and Eisman, J.A. (1995). Effects of estrogen exposure and reproductive factors on bone mineral density and osteoporotic fractures. *J. Clin. Endocrinol. Metab.* **80**, 2709–2714.

Ott, S.M., Lipkin, E.W., and Newell-Morris, L. (1999). Bone physiology during pregnancy and lactation in young macaques. *J. Bone Miner. Res.* **14**, 1779–1788.

Pavelka, M.S., and Fedigan, L.M. (1991). Menopause: A comparative life history perspective. *Yearb. Phys. Anthropol.* **34**, 13–38.

Phillips, A.J., Ostlere, S.J., and Smith, R. (2000). Pregnancy-associated osteoporosis: Does the skeleton recover? *Osteoporos Int.* **11**, 449–454.

Pollard, T.M. (1999). Sex, gender and cardiovascular disease. In T.M. Pollard and S.B. Hyatt (eds) Sex, gender, and health. Cambridge University Press, Cambridge, pp. 53–74.

Poulsen, L.W., Qvesel, D., Brixen, K., Vesterby, A., and Boldsen, J.L. (2001). Low bone mineral density in the femoral neck of medieval women: A result of multiparity? *Bone* **28**, 454–458.

Rodin, A., Dunca, A., Quartero, W.P., Pisofidis, G., Mashiter, G., Whitaker, K., Crook, D., Stevenson, J.C. *et al.* (1989). Serum concentrations of alkaline phosphatase isoenzymes and osteocalcin in normal pregnancy. *J. Clin. Endo. Metab.* **68**, 1123–1127.

Seki, K., Makimura, N., Mitsui, C., Hirata, J., and Nagata, I. (1991). Calcium-regulating hormones and osteocalcin levels during pregnancy: A longitudinal study. *Am. J. Obstet. Gynecol.* **164**, 1248–1252.

Shahtaheri, S.M., Aaron, J.E., Johnson, D.R., and Paxton, S.K. (1999a). The impact of mammalian reproduction on cancellous bone architecture. *J. Anat.* **194**, 407–421.

Shahtaheri, S.M., Aaron, J.E., Johnson, D.R., and Purdie, D.W. (1999b). Changes in trabecular bone architecture in women during pregnancy. *Br. J. Obstet. Gynaecol.* **106**, 432–438.

Silber, M., Larsson, B., and Uvnas-Moberg, K. (1991). Oxytocin, somatostatin, insulin and gastrin concentrations vis-a-vis late pregnancy, breastfeeding and oral contraceptives. *Acta. Obstet. Gynecol. Scand.* **70**, 283–289.

Sowers, M. (1996). Pregnancy and lactation as risk factors for subsequent bone loss and osteoporosis. *J. Bone Miner. Res.* **11**, 1052–1060.

Sowers, M., Clark, M.K., Hollis, B., Wallace, R.B., and Jannausch, M. (1992). Radial bone mineral density in pre- and perimenopausal women: A prospective study of rates and risk factors for loss. *J. Bone Miner. Res.* **7**, 647–657.

Sowers, M., Corton, G., Shapiro, B., Jannausch, M.L., Crutchfield, M., Smith, M.L., Randolph, J.F., and Hollis, B. (1993). Changes in bone density with lactation [see comments]. *JAMA* **269**, 3130–3135.

Sowers, M., Eyre, D., Hollis, B.W., Randolph, J.F., Shapiro, B., Jannausch, M.L., and Crutchfield, M. (1995). Biochemical markers of bone turnover in lactating and nonlactating postpartum women. *J. Clin. Endocrinol. Metab.* **80**, 2210–2216.

Sowers, M.F., Scholl, T., Harris, L., and Jannausch, M. (2000). Bone loss in adolescent and adult pregnant women. *Obstet. Gynecol.* **96**, 189–193.

Specker, B.L., Tsang, C., and Ho, M. (1991). Changes in calcium homeostasis over the first year postpartum: Effect of lactation and weaning. *Obstet. Gynecol.* **78**, 56–62.

Sperling, S., and Beyene, Y. (1997). A pound of biology and a pinch of culture or a pinch of biology and a pound of culture? The necessity of integrating biology and culture in reproductive studies. In L. Hager (ed.) Women in human evolution. Routledge, New York, pp. 137–152.

Strassmann, B.I. (1997). The biology of menstruation in homo sapiens: Total lifetime menses, fecundity, and non-synchrony in a natural-fertility population. *Current Anthropology* **38**, 123–129.

Stuart-Macadam, P. (1995). Breastfeeding in prehistory. In P. Stuart-Macadam and K.A. Dettwyler (eds) *Breastfeeding: Biocultural Perpsectives.* Aldine de Gruyter, New York.

Stuart-Macadam, P. and Dettwyler, K.A. (ed.) (1995). *Breastfeeding: Biocultural Perspectives.* Aldine de Gruyter, New York.

Szulc, P., and Delmas, P.D. (1995). Is there a role for vitamin K deficiency in osteoporosis? In P. Burckhardt and R.P. Heaney (eds) *Nutritional Aspects of Osteoporosis '94.* Ares-Serono Symposia, Rome, pp. 357–365.

Treloar, A.E. (1974). Menarche, menopause, and intervening fecundability. *Human Biology* **46**, 89–107.

Vogel, M., Hahn, M., Caselitz, P., Woggan, J., Pompesius-Kempa, M., and Delling, G. (1990). Comparison of trabecular bone structure in man today and an ancient population in Western Germany. In H.E. Takahashi (ed.) *Bone Morphometry.* Nishimura, Japan, pp. 220–223.

Von Endt, D.W., and Ortner, D.J. (1984). Experimental effects of bone size and temperature on bone diagenesis. *J. Arch. Sci.* **11**, 247–253.

Weaver, D.S. (1998). Osteoporosis in the bioarchaeology of women. In A. Grauer and P. Stuart-Macadam (eds) *Sex and Gender in Paleopathological Perspective.* Cambridge University Press, Cambridge, pp. 27–46.

Whytehead, R. (1986). The excavation of an area within a Roman cemetery at West Tenter Street, London E1. *Transactions of the London and Middlesex Archaeological Society* **37**, 23–68.

Widstrom, A.M., Winberg, J., Werner, S., Hamberger, B., Eneroth, P., and Uvnas-Moberg, K. (1984). Suckling in lactating women stimulates the secretion of insulin and prolactin without concomitant effects on gastrin, growth hormone, calcitonin, vasopressin or catecholamines. *Early Hum. Dev.* **10**, 115–122.

Yamaga, A., Taga, M., Minaguchi, H., and Sato, K. (1996). Changes in bone mass as determined by ultrasound and biochemical markers of bone turnover during pregnancy and puerperium: A longitudinal study. *J. Clin. Endocrinol. Metab.* **81**, 752–756.

Yamamoto, N., Takahashi, H.E., Tanizawa, T., Kawashima, T., and Endo, N. (1994). Bone mineral density and bone histomorphometric assessments of postpregnancy osteoporosis: A report of five patients. *Calcif. Tissue Int.* **54**, 20–25.

Zeni, S.N., Di Gregorio, S., and Mautalen, C. (1999). Bone mass changes during pregnancy and lactation in the rat. *Bone* **25**, 681–685.

8

Functional Adaptation and Fragility of the Skeleton

R. Bruce Martin

1. Introduction

It is human nature that our perspectives on various subjects are colored by expectations derived from previous experiences, and this includes our attempts to understand the physiology and pathology of the skeleton. Medical students, having studied biochemistry far more than mechanics, often regard the skeleton as a static, mechanical framework on which are hung all the more interesting, biochemical parts of the body. In this view, the only physiologically interesting role of the skeleton is as a calcium reservoir, and beyond that its medical significance is summarized by the word "fractures." Anthropology students, on the other hand, learn to value the skeleton as the part of the body that survives death, decay, and geological storage. A surviving bone may be examined at great length to try to elicit the behaviors, diet, illnesses, and other characteristics of its former owner. To obtain a more complete understanding of the role and function of the skeleton from any perspective, perhaps we should all try to see the skeleton from a bone's own standpoint. This Chapter attempts to do that in the light of new developments in bone biology and mechanics that are of great consequence for both medicine and anthropology.

While the skeleton plays an important role in mineral homeostasis, it is primarily a mechanical organ, as the medical student suspected. However, this is hardly a simple obligation, and the skeleton is far from static. Instead, it is homeostatic: that is, bone biology changes skeletal structure in response to the organism's activities so as to maintain the tissue-level effects of these activities at a tolerable level. The word "adaptation" in this Chapter's title refers to this homeostatic capacity: the ability of bone cells to sense mechanical loading day-by-day and change bone structure in ways that preserve skeletal function and increase the organism's ability to survive. (It is important to point out that we are speaking here of a somatic adaptation, not an evolutionary adaptation involving genetic modulation of skeletal structures. However, these two kinds of adaptation are interrelated, and we shall return to this subject later in the Chapter.)

R. Bruce Martin • Department of Orthopaedics, University of California at Davis School of Medicine.

Bone Loss and Osteoporosis: An Anthropological Perspective, edited by Sabrina C. Agarwal and Sam D. Stout. Kluwer Academic/Plenum Publishers, New York, 2003.

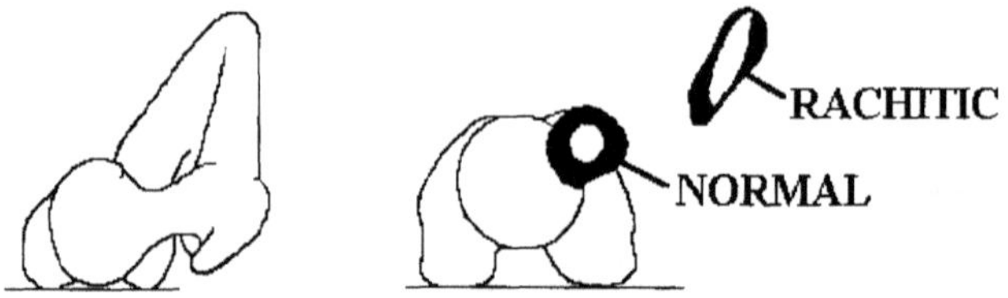

Figure 8.1. Sketch of a rachitic femur viewed proximal-to-distal (left) and the shape and location of its midshaft cross-section as compared to that of a normal femur (right). The location of the rachitic femur's cross-section is displaced relative to the femoral head and distal condyles because the bone was extremely bowed. Modified from Pauwels (1980), with permission.

It is difficult to discuss "mechanical adaptation" of bone without mentioning the name of Julius Wolff, the German surgeon who popularized the concept that the skeleton adapts itself to mechanical forces, so that this concept is now called "Wolff's Law" (Wolff, 1892a,b). However, the wider history of this concept is interesting and informative because others made more penetrating observations than Wolff. As reviewed by Roesler (1981, 1987), the 19th century literature established two central concepts as important in somatic skeletal adaptation. First is the idea of optimizing bone strength with respect to weight, and second is the concept that this process involves self-regulation of bone structure by cells responding to a mechanical signal. Several authors contributed to these ideas, but prominent among them was Roux (1881), who proposed that the construction of mechanically efficient bony architectures is carried out by bone cells responding to a mechanical *functional stimulus*. Not surprisingly, this concept emerged simultaneously with Claude Bernard's introduction of the idea of physiologic homeostasis.

What do we mean when we assert that bone homeostatically adapts itself to mechanical demands? The concept is often illustrated by the same observations that were pointed out historically. First, the *amount* of calcified tissue in a region of the skeleton is in some degree proportional to the *magnitude* of its loading. Secondly, the *shape* of a skeletal region is governed by the *directionality* of the applied forces. The classic examples are, for the effect of load magnitude, smaller, thinner, and more porous bones in paralyzed limbs; and for the effect of load direction, the organization of cancellous bone into trabecular arcades that seem arranged so as to keep the bony stresses within a physiologic limit using a minimal amount of tissue. An alternative example of the effect of load direction would be the asymmetrical shape of a long bone cross-section when bending habitually occurs in a particular direction (Figure 8.1). In addition to *adapting* bones to changing functional demands, bone biology is also responsible for *maintaining* bone tissue against the debilitating effects of fatigue damage. Such damage, incurred during normal activities, could, in the long run and absent of remodeling, make bone as fragile as a serious bone disease such as osteogenesis imperfecta.

2. Mechanisms of Functional Adaptation

What are the mechanisms by which such adaptations can be accomplished? There are two parts to this question, the first dealing with the sensors, and the second with the effectors. The latter is addressed first because the answer is more certain.

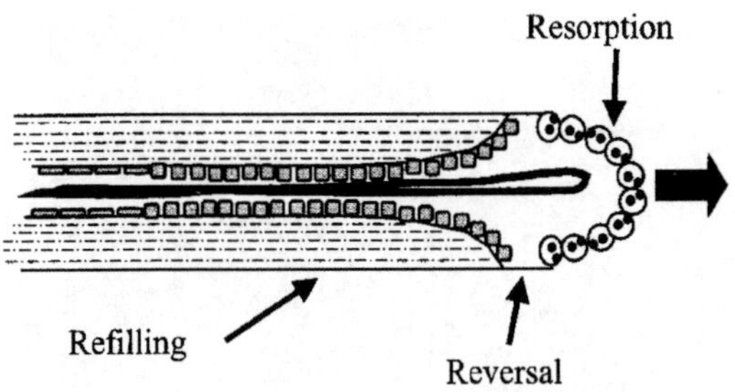

Figure 8.2. Schematic diagram of a BMU seen in longitudinal section as it tunnels from left to right through cortical bone. The three stages of the remodeling cycle at a particular location in the bone are indicated: resorption by osteoclasts, reversal as osteoclasts leave the scene, and refilling by osteoblasts. A typical BMU advances approximately 40 μm/day and creates a cylindrical osteonal bone structural unit about 200 μm in diameter and perhaps 5 mm long.

2.1. Effector Cells

The effectors are obviously the cells that remove (osteoclasts) and add (osteoblasts) bone tissue. It is not quite so simple, however, because these cells may operate either independently or in concert. In bone *modeling*, each cell type operates independently on a periosteal, endosteal, or trabecular bone surface, adding or removing material. In bone *remodeling*, the two cell types work together in teams called Basic Multicellular Units (BMUs), with osteoclasts removing bone and osteoblasts following them to replace (more-or-less) the resorbed bone (Figure 8.2). Modeling activities can make a bone larger or smaller, or change its shape, by sculpting its surfaces. While in principle remodeling could function similarly by arranging an imbalance between resorption and formation in each BMU, it seems that most remodeling serves to "turn over" bone tissue by more-or-less replacing the removed material. In cortical bone, this involves tunneling and slightly incomplete refilling to form a secondary osteon with its central Haversian canal. In cancellous bone, or on other bone surfaces, BMUs form a "hemi-osteon" by resorbing a trench and refilling it (Parfitt, 1994).

2.2. Sensor Cells

It is becoming increasingly clear that osteocytes and bone lining cells (BLCs) form a syncytium that functions as the "mechanosensor" responsible for bone's ability to adapt to changes in mechanical loading (Skerry *et al.*, 1989; Lanyon, 1993; Aarden *et al.*, 1994; Weinbaum *et al.*, 1994; Donahue, 1998; Knothe-Tate *et al.*, 2000; Martin, 2000). Osteocytes are osteoblasts that became buried in the bone matrix during bone formation. BLCs are osteoblasts that did not become buried, or apoptose at the cessation of bone formation, and ended up as flattened cells attached to the bone surface. During bone formation, osteoblasts are connected to one another via cell processes and gap junctions. As osteoblasts are converted to osteocytes they maintain these connections, both to previously buried osteocytes and to the remaining adjacent osteoblasts, with the passageways called canaliculi forming about the cell processes as they are entombed. When bone formation ceases at a location, and the last osteoblasts differentiate to become the residual BLCs on

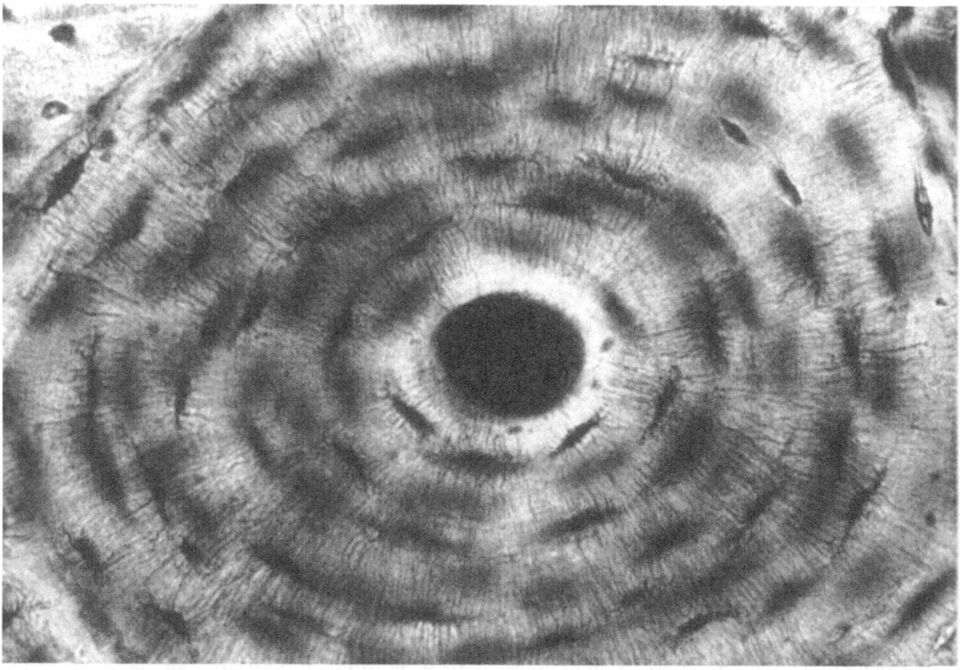

Figure 8.3. Photomicrograph of an osteon in cross-section showing its network of osteocyte lacunae (dark ellipses) connected by canaliculi (fine dark lines radiating from lacunae) that penetrate all regions of the tissue. Undemineralized cross-section from an equine metacarpal, stained *en bloc* in basic fuchsin; field width approximately 200 μm.

the now inactive bone surface, these cells inherit the many connections to the system of osteocytes in the adjacent bone matrix. The result is that all healthy bone matrix is inhabited by a syncytium of osteocytes, BLCs, and their connecting processes that permeates every cubic millimeter of the subjacent bone (Figure 8.3).

2.3. Strain and the Mechanostat

Just as a thermostat controls a furnace to regulate temperature in a room, a "mechanostat" is thought to regulate bone structure. Imagine a small cube of cortical bone within a long bone diaphysis. When the bone is loaded, the size and shape of this volume may change. Fractional changes in the cube's dimensions are known as *strains. In vivo* measurements in a variety of animals show that the greatest bone strains during various activities are of similar magnitudes across species. These local deformations can be measured by attaching a small gauge to the bone surface and electrically measuring its fractional change in length (strain) under load. Peak strains are typically no more than 0.003000 mm/mm, alternatively called 3,000 microstrain. More common functional strain values are a few hundred microstrain, and fracture occurs at about 25,000 microstrain. The mechanostat is the hypothetical physiologic system that controls strain by making bones more or less robust.

A working theory of current interest proposes that strains produced by skeletal loading force bone fluid through the system of canaliculi, and these fluid flows act on the osteocytes to generate integrated signals within the syncytium. These signals are compared to a "set point" that is somehow manifest in the osteocyte-BLC syncytium, and when an error of sufficient magnitude is detected, BLCs activate appropriate modeling or remodeling responses to add or remove bone, thereby reducing or increasing bone strain (Weinbaum *et al.*, 1994; Turner and Forwood, 1995; Donahue, 1998).

An alternative view is that strain in bone is required to nourish osteocytes by "pumping" nutrients through the canalicular network, and lack of nutrition results in a "signal" for a disuse response. A plausible hypothesis is that osteocytes in under-strained bone suffer apoptosis for lack of nutrition, and when this situation is sensed by the BLCs, appropriate modeling and/or remodeling response is activated, resulting in loss of bone. Conversely, mechanical overload may produce microscopic damage, called "microdamage" or "microcracks," that similarly cause osteocyte apoptosis and the activation of appropriate modeling and remodeling responses (Verborgt *et al.*, 2000).

Several authors have suggested rules by which specific adaptive changes in cortical bone *shape*, and trabecular bone *architecture*, are effected by modeling and/or remodeling; these are reviewed in Martin *et al.* (1998). However, it has been very difficult to experimentally verify these hypothetical rules, and they will not be discussed here. Instead, we turn our attention to current concepts about the mechanisms by which modeling and remodeling alter bone *mass* in response to variations in the magnitude of mechanical loading.

2.4. The Two Poles of Adaptation

If we ignore the difficult problem of how bones adapt their shapes to suit the directionality of the mechanical loading that they experience, and consider only how they adjust their mass or size in response to the magnitude of loading, then we have a simpler, bi-polar situation: loading can be sub-normal, resulting in a "disuse state," or super-normal, producing overload and damage in the tissue.

2.4.1. Disuse: Subnormal Loading

When loading of a bone is reduced, three responses are observed. First, the rate of intracortical remodeling is increased (Schaffler, 1990). This increases the intracortical "remodeling space" in the form of BMU resorption and refilling spaces (Figure 8.4). Individually, each of these spaces is temporary, but as long as the remodeling rate is elevated, the additional active BMUs will increase the bone's porosity. This will make the bone less stiff, and increase the strain back toward the normal level.

In addition, modeling in the form of resorption is typically activated on the endosteal and trabecular surfaces (Li *et al.*, 1990). (For reasons not yet understood, this response seems to occur on surfaces next to marrow.) This decreases the bone's cross-sectional area, making it less robust, and increases the strain level back to normal. Finally, if the bone is in a growing animal, the rate of periosteal bone formation will diminish (Uhthoff, 1982), which over time will produce a bone that is smaller and less stiff, and again serve to return strains to normal values.

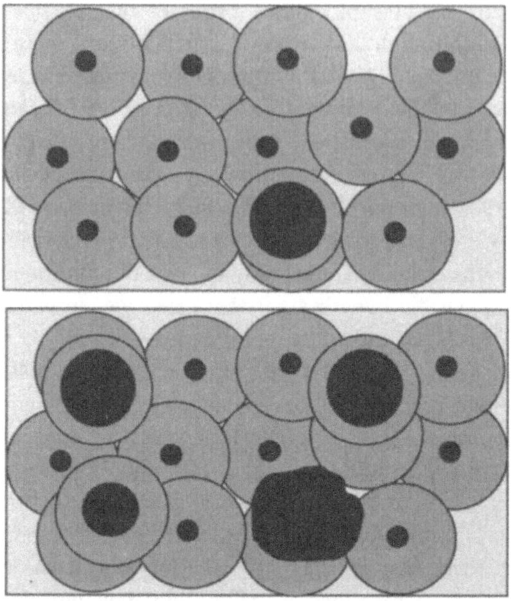

Figure 8.4. Diagram illustrating how an increase in the rate of osteonal remodeling amplifies the porosity of the bone; this also reduces the stiffness of the bone tissue.

2.4.2. Overuse: Supernormal Loading

When a bone experiences elevated loading, three responses are again observed (Woo *et al.*, 1981; Heinonen *et al.*, 2001). First, whether or not the bone is in a growing animal, the rate of periosteal bone formation will increase, which will reduce strain by producing a larger, stiffer bone. Second, osteoblastic modeling may also add bone to the endosteal and trabecular surfaces, increasing the bone's stiffness and decreasing strain. Finally, activation of intracortical remodeling will be *increased*, just as in the case of disuse. This seems illogical at first, but it serves the important function of removing fatigue damage caused by the elevated strain. That is, when a BMU is initiated in the vicinity of, and tunnels through, a site of fatigue damage, it removes and replaces everything in its path with new, undamaged bone, including any sort of physical damage. However, this removal of damage bears a cost: an increase in intracortical porosity, as in the case of disuse, that will exacerbate the elevated bone strain. The modeling responses on the bone surfaces, particularly the periosteal response, must compensate for this. When the overload is severe, the periosteal response accelerates and forms woven bone. If strains cannot be brought under control, a "stress fracture" occurs due to the combination of fatigue damage and the porosity produced by the remodeling response (Martin, 1995, 2001c).

3. Skeletal Maintenance

In the preceding paragraph on supernormal loading we came within sight of a boundary between what we have called "adaptation" and a different function of remodeling that is better called "maintenance." The difference between these functions is subtle but important. "Adaptation" of an organ implies that it was initially fit for its functional demands, but those demands changed, and adaptive modeling processes changed the organ to better fit the altered demands. That is what the mechanostat achieves by modeling and remodeling bones subjected to sub- and supernormal loading. However, remodeling goes on virtually all the time for the *maintenance* of a skeleton that is subjected to a constant routine of loading, day after day. The reason an adapted bone needs to remodel is that the strain level determined by the mechanostat is high enough that fatigue damage constantly forms and must be removed to avoid fatigue failure. Let us explore this concept in more detail.

Historically, the function of bone remodeling has been debated by proponents of two principal theories (Lacroix, 1971). In the 19th century it was proposed that remodeling served to alter the internal structure of bone to provide for better mechanical strength. Subsequently, in the first half of the 20th century, following the discovery of parathyroid hormone and the necessity of maintaining serum calcium within a narrow range of values, it was proposed that remodeling was a mechanism for transporting calcium between bone and interstitial fluid. Since then, surgeons and biomechanicians have been the principal advocates of the former theory, while endocrinologists and biologists have supported the metabolic theory. However, in recent years the role of remodeling in calcium homeostasis has been challenged, primarily because of evidence that most calcium transport in and out of bone occurs across bone surfaces that are quiescent rather than remodeling (Parfitt, 1993; Talmage *et al.*, 2000).

3.1. Fatigue Damage Activates Remodeling

At the same time, increasing attention has been drawn to the role of remodeling in removing fatigue damage, a concept introduced by Frost (1960). In fact, there is compelling evidence that fatigue damage of varying kinds, including "microcracks" about 100 μm long, occurs when bone is loaded to physiologic strain levels, and that such damage activates remodeling (Burr *et al.*, 1985, 1997; Mori and Burr, 1993; Bentolila *et al.*, 1998; Verborgt *et al.*, 2000). When one experimentally produces fatigue microcracks in living bone, new osteonal BMUs are initiated in spatial and temporal proximity to them. This is true even in rats, which do not usually remodel their cortical bone. While remodeling is also activated in a disuse state (Li *et al.*, 1990; Schaffler, 1990), and in estrogen deficiency (Wronski *et al.*, 1985; Dannucci *et al.*, 1987), the principal basis for remodeling in a skeleton not affected by these conditions may be fatigue damage (Martin, 2002). Furthermore, it is known that when normal remodeling in dogs is reduced by treatment with bisphosphonates, microdamage accumulates in significant amounts (Mashiba *et al.*, 2000).

These observations strongly suggest that remodeling is important for the maintenance of a skeleton in the face of constantly accumulating fatigue damage incurred during normal use. This hypothesis is also supported by data showing that the intensity of osteonal remodeling correlates with distinctive patterns of locomotion (Schaffler and Burr, 1984) and intensity of exercise (Burr *et al.*, 1995). One might well ask why this should be the case; why not simply make bones bigger, so that the strains are lower and such microcracks do not form? The writer proposes that the answer to this question lies in the evolutionary value of reducing skeletal weight.

3.2. Remodeling Reduces Skeletal Weight

Bone is heavy. The density of bone tissue is about 2 g/ml, approximately twice that of other tissues. Of course, bone is heavy because it is mineralized, and it is mineralized in order that it may support compressive loads. While in most animals the skeleton only weighs a small fraction of body weight (about 6% in humans), it nevertheless is an important determinant of speed, agility, and metabolic energy requirements. This is because of the close functional relationship between bone and muscle. If a bone is heavier, more muscle is required to move it at a given speed, and increased muscle and bone mass require that other organs be larger to supply their metabolic needs. Conversely, reducing skeletal weight implicitly allows the rest of the body to be lighter as well. Of course, one may point to elephants, dinosaurs, and other large vertebrates as evidence that a large body is not necessarily incompatible with evolutionary fitness, but the observation remains that the evolutionary fitness of vertebrates is broadly dependent on speed, agility, and metabolic efficiency.

Indeed, it can be argued that the need for light bones and the control of fatigue damage is greatest in the largest vertebrates. One who understood the physics behind this argument was Galileo Galilei, who observed that [quoted by Haldane (1956); see also Thompson (1956)]:

> ... it would be impossible to build up the bony structures of men, horses, or other animals so as to hold together and perform their normal functions if these animals were to be increased enormously in height; for this increase in height can be accomplished only by employing a material which is harder and stronger than usual, or by enlarging the size of the bones, thus changing their shape until the form and appearance of the animals suggest a monstrosity.

In the quote, the word "size" refers to the diameters of limbs and bones *in proportion to their lengths*.

3.3. Responsive versus Permissive Remodeling

It is useful to consider that there are two ways in which remodeling achieves a lighter, more compact skeleton (Figure 8.5). One of these mechanisms is *responsive* and the other is *permissive*. First, as noted in Section 2.4.1, when the mechanostat determines that bone strain is below the set point, it activates remodeling as one means of removing bone (the other being modeling by osteoclasts working independently of osteoblasts). This is the *responsive* mechanism for keeping bones light relative to the loads they experience, as originally described by Frost (1987). However, the mechanostat is set relatively high, so that equilibrium strains are substantial and fatigue damage is produced at a rate that would lead to fatigue failure in a fraction of the animal's lifetime if allowed to accumulate. This is where *permissive* remodeling functions. The continuous, automatic remodeling of bone whenever and wherever such damage occurs prevents the accumulation of fatigue damage and makes the effective fatigue life, if not infinite, at least longer than the animal's expected lifetime. To reiterate, *responsive remodeling* activated by strains below the mechanostat set point keeps the skeleton light and gracile, and *permissive remodeling* activated by fatigue damage allows the light, gracile skeleton to last a lifetime.

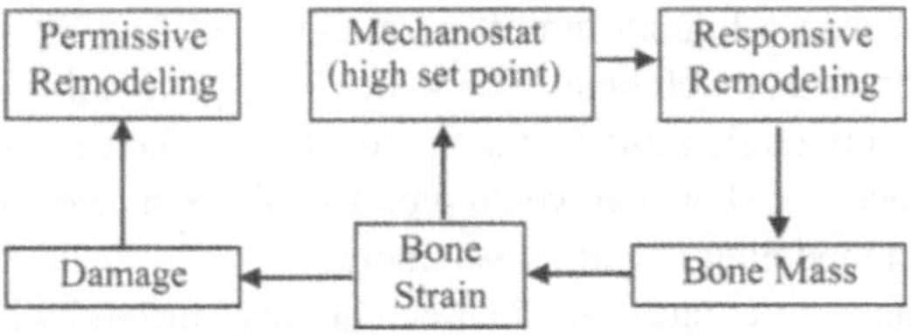

Figure 8.5. The roles of permissive and responsive remodeling in achieving a light skeleton. The mechanostat is set to a relatively high strain. When the bone strain is below this level, a disuse state is perceived and responsive remodeling is activated (along with resorptive modeling) to reduce bone mass. When the actual strain is at the desired level, the resulting fatigue damage activates permissive remodeling that prevents its accumulation.

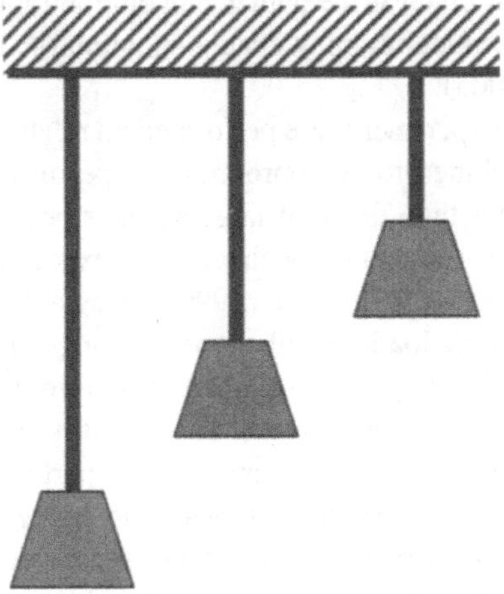

Figure 8.6. Schematic diagram illustrating an experiment by Leonardo da Vinci which demonstrated that longer specimens of iron wire are weaker. Each wire had the same diameter but their lengths varied. They were loaded by successively larger amounts of weight until they broke. Fracture loads were greater for shorter wires than for longer wires. For a given load, stress and strain were independent of length because the wires had similar cross-sectional areas and stiffnesses. The diminishment of strength was caused by longer wires having more volume, and therefore a greater probability of containing a flaw capable of initiating a fracture.

3.4. The Volume Effect on Strength and Fatigue Life

There is another reason why reducing the size of bones is important. This can be illustrated by an experiment performed by Leonardo da Vinci which demonstrated that larger structures fail at a lower strain than smaller structures (Hertzberg, 1996). Da Vinci showed this by testing the tensile strengths of groups of iron wires of identical diameter but varying lengths (Figure 8.6). Because the strain was the same throughout each wire, the only difference between the groups was the volume of material that was tested, and the strengths were inversely proportional to the volumes. This is because fractures are initiated at flaws in the material, and larger volumes are more likely to have more, and larger, defects. This principle applies to fatigue strength as well, and to bone as well as other materials (Taylor *et al.*, 1999). Thus, a rat femur will have many fewer flaws and a much greater fatigue life than a human femur repeatedly loaded to the same peak strain and containing 1,000 times as much bone. The writer believes that this is why small animals, like rats and mice, only rarely remodel their cortical bone: there is so little material in their bones that the chance of a flaw that would produce microdamage under physiologic loading, and initiate a remodeling response, is remote.

Of course, most vertebrates find their evolutionary niches by being bigger than rats, and their bones remodel. It would seem that during the course of vertebrate evolution, there were at least two options for dealing with the problem of fatigue of bone. The first was to have very robust bones with such low levels of physiologic strain that fatigue damage would be rare and the fatigue life longer than the animal's lifetime. The other option was to "arrange" for osteoclasts and osteoblasts to form BMUs and remodel away fatigue damage as it develops. This would mean that bones could be much lighter and more gracile, and it is clear that this was the path that evolution followed. A simple model of this situation suggests that remodeling may enable an animal to reduce its skeletal weight by 20% or more (Martin, 2003).

Most bone fatigue experiments are performed on relatively small specimens cut from the whole bone and machined to an appropriate shape. Just as the fatigue lives of small animals' bones are greater than those of large animals because of the volume effect, the fatigue lives of small experimental specimens are expected to be substantially longer than those of the whole bones (Taylor *et al.*, 1999). Using a finite element model of a human tibia subjected to physiologic loading without remodeling, Taylor and Kuiper (2001) found that fatigue data for small test specimens, when applied to the tibial model, predicted that the fatigue life would be only about 3 years. This result is consistent with the concept that fatigue damage removal by remodeling is an essential part of bone biology. That is, bones are usually sized so that they experience strains large enough to cause fatigue failure in a small fraction of a typical mammal's lifetime if damage is not constantly being removed by remodeling. The advantage gained is a significantly lighter skeleton.

3.5. Somatic versus Evolutionary Adaptation

As we have seen, bones adapt their structure to variations in mechanical loading, particularly during growth and development, but also throughout life. However, skeletal morphometry is also governed by a basic genetic plan for each species, and for subsets of species. For example, speaking of adults, a dachshund's skeleton is always going to be very different from a greyhound's, no matter how much one might manipulate their activities so as to change the strains in their bones and the resulting bone structure. There has been much debate about the relationships between skeletal mechanical adaptability and genetic determinants of skeletal architecture. For example, the angle of femoral neck anteversion is substantially greater in people of Polynesian ancestry than in those of European ancestry (Houghton, 1980). Presumably, this could be because the genes coding for certain aspects of skeletal development are different in these two groups of people. However, it could also conceivably be due to a culturally determined behavioral trait, such as squatting, that affects the habitual loading of the hip joint. Another possibility is that genetic selection for another anatomical characteristic altered the loading across the hip joint. For example, Houghton has suggested that Polynesians' long voyages of migration in open canoes selected for people with large, muscular bodies because of the thermodynamic advantages that this conferred in the face of exposure to the elements. A theory could be constructed that the forces about the hip joint are altered by this musculature and this produces the observed anteversion by somatic rather than genetic adaptation. The point here is that genetic and somatic adaptability operate simultaneously, and it therefore can be very difficult to sort out their individual effects.

However, and by the same token, genetic and somatic adaptations can assist one another, as Bateson (1987) has discussed at some length. The idea here is that while genetic mutations sometimes introduce an anatomic or physiologic change that provides some survival advantage for individuals of a species living in a certain environment, there are usually going to be disadvantages associated with the change as well, and somatic adaptations may ameliorate these disadvantages to the point that the advantage prevails. For example, suppose a genetic anomaly occurred in a prey species that raised the mechanostat set point to a higher strain. That would cause the long bones to be thinner and more gracile. This could allow the animal to run faster for longer periods of time using a given amount of metabolic energy. However, it would also cause the strains in these bones to be correspondingly greater (so as to match the set point), and this in turn would increase the rate of fatigue damage formation. The somatic adjustment permitting this would be an increase in the remodeling rate and the associated damage removal rate.

With these possibilities in mind, one cannot assume that such skeletal differences as those between Neanderthals and modern humans represent only genetic or somatic adaptation. The differences seem more likely to represent a complementary mixture of both kinds of adaptation.

4. Skeletal Fragility

If one accepts the premise that minimizing skeletal weight confers evolutionary advantages, and that mechanisms for achieving this are built-in to bone biology, then it follows that bone fragility is a relative term and the skeleton is constantly at some risk of becoming light to the point of excessive fragility. The putative existence of a mechanostat set point in the genetic coding of bone cells implies that variations in this coding will cause some individuals to have bones of increased gracility, and others of greater robusticity. The mean value of this set point within the population of a particular species should be determined by the relative survivability of individuals having exceptionally high or low set points *in the context of other factors*. In this context, skeletal fragility is but the other side of skeletal lightness, and not an absolute state of inferiority.

Of course, skeletal fragility may vary for many other reasons than variations in the individual's genetically determined mechanostat set point. Obviously, diseases may render the skeleton frail in various ways, such as a tumor that disrupts structure, or Paget's disease, in which a virus is thought to cause a pathologically aggressive and faulty form of remodeling. However, two other causes of fragility are of broader anthropological interest. First, the problem may be a genetic error in the coding for a component of bone tissue. The archetypical example of this would be osteogenesis imperfecta, a group of bone diseases caused by a variety of defects in the coding for Type I collagen, and leading to skeletal fragility of great variability, depending on the particular error. Similarly, variants of the genetic coding for other structural molecules, such as proteoglycans, may affect bone's mechanical properties. Such errors in the composition of the bone tissue will frequently involve weakness in fatigue and be manifest as excessive microdamage and its associated remodeling. Thus, the concept of fatigue damage removal by remodeling as basic to bone biology is also important in understanding the fragility of pathologic bone. Furthermore, it is useful to hypothesize that the severity of the effects of these errors approximates a continuum, from being lethal at birth to slight variabilities in bone mechanical properties throughout life. At the latter end of the scale, whether or not an individual's skeletal phenotype is "good" or "bad" may be largely circumstantial. For example, a particular individual may have bones that resist traumatic fracture exceptionally well, but are more susceptible to fatigue damage. From an evolutionary perspective the question of phenotypic superiority then becomes dependent on the environmental circumstances that the skeleton faces, including cultural as well as physical features. The significance of these kinds of genetically-determined fragilities and variabilities may be magnified in small population groups.

These concepts regarding the genetic determinants of an individual's bone strength do not address the causes of skeletal fragility of greatest interest in modern society: age-related and menopause-related bone loss. There are a number of possible contributors to age-related bone loss, including reduced activity among older individuals and age-related diminishment of steroid levels in men as well as women. Because age-related bone loss is more severe in women than in men, the emphasis here will be on the fundamental connection between estrogen and the mechanostat, and its postmenopausal implications.

4.1. The Mechanostat and Sexual Dimorphism

It has long been clear that sex hormones influence skeletal growth and development, and in recent years more has been learned about the basics of sexual dimorphism and its relationship to the mechanostat. Studies in rats show that testosterone and estrogen act on the growth plate to accelerate and diminish, respectively, longitudinal bone growth, so that males are generally larger than females. These two hormones also act differentially on the endosteal and periosteal surfaces: testosterone increases periosteal bone formation and estrogen increases endosteal bone formation (Turner *et al.*, 1989, 1990a,b). Broadly speaking, this distinction has fundamental effects on skeletal size, strength, and adaptability in male and female vertebrates.

These gender-specific modeling effects are consistent with the results of Garn's (1970) early studies of endosteal and periosteal apposition in the cortex of the human metacarpal (Figure 8.7). In men, there is a steady increase in both periosteal and endosteal radius during growth, following which there is a steady state until middle age, when slow radial expansion occurs both periosteally and endosteally. (There is some indication that these trends reverse themselves in old age.) In females, on the other hand, the endosteal expansion during growth is interrupted and reversed at menarche (MA), so that substantial bone is added to the endosteal surface as circulating estrogen levels rise during the final years of puberty. This bone is retained until the age of menopause (MP), when it begins to steadily resorb. These data for humans are consistent with the rat data, at least insofar as both indicate that estrogen acts to cause bone formation on the endosteal surface, but not on the periosteal surface.

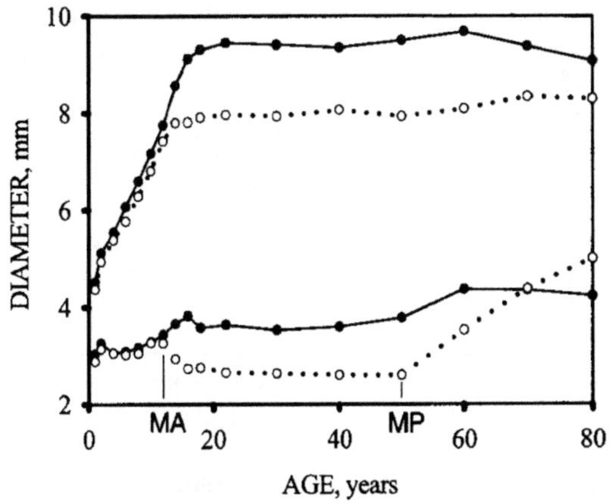

Figure 8.7. Graph showing how the endosteal and periosteal diameters of the human third metacarpal bone change as functions of age in males (solid lines) and females (dotted lines). After data by Garn (1970) and a similar graph by Turner (1991).

4.2. Mechanical Priorities in Male and Female Bones

The fact that males add bone to the periosteal surface and females to the endosteal surface during puberty has important mechanical implications. The resistance of long bone cortices to bending and torsion is proportional to a geometric variable known as the "second moment" of the cross-sectional area. Simply put, this means that material far from the center of the bone cross-section contributes substantially more toward stiffness and strength than material near the center. Because the medullary canal is at the center of the bone, and the periosteal membrane defines the limit of a bone's cross-section, these anatomic features acquire mechanical significance. By promoting periosteal formation, testosterone builds bone strength more than estrogen. On the other hand, by promoting endosteal bone formation, estrogen adds bone that is of less mechanical consequence *if it is lost*. This is important because the bone added to girls' endosteal surfaces during puberty is resorbed during times of bone loss associated with reproduction, including lactation, disuse, and following menopause. Thus, this system may be seen as a compromise between the mechanical and metabolic demands on the skeletons of female mammals. (Similar but more complex endocortical compromises occur in vertebrate mothers that lay eggs with calcified shells and therefore experience even more critical calcium demands.)

4.3. Estrogen and the Mechanostat Set Point

Now consider another set of data. Figure 8.8 shows how whole body bone mineral content (BMC) and lean body mass (LBM) increase with age in girls and boys (Schiessl *et al.*, 1998). Each point on the graph represents the means of these two variables for a group of children of the same age and gender. One sees that BMC increases in linear proportion to LBM throughout skeletal development in boys, consistent with the observation that most bone loading is due to muscle forces, which are approximately proportional to LBM. However, the corresponding plot for girls shows a distinct increase in slope near the

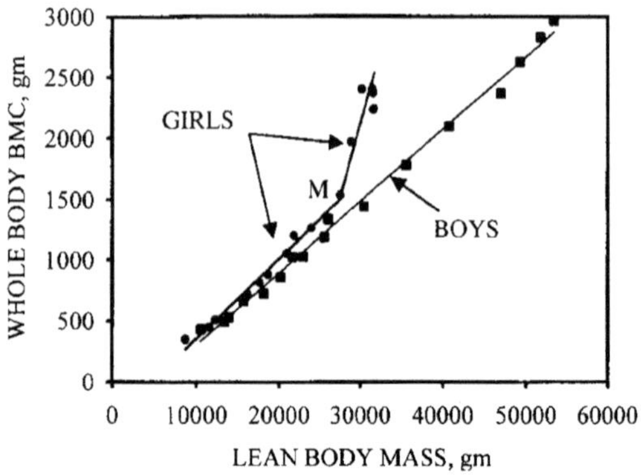

Figure 8.8. Graph showing the relationship between whole body bone mass and LBM in girls and boys as they grow to skeletal maturity. Each point represents a group of girls or boys of similar age. Boys exhibit a linear increase in bone mass as increasing muscle mass applies more and more force to the skeleton. Girls' bone mass increases in similar proportionality until the age of menarche (M), when the slope becomes steeper. Data re-plotted from Scheissl *et al.* (1998).

onset of puberty, when estrogen levels rise. This result is consistent with Frost's (1992) hypothesis that estrogen acts to lower the set point of the skeleton's mechanostat control system for strain, increasing the bone mass associated with normal loading. (It is noteworthy that the descriptions of gender distinctions in age-related bone mass and structure presented in this Chapter are consistent with data for subadult human ribs reported by Streeter and Stout, Chapter 6, this volume.)

Frost's hypothesis is further supported by data showing that mechanical loading and estrogen act synergistically on collagen synthesis in cultured rat ulnas (Cheng *et al.*, 1996), and more recent data indicating that estrogen and mechanical strain act through a common pathway in osteoblast-like cells (Zaman *et al.*, 2000). In these experiments, when estrogen was present, less mechanical stimulus was required for a given response. If this fundamental property is present in functional osteocytes and osteoblasts, a mechanism for estrogenic control of the mechanostat set point is at hand. It is postulated that the cells of the osteocyte-bone lining cell syncytium have internal estrogen receptors, and when estrogen binds to these receptors in sufficient quantities, the transduction of mechanical strain into modeling and remodeling responses on adjacent bone surfaces is altered. In the terminology of control theory, the "set point" of the system is altered, so that the equilibrium strain is decreased. Consequently, bone is added and bone strains fall to match the set point. However, there is apparently an as yet undefined aspect of this system that causes this response to occur primarily on bone surfaces in contact with marrow, so that bone is added endosteally rather than periosteally. This bone is then available to be resorbed during lactation and provide calcium to the child's skeleton.

4.4. Menopause, the Set Point, and Postmenopausal Fragility

Subsequently, at menopause, when circulating estrogen levels decline, the mechanostat set point would be expected to rise. This would make what were previously "normal" bone strains lower than the set point, and the response would be essentially the same as that in a disuse state. Thus, this theory provides a straight-forward explanation for postmenopausal bone loss. It also reflects on the question of the evolutionary forces that led to the virtually unique phenomenon of menopause in humans. In one way or another, theories of menopause are based on the concept that limiting the child-bearing portion of women's lives improved their ability to pass their genes on to future generations (Bogin and Smith, 1996; Hawkes *et al.*, 1998; Peccei, 2001). Apparently, the advantages of menopause, whatever they may have been, outweighed the disadvantages of postmenopausal bone loss.

The etiology of postmenopausal fracturing in our own time is bound up with such ancillary factors as calcium-deficient diets and minimal load-bearing exercise. Surely, the nutritional and skeletal loading conditions under which menopause evolved must have been quite different, and one can think of additional reasons why the significant problem that postmenopausal fractures present in modern society may not have existed during the evolution of menopause. Almost certainly, postmenopausal activity levels would have been greater than in today's society, so that the difference between the postmenopausal, estrogen-deficient set point and the daily strain stimulus would not have been so great as for modern women, and less bone would have been lost as estrogen levels declined. Also, the demands of lactation on female's skeletons may have been substantially greater than today, due to more pregnancies and/or longer nursing periods, further diminishing the relative disadvantage of later postmenopausal bone loss. In any case, the concept of estrogen and mechanical loading acting on bone mass through a common pathway provides an important avenue for thinking about the skeletal factors that would have been at work during the evolution of menopause.

5. Summary

This chapter has presented the author's interpretation of some of the current thinking about functional adaptability and fragility of the skeleton. Two key concepts have been emphasized. First, because bone is substantially heavier than other tissues, it is advantageous to closely control skeletal weight. This is achieved by adaptive bone modeling and remodeling under the control of a so-called mechanostat, a physiological device that is distributed throughout all bone tissue in the form of the osteocyte-bone lining cell syncytium. However, as evolutionary pressures for reducing skeletal weight drove the mechanostat strain set point upward, the result was fatigue damage that strongly limited the skeleton's functional lifetime. Vertebrates solved this problem by remodeling bone to remove fatigue damage as it occurs, and this is the second key concept. Together, these physiologic systems for modeling and remodeling constitute the fundamental machinery of bone biology.

The advantage of having a light skeleton is constantly threatened by the disadvantage of its relative fragility. Thus, a third key concept is that skeletal fragility is not just a problem of pathology, but is a fundamental risk inherent when a system functions at the edge of a safe domain. Along with the other genomic perturbations that vertebrate species exhibit in the process of evolving ways to better compete for their existence, the skeleton is constantly being pushed toward and away from this edge by variations in its structural, adaptive, and maintenance physiology. Some cases of skeletal fragility must represent instances in which a genomic determinant of skeletal lightness was pushed too far. Certainly, this has occurred in evolving humans as much as in other vertebrates.

Competing physiologic demands are obviously different in males and females, and these are manifest in the skeleton as much as any other organ system. Vertebrate reproduction requires the pregnant female to transfer a substantial portion of her skeletal resources to her offspring, and this demand is increased by lactation in mammalian females. It is becoming clear that part of the physiologic system that enables this is a mechanism by which estrogen acts on the pubertal female's mechanostat to store bone material over and above that needed for mechanical function. This extra bone is placed where it has minimal mechanical usefulness, so that the mechanical consequences of its loss are minimized. Furthermore, the loss is temporary because when the demands of each child's pregnancy and lactation have ceased, estrogen drives the mechanostat to add extra bone once again.

Whatever the advantages were that led to the evolution of menopause in human females, the fact that this change of state included a severe diminishment in estrogen production meant that postmenopausal bone loss would occur. Even though the lost bone is primarily from endosteal and trabecular surfaces, where the mechanical consequences are less serious than periosteal bone loss would be, the long-term effects are, in many modern women, disastrous. An important question for anthropologists is, "To what extent was this true in the long and varied history of human societies, and what adaptive calculus allowed the postmenopausal changing of the mechanostat set point to be permissible in the evolution of menopause?"

Acknowledgments

This work was supported by NIH grants AR 41644 and AR 47205, and by the Doris Linn Chair of Bone Biology.

References

Aarden, E.M., Burger, E.H., and Nijweide, P.J. (1994). Function of osteocytes in bone. *Bone* **55**, 287–299.

Bateson, G. (1987). *Steps to an Ecology of Mind.* Jason Aronson Inc., Northvale, NJ.

Bentolila, V., Boyce, T.M., Fyhrie, D.P., Drumb, R., Skerry, T.M., and Schaffler, M.B. (1998). Intracortical remodeling in adult rat long bones after fatigue loading. *Bone* **23**, 275–281.

Bogin, B. and Smith, B.H. (1996). Evolution of the human life cycle. *Am. J. Hum. Biol.* **8**, 703–716.

Burr, D.B., Forwood, M.K., Fyhrie, D.P., Martin, R.B., Schaffler, M.S., and Turner, C.H. (1997). Bone microdamage and skeletal fragility in osteoporotic and stress fractures. *J. Bone Miner. Res.* **12**, 6–15.

Burr, D.B., Martin, R.B., Schaffler, M.B., and Radin, E.L. (1985). Bone remodeling in response to *in vivo* fatigue microdamage. *J. Biomech.* **18**, 189–200.

Burr, D.B., Yoshikawa, T., and Ruff, C.B. (1995). Moderate exercise increases intracortical activation frequency in old dogs. *Trans. Orthop. Res. Soc.* **20**, 204.

Cheng, M.Z., Zaman, G., Rawlinson, S.C., Suswillo, R.F., and Lanyon, L.E. (1996). Mechanical loading and sex hormone interactions in organ cultures of rat ulna. *J. Bone Miner. Res.* **11**, 502–511.

Dannucci, G.A., Martin, R.B., and Patterson-Buckendahl, P. (1987). Ovariectomy and trabecular bone remodeling in the dog. *Calcif. Tissue Int.* **40**, 194–199.

Donahue, H.J. (1998). Gap junctional intercellular communication in bone: A cellular basis for the mechanostat set point. *Calcif. Tissue Int.* **62**, 85–88.

Frost, H.M. (1960). Presence of microscopic cracks in vivo in bone. *Henry Ford Hosp. Med. Bull.* **8**, 25–35.

Frost, H.M. (1987). Bone "mass" and the "mechanostat": A proposal. *Anat. Rec.* **219**, 1–9.

Frost, H.M. (1992). The role of changes in mechanical usage set points in the pathogenesis of osteoporosis. *J. Bone Miner. Res.* **7**, 253–261.

Garn, S.M. (1970). *The Earlier Gain and the Later Loss of Cortical Bone.* Charles C. Thomas, Springfield, IL.

Haldane, J.B.S. (1956). On being the right size. In J.R. Newman (ed.), *The World of Mathematics.* Simon and Shuster New York, pp. 952–956.

Hawkes, K., O'Connell, J.F., Jones, N.G.B., Alverez, H., and Charnov, E.L. (1998). Grandmothering, menopause, and the evolution of human life histories. *Proc. Natl. Acad. Sci.* **95**, 1336–1339.

Heinonen, A., Sievanen, H., Kyrolainen, H., Perttunen, J., and Kannus, P. (2001). Mineral mass, size, and estimated mechanical strength of triple jumpers' lower limb. *Bone* **29**, 279–285.

Hertzberg, R.W. (1996). *Deformation and fracture mechanics of engineering materials.* John Wiley and Sons, New York.

Houghton, P. (1980). *The First New Zealanders.* Hodder and Stoughton, Auckland.

Knothe-Tate, M.L., Steck, R., Forwood, M.R., and Niederer, P. (2000). In vivo demonstration of load-induced fluid flow in the rat tibia and its potential implications for processes associated with functional adaptation. *J. Exp. Biol.* **203**, 2737–2745.

Lacroix, P. (1971). The internal remodeling of bones. In G.H. Bourne (ed.), *The Biochemistry and Physiology of Bone.* Academic Press, New York.

Lanyon, L.E. (1993). Osteocytes, strain detection, bone modeling and remodeling. *Calcif. Tissue Int.* 53 (suppl.), S102–S106.

Li, X.J., Jee, W.S.S., Chow, S.Y., and Woodbury, D.M. (1990). Adaptation of cancellous bone to aging and immobilization: A single photon absorptiometry and histomorphometric study. *Anat. Rec.* **227**, 12–24.

Martin, R.B. (1995). A mathematical model for fatigue damage repair and stress fracture in osteonal bone. *J. Orthop. Res.* **13**, 309–316.

Martin, R.B. (2000). Toward a unifying theory of bone remodeling. *Bone* **26**, 1–6.

Martin, R.B. (2002). Is all cortical bone remodeling initiated by microdamage? *Bone* **30**, 8–13.

Martin, R.B. (2003). Fatigue damage, remodeling, and the minimization of skeletal weight. *Journal of Theoretical Biology* **220**, 271–276.

Martin, R.B. (2001c). The role of bone remodeling in preventing or promoting stress fractures. In D.B. Burr and C. Milgrom (eds), Musculoskeletal fatigue and stress fractures. CRC Press, Boca Raton, FL, pp. 183–201.

Martin, R.B., Burr, D.B., and Sharkey, N.S. (1998). Skeletal Tissue Mechanics. Springer-Verlag, New York.

Mashiba, T., Hirano, T., Turner, C.H., Forwood, M.R., Johnston, C.C., and Burr, D.B. (2000). Suppressed bone turnover by bisphosphonates increases microdamage accumulation and reduces some biomechanical properties in dog rib. *J. Bone Miner. Res.* **15**, 613–620.

Mori, S. and Burr, D.B. (1993). Increased intracortical remodeling following fatigue damage. *Bone* **14**, 103–109.

Parfitt, A.M. (1993). Calcium homeostasis. In G.R. Mundy and Martin T.J. (eds), *Physiology and Pharmacology of Bone.* Springer-Verlag, Berlin, pp. 1–65.

Parfitt, A.M. (1994). Osteonal and hemi-osteonal remodeling: The spatial and temporal framework for signal traffic in adult human bone. *J. Cell. Biochem.* **55**, 273–286.

Pauwels, F. (1980). *Biomechanics of the Locomotor Apparatus. Contributions on the Functional Anatomy of the Locomotor Apparatus.* Springer-Verlag, New York.

Peccei, J.S. (2001). A critique of the grandmother hypotheses: Old and new. *Am. J. Hum. Biol.* **13**, 434–452.

Roesler, H. (1981). Some historical remarks on the theory of cancellous bone structue (Wolff's law). In S.C. Cowin (ed.), *Mechanical Properties of Bone.* American Society of Mechanical Engineers, New York, pp. 27–42.

Roesler, H. (1987). The history of some fundamental concepts in bone biomechanics. *J. Biomech.* **20**, 1025–1034.

Roux, W. (1881). *Der zuchtende Kampf der Teile, oder die 'Teilauslese' im Organismus (Theorie der 'funktionellen Anpassung').* Wilhelm Engelmann, Leipzig.

Schaffler, M.B. (1990). Immobilization induced bone loss: quantitative histological studies of cortical bone resorption. *Trans. Orthop. Res. Soc.* **15**, 187.

Schaffler, M.B. and Burr, D.B. (1984). Primate cortical bone microstructure: Relationship to locomotion. *Am. J. Phys. Anthropol.* **65**, 191–197.

Schiessl, H., Frost, H.M., and Jee, W.S.S. (1998). Estrogen and bone-muscle strength and mass relationships. *Bone* **22**, 1–6.

Skerry, T.M., Bitensky, L., Chayen, J., and Lanyon, L.E. (1989). Early strain-related changes in enzyme activity in osteocytes following bone loading *in vivo. J. Bone Miner. Res.* **4**, 783–788.

Talmage, R.V., Lester, G.E., and Hirsch, P.F. (2000). Parathyroid hormone and plasma calcium control: An editorial. *J. Musculoskeletal Neuronal Interactions* **1**, 121–126.

Taylor, D. and Kuiper, J.-H. (2001). The prediction of stress fractures using a "stressed volume" concept. *J. Orthop. Res.* **19**, 919–926.

Taylor, D., O'Brien, F., Prina-Mello, A., Ryan, C., O'Reilly, P., and Lee, T.C. (1999). Compression data on bovine bone confirms that a "stressed volume" principle explains the variability of fatigue strength results. *J. Biomech.* **32**, 1199–1203.

Thompson, D.A.W. (1956). On Magnitude. In J.R. Newman (ed.), *The World of Mathematics*. Simon and Shuster, New York, 1001–1046.

Turner, C.H. (1991). Editorial: Do estrogens increase bone formation? *Bone* **12**, 305–306.

Turner, C.H. and Forwood, M.R. (1995). What role does the osteocyte network play in bone adaptation? *Bone* **16**, 283–285.

Turner, R.T., Colvard, D.S., and Spelsberg, T.C. (1990a). Estrogen inhibition of periosteal bone formation in rat long bones: Down-regulation of gene expression for bone matrix proteins. *Endocrinology* **127**, 1346–1351.

Turner, R.T., Hannon, K.S., Demers, L.M., Buchanan, J., and Bell, N.H. (1989). Differential effects of gonadal function on bone histomorphometry in male and female rats. *J. Bone Miner. Res.* **4**, 557–563.

Turner, R.T., Wakley, G.K., and Hannon, K.S. (1990b). Differential effects of androgens on cortical bone histomorphometry in gonadectomized male and female rats. *J. Orthop. Res.* **8**, 612–617.

Uhthoff, H.K. (1982). The influence of mechanical factors of the activity of the three bone envelopes. *Acta Orthop. Belg.* **48**, 563–575.

Verborgt, O., Gibson, G.J., and Schaffler, M.B. (2000). Loss of osteocyte integrity in association with microdamage and bone remodeling after fatigue in vivo. *J. Bone Miner. Res.* **15**, 60–67.

Weinbaum, S., Cowin, S.C., and Zeng, Y. (1994). A model for the excitation of osteocytes by mechanical loading-induced bone fluid shear stresses. *J. Biomech.* **27**, 339–360.

Wolff, J. (1892a). *Das Gasetz der Transformation der Knochen*. Hirschwald, Berlin.

Wolff, J. (1892b). *The Law of Bone Remodeling*. Springer-Verlag, Berlin.

Woo, S.L.Y., Gomez, M.A., Amiel, D., Ritter, M.A., Gelberman, R.H., and Akeson, W.H. (1981). The effects of exercise on the biomechanical and biochemical properties of swine digital flexor tendons. *J. Biomech. Eng.* **103**, 51–56.

Wronski, T.J., Lowry, P.L., Walsh, C.C., and Ignaszewski, L.A. (1985). Skeletal alterations in ovariectomized rats. *Calcif. Tissue Int.* **37**, 324–328.

Zaman, G., Cheng, M.Z., Jessop, H.L., White, R., and Lanyon, L.E. (2000). Mechanical strain activates estrogen response elements in bone cells. *Bone* **27**, 233–239.

9

Effects of Vitamin D on Bone and Natural Selection of Skin Color: How Much Vitamin D Nutrition are We Talking About?

Reinhold Vieth

1. Introduction

Until the 1990s, the criterion for appropriate vitamin D nutrition was simply the absence of overt rickets or osteomalacia (Blumberg *et al.*, 1963). Now, circulating 25-hydroxyvitamin D [25(OH)D] concentrations are the appropriate measure of vitamin D nutritional status (Standing Committee on the Scientific Evaluation of Dietary Reference Intakes, 1997). It is now possible to make more quantitative comparisons of vitamin D nutrition through primate and human evolution, and to draw inferences about how differences in vitamin D nutrition may have affected susceptibility to disease.

Authentic vitamin D comes in two forms, vitamin D_3 and D_2. Vitamin D_2, ergocalciferol, can be synthesized by exposing a fat extract of yeast to UV light. However, no metabolite of vitamin D_2 is normally detectable in the blood of humans or primates (Marx *et al.*, 1989; Trang *et al.*, 1998). The present discussion focuses on vitamin D_3, cholecalciferol, the natural, physiological form of vitamin D in mammals. Vitamin D_3 (from here on, vitamin D) is the natural, and more potent form of vitamin D in all primate species including humans (Marx *et al.*, 1989; Trang *et al.*, 1998). Vitamin D is the raw material for production of the hormone 1,25-dihydroxyvitamin D, synthesized and released by the kidney according to the needs of calcium homeostasis (Figure 9.1). For this, vitamin D itself plays a role as a structural substrate; similar to the way cholesterol is the structural raw material for other steroid hormones. For vitamin D, the intervening metabolite, 25(OH)D, is synthesized in liver mitochondria and liver microsomes. 25(OH)D has a biological half-life of about 2 months, and is thought to be relatively inactive. Because of these features,

---

Reinhold Vieth • Department of Laboratory Medicine and Pathobiology, University of Toronto, and Mount Sinai Hospital, Toronto.

Bone Loss and Osteoporosis: An Anthropological Perspective, edited by Sabrina C. Agarwal and Sam D. Stout. Kluwer Academic/Plenum Publishers, New York, 2003.

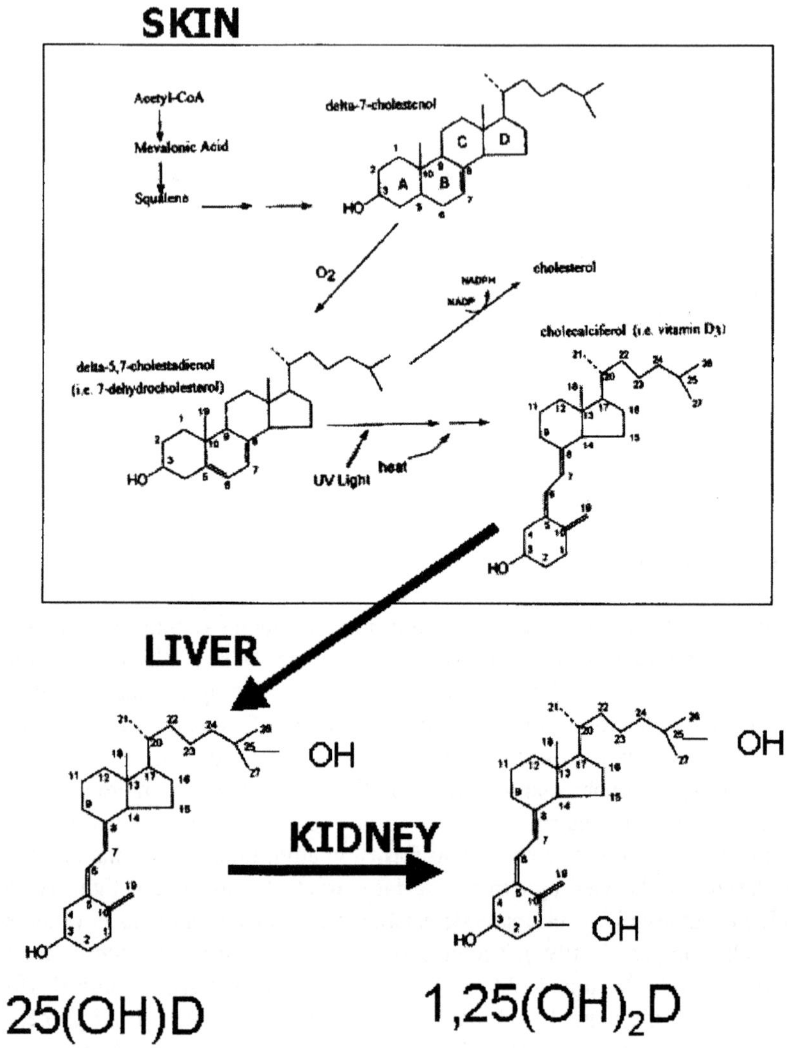

Figure 9.1. The skin of mammals actively synthesizes cholesterol. 7-dehydrocholesterol is an immediate precursor of cholesterol. 7-dehydrocholesterol present within the skin and in the oils secreted by skin is unstable. Part of the molecule breaks open during exposure to ultraviolet B light (285–310 nm), and this results in the nonenzymic generation of cholecalciferol. Within 1–3 days, the vitamin D is acted upon by 25-hydroxylase enzyme in the liver to produce 25(OH)D, the inactive, long-term storage form of vitamin D. The kidney uses some 25(OH)D to generate the hormone, $1,25(OH)_2D$, the levels of which are about 1,000 fold lower than those of 25(OH)D. The circulating level of hormone is regulated independently of vitamin D nutrition, and increases in response to the need for calcium. $1,25(OH)_2D$ stimulates the active transport of calcium through the intestinal mucosa. Recently, 25(OH)D-1-hydroxylase has been found in other tissues, and its presence may provide a mechanism through which the vitamin D nutrition can affect aspects of health beyond just calcium homeostasis.

25(OH)D has recently been acknowledged as the acceptable way to assess vitamin D nutritional status (Standing Committee on the Scientific Evaluation of Dietary Reference Intakes, 1997).

Primates do not normally need vitamin D in their food, because sufficient sunlight makes it impossible to become vitamin D deficient. For humans, the "evolution" of vitamin D into a nutrient stems from the shift of humans away from the equator, from increased pollution, and from the cultures that avoid exposing skin surface to sunshine. This includes the use of clothing.

Vitamin D may have been a primordial steroid-like hormone in living things, and its effect was to signal exposure to ultraviolet light. Essentially all fungi, plants, and animals produce provitamin D, molecules that can become vitamin D (Holick, 1992). These are converted to previtamin D by exposure to sunlight (ultraviolet light B, 215–240 nm). Species of all vertebrate classes require vitamin D, and this must be metabolized to $1,25(OH)_2D$ before it exhibits biological activity (Henry and Norman, 1975; Holick, 1992).

2. Skin and Vitamin D Uptake

The skin is a major site of cholesterol synthesis. Cholesterol and its precursors are required for integrity of skin-cell membranes, and they are components of the oil secreted by skin into fur and hair. Vitamin D is generated in the skin by an unregulated process that involves only the dermal enzymes needed to synthesize cholesterol. Most of the vitamin D that is used for vitamin supplements and for milk fortification is derived from a form of fur—the lipid obtained from the defatting of lamb and sheep wool. This fat extract is exposed to UV, and the vitamin D is purified for nutritional use. When 7-dehydrocholesterol, a precursor in the synthetic path to cholesterol, is exposed to ultraviolet B light, the B-ring of the steroid molecule is split open between carbon 9 and carbon 10, to produce a secosteroid (a fractured steroid). It takes about 24 hr for this previtamin D to isomerize spontaneously into the mature vitamin D_3 that is useful for the body. If there is sustained exposure to ultraviolet light, the previtamin D and vitamin D in skin deteriorate to tachysterol and other compounds. This photodecomposition explains why excess sun exposure does not cause vitamin D intoxication. It takes 1–4 days after sun exposure before increases in vitamin D are apparent in the circulation (Haddad *et al.*, 1993).

As humans age, the skin loses capacity for vitamin D production because its rate of cholesterol synthesis is less. In people over 70 years of age, a given amount of sun exposure may generate only a fourth of the vitamin D achieved in young individuals. Furthermore, the intensity of ultraviolet light from the sun diminishes during winter months. For example at the latitude of Boston (42°N), there is not enough outdoor ultraviolet intensity between November and February to generate any vitamin D in the skin, and this phenomenon is worse at higher latitudes (Webb *et al.*, 1988).

Absorption of vitamin D generated within the skin into the blood is facilitated by a concentration of a vitamin D-binding protein (DBP) that exists at remarkably high concentration, compared to specific carriers for lipid-soluble hormones (Bikle and Pillai, 1993; Vieth, 1994). If vitamin D is consumed orally, it is absorbed as if it were cholesterol, in chylomicrons that deliver lipids to adipose tissue, and from which chylomicron remnants are cleared by the liver, making vitamin D available for metabolism (Haddad *et al.*, 1993).

Eventually, all vitamin D and its metabolites circulate bound to DBP, a protein that can be taken up selectively by the kidney and probably some other tissues expressing megalin, which is a translocating protein and a member of the low density lipoprotein (LDL) receptor family (Nykjaer *et al.*, 1999). Still, much of the 25(OH)D and $1,25(OH)_2D$ enters cells by diffusion of that small proportion of the seco-steroid present in the unbound, "free" form. This follows the classic model by which other fat-soluble hormones also enter target tissues (Vieth, 1994).

2.1. Metabolism of Vitamin D

Enzymes in human liver microsomes and mitochondria convert vitamin D to 25(OH)D. The concentration of this metabolite reflects vitamin D nutritional status. The kidney functions as an endocrine gland synthesizing and secreting the hormone, $1,25(OH)_2D$. Production of $1,25(OH)_2D$ is stimulated by low circulating calcium, low phosphate, and high parathyroid hormone (PTH). $1,25(OH)_2D$ stimulates the active transport of calcium through intestinal mucosa. Together with calcium, $1,25(OH)_2D_3$ suppresses the parathyroid gland. Together with PTH, $1,25(OH)_2D$ regulates both bone resorption and bone formation, thereby maintaining normal bone and mineral physiology.

Normal $1,25(OH)_2D$ production rates range between 0.2 and 2 μg per day. The RDA for vitamin D from infants to adults under 50 years is 2.5 μg per day (200 IU/day) (Standing Committee on the Scientific Evaluation of Dietary Reference Intakes, 1997), but the evidence points to a far higher total need for vitamin D in adults, from both sun and diet (Vieth, 1999).

3. What is a Lack of Vitamin D?

The clinical decision level for poor vitamin D nutrition is a low 25(OH)D, less than 25 nmol/L (10 ng/mL). Levels below this are considered diagnostically causal of rickets and osteomalacia. The published 25(OH)D levels in children with frank nutritional rickets range as high as 20 nmol/L (8 ng/mL) (Chesney *et al.*, 1981; Garabedian *et al.*, 1983). However, milder forms of vitamin D "insufficiency" are starting to be recognized. In particular, the consequence of long-term vitamin D insufficiency is osteoporosis (Heaney, 1999), a long-term negative balance in the equilibrium of calcium with the skeleton.

It is wrong to assume that simply because individuals live at southern latitudes, they need less vitamin D supplementation—some people actively avoid exposing skin to the sun, and the supply of dermal vitamin D is a function of sun exposure and amount of skin surface exposed.

Calcium metabolism reflects only one aspect of vitamin D action. In cell culture systems *in vitro*, $1,25(OH)_2D$ acts on many tissues that are not related to calcium metabolism, including the hematopoietic and lymphatic systems, skeletal muscle, vascular smooth muscle, skin, reproductive tissues, the brain, and spinal cord

(Walters *et al.*, 1992; McGrath, 2001). Several tissues possess 25(OH)D-1-hydroxylase; therefore, they have the ability to produce their own $1{,}25(OH)_2D$ (Hewison *et al.*, 2000). This hormone production capability for local regulation of cellular activity is known as a paracrine control system (Dusso *et al.*, 1990; Hewison *et al.*, 2000). Such paracrine mechanisms can explain why vitamin D nutrition is related to various cellular mechanisms and their effects on many aspects of human health (Table 9.1). Walters *et al.* (1992) have concluded "vitamin D deficiency is a heterogeneous collection of physiologic conditions". In the most general sense, vitamin D deficiency is a state in which the supply of vitamin D is not sufficient for the optimal operation of at least one function that depends upon it.

Table 9.1. Diseases Known to be, or Implicated as being Prevented by Greater Vitamin D Nutrition or Skin UV Exposure

Disease	Type of evidence supporting the association	Reference
Rickets	Long established, causal, and preventive	
Osteomalacia	Long established, causal, and preventive	
Osteoporosis	Direct, controlled studies that vitamin D prevents loss of bone density and lessens fracture risk	Chapuy *et al.*, 1992; Dawson-Hughes *et al.*, 1991; Dawson-Hughes *et al.*, 1997
Blood-pressure regulation	Epidemiological and interventional data	Krause *et al.*, 1998; Pfeifer *et al.*, 2000; Rostand, 1997
Risk of diabetes	Epidemiological and case-control data	Eva, 1999; Stene *et al.*, 2000
Progression osteoarthritis	Epidemiological, cross-sectional studies	Lane *et al.*, 1999; McAlindon *et al.*, 1996
Diminished intra-uterine growth	Presumed effect	Fuller, 2000
Resistance to pneumonia	Epidemiological association with rickets	Muhe *et al.*, 1997
Multiple sclerosis, occurrence and progression	Epidemiological data and lab effects on tissue	Embry *et al.*, 2000; Hayes *et al.*, 1997; Mahon *et al.*, 2001
Prevention of tuberculosis,	Epidemiological data and lab effects on tissue	Chan, 2000; Douglas *et al.*, 1998
Protection against cancers		
Breast	Epidemiological data and lab effects on tissue	Garland *et al.*, 1999
Prostate	Epidemiological and lab effects on tissue	Hsu *et al.*, 2001; Schwartz *et al.*, 1997; Schwartz *et al.*, 1998
Large bowel	Epidemiological and cross-sectional data based on latitude and serum 25(OH)D	Garland *et al.*, 1999

There is growing epidemiological evidence, which amounts only to circumstantial evidence at this time, that vitamin D nutrition affects many diseases not previously associated with this nutrient. These diseases are summarized in Table 9.1. The list is so long that it is probably hard for some readers to believe that one nutrient could have so much attributed to it. However, vitamin D is a very unusual nutrient. It's most abundant form in the circulation, 25(OH)D, serves as the raw material that many tissues need for paracrine hormone control of their own cellular functions. Furthermore, the capacity for $1,25(OH)_2D$ production by the kidney and other tissues is not just a function of the amount of 1-hydroxylase enzyme. *In vivo* $1,25(OH)_2D$ production is determined by mass action. For example, a doubling in the concentration of 25(OH)D results in double the rate at which a given amount of 1-hydroxylase produces the hormone (Vieth *et al.*, 1990). I am not aware of any other hormone-generating system so severely limited by the supply of substrate, except in the case of severe iodine deficiency, and its effect on thyroid hormone production. The situation where vitamin D supply became limiting to production of the hormone made from it did not exist during early human development. Sunshine was never lacking, and it is certain that humans were not designed through evolution to wear clothes. Exposure of the face and hands exposes a mere 5% of our skin surface area, and many modern humans avoid exposing even that to the sun. If the sun provides a nutrient, most of us are depriving ourselves of it. Because this is so prevalent, we assume this to be our normal state of vitamin D nutrition.

4. "Normal" Requirements for Calcium and Vitamin D

Vitamin D and calcium are the key nutrients favoring bone growth and preservation throughout life. Calcium alone has never been shown to prevent fractures. However, calcium combined with 17.5–20 μg/d vitamin D, results in lower fracture risk in the elderly (Chapuy *et al.*, 1992; Dawson-Hughes *et al.*, 1997). When elderly people previously deficient in vitamin D are given an annual injection of vitamin D, they have fewer fractures (Heikinheimo *et al.*, 1992). Aside from benefits to bone density, the reduction in fractures with vitamin D supplementation is attributed to improved neuromuscular function, better balance, and fewer falls (Pfeifer *et al.*, 2000). The latter actions of vitamin D have no direct connection with calcium or bone.

Higher vitamin D supplies than what prevails in modern times are probably normal for our species. Consensus holds that modern humans originated in equatorial Africa, were exposed to abundant sunshine and wore no clothing. The calcium intakes of prehistoric humans have been estimated by Eaton and Nelson to be over 1,500 mg/day, who contend that such calcium supplies represent the natural paradigm for humans (Eaton and Nelson, 1991). However, these Paleolithic calcium intakes are difficult to maintain in the modern world. Adults must consume dairy products, or take calcium supplements merely to maintain the kinds of calcium intakes now regarded as "adequate," based on dietary recommendations (Standing Committee on the Scientific Evaluation of Dietary Reference Intakes, 1997). However, the practice of milk consumption into adulthood is unusual for any species, and for humans it is a relatively recent phenomenon. It would seem more likely that like any other nutrient throughout human history, calcium nutrition was highly variable, affected by region, seasonal food supply, and dietary and cultural preferences

(Nestle, 2000). Perhaps such high dietary intakes would not be necessary if the supply of vitamin D were greater. I propose that the high requirements that modern adults have for calcium are because of the need to compensate for a severe lack of vitamin D compared to their evolutionary paradigm.

5. Fur-Bearing Primates Obtain Vitamin D by Mouth

In contrast to the unreliable supply of just about any other nutrient during primate evolution, there can be no doubt that the state of vitamin D "nutrition" must have been far greater than what prevails in modern times. This kind of statement could not have been made until recently, because there was no widely acknowledged way to characterize the status of vitamin D nutrition. However, the consensus is now established that the circulating concentration of 25(OH)D is the primary measure of vitamin D nutritional status (Standing Committee on the Scientific Evaluation of Dietary Reference Intakes, 1997). Because of this, we can use modern data to infer what the 25(OH)D concentrations would have been in early humans. From this, we can estimate what the effective daily supply of vitamin D would have been during early human evolution.

At the low latitudes natural to all primates, sunlight penetrates the atmosphere with enough UVB light all year to disrupt 7-dehydrocholesterol molecules in the skin, and produce cholecalciferol (vitamin D) (Holick *et al.*, 1981). In all studies of healthy non-human primates, circulating 25(OH)D concentrations exceed 80 nmol/L (Ott *et al.*, 1999) (Table 9.2) (Vieth *et al.*, 1987; Marx *et al.*, 1989; Gacad and Adams, 1992; Kewenig *et al.*, 1999). New World primates given sun exposure attain circulating 25(OH)D in excess of 500 nmol/L (Gacad and Adams, 1992). Similarly, Rhesus macaques, from the Old World, and raised outdoors in Puerto Rico have average 25(OH)D concentrations of more than 500 nmol/L (Vieth *et al.*, 1987). I do not mean to imply that the data on monkeys should apply to humans, but to highlight the earlier trend of high 25(OH)D levels toward the evolution of humans. There have been severe difficulties with rickets in captive apes and monkeys, and to overcome the problem, commercial diets for captive primates contain far more vitamin D than do human diets (Fiennes, 1974; Vieth *et al.*, 1987).

The high 25(OH)D concentrations, and relatively high vitamin D requirements of apes and monkeys are understandable in light of their biology—their body surface area relative to mass is generally greater than for humans, and they are inveterate groomers, consuming by mouth the vitamin D generated from the oils secreted by skin into fur. Although much of the vitamin D produced within human skin is absorbed directly, birds and fur-bearing animals acquire most of their vitamin D orally, as they groom themselves (Bicknell and Prescott, 1946; Carpenter and Zhao, 1999). Vitamin D is generated from the oily secretions of skin into fur. The oral consumption of UV-exposed dermal excretion is the way many animals acquire the "nutrient," vitamin D. Although Fraser (1983) has argued that dermal absorption of vitamin D may be more natural, what we know from animals indicates that oral consumption is equally physiological. Since vitamin D can be extracted from UV-exposed human sweat and skin secretions (Bicknell and Prescott, 1946), it is also reasonable to think that early humans obtained some of their vitamin D by mouth as well, by licking the skin.

Table 9.2. Circulating Concentrations of 25(OH)D in Non-human Primates and in Modern Adults with Abundant Sun Exposure

	25(OH)D Mean values nmol/L	Reference
Non-human primates		
Rhesus Macaques, outdoor	500	Vieth *et al.*, 1987
Rhesus Macaque	322.5	Ott *et al.*, 1999
Rhesus Macaque	362.5	Kewenig *et al.*, 1999
Old World, No UV	110	Marx *et al.*, 1989
Old World, No UV	170	Marx *et al.*, 1989
New World, No UV	140	Marx *et al.*, 1989
New World, No UV	150	Marx *et al.*, 1989
New World, pre-UV	87.5	Gacad and Adams, 1992
New World, post-UV	575	Gacad and Adams, 1992
New World	335	Adams *et al.*, 1985
Old World (gorilla, orangutang)	82.5	Adams *et al.*, 1985
Humans under sunny conditions		
Puerto Rico, hospital personnel	105	Haddock *et al.*, 1982
Puerto Rico farmers	135	Haddock *et al.*, 1982
St. Louis, USA, lifeguards	163	Haddad and Kyung, 1971
Israel lifeguards	148	Better *et al.*, 1980

To estimate the circulating 25(OH)D concentrations prevalent in humans of the late Paleolithic period, we need to focus on people in sun-rich environments who regularly expose most of their skin surface to the sun. Lifeguards in the United States and in Israel, as well as farmers in the Caribbean all exhibit serum 25(OH)D concentrations greater than 100 nmol/L (Haddock *et al.*, 1982) (Table 9.2) (Haddad and Kyung, 1971; Better *et al.*, 1980). Furthermore, even regular short periods in sun-tan parlors consistently raise serum 25(OH)D to beyond 80 nmol/L (Dent *et al.*, 1973; Stamp *et al.*, 1977; Mawer *et al.*, 1984; Varghese *et al.*, 1989; Matsuoka *et al.*, 1990; Falkenbach *et al.*, 1993; Krause *et al.*, 1998). The synthesis of vitamin D is a self-limiting chemical reaction whereby equilibrium is achieved between production of precursors that will become vitamin D, and the photocatalytic breakdown of these precursors and vitamin D into inactive molecules (Webb *et al.*, 1989). Skin color does not affect the amount of vitamin D that can be generated. However, darker skin requires longer exposure. Very black skin requires about 1.5 hr, or six times longer than white skin, to reach the equilibrium for vitamin D production (Holick *et al.*, 1981). At least four studies show that UV exposure of the full skin surface of an adult is equivalent to a vitamin D consumption of about 250 ug (10,000 IU/d) (Stamp, 1975; Davie *et al.*, 1982; Holick, 1995; Chel *et al.*, 1998).

At latitudes beyond 40°, the angle of the sun is so low for much of the year, that UVB light penetration to the earth's surface is minimal. For much of the rest of the year UV intensity is much lower than at tropical latitudes (Webb *et al.*, 1988). At high latitudes, black skin would need substantially more than 1.5 hr to achieve the yield of vitamin D they could attain more readily at lower latitudes. Even if modern humans do live in sunny climates, they are not ensured of a desirable serum 25(OH)D concentration. Culture, clothing, and shelter minimize the natural production of vitamin D by skin. Consequently 25(OH)D concentrations for populations in the Middle East tend to be even lower than they are for people living in America or Europe (Sedrani *et al.*, 1983; Al Arabi *et al.*, 1984; Fonseca *et al.*, 1984; Fuleihan and Deeb, 1999; Alagol *et al.*, 2000). These differences in vitamin D nutrition are not attributable to fortification of milk, because this is not permitted in most European countries.

Since early human evolution occurred under UV-rich conditions, typical 25(OH)D concentrations were surely higher than 100 nmol/L. Levels like this are now seen only in lifeguards and farmers. This range of 25(OH)D concentration reflects an adult vitamin D input of 200–500 μg/day (Vieth, 1999). Since our genome was selected through evolution under these conditions, it should be evident that our biology was optimized for a vitamin D supply far higher than what we currently regard as normal. The question of whether such high levels of vitamin D nutrition actually make a difference to human health needs to be addressed with further research involving controlled prospective studies of vitamin D supplementation.

6. Vitamin D Deficiency Affecting Genetic Selection for Lighter Skin Color

In a biological sense, all modern humans belong to a species designed by evolution and natural selection to be native to the environment of the Horn of Africa. Deeply pigmented skin is probably the natural, default color (Sturm *et al.*, 1998; Jablonski and Chaplin, 2000). Dark skin protects against skin cancer, and preserves the function of sweat glands needed for thermoregulation. Moreover, dark skin protects circulating micronutrients, especially folic acid, from photodegradation. Folic acid is needed to ensure an intact fetal neural tube (Jablonski and Chaplin, 2000), and thus dark skin would have been prevalent because natural selection favored it for survival and reproduction.

As the first human populations migrated out of Africa, the vitamin D supplies declined because of less ultraviolet light exposure. Among populations across the Old World, there is a striking correlation between skin reflectivity (whiteness of skin) and latitude (Relethford, 1997; Jablonski and Chaplin, 2000). Among White children living in Great Britain, rickets was observed in at least one third of children tested by all large public health studies reported between 1868 and 1935 (Harris, 1956). If it had been children with dark skin in Great Britain or northern Europe prior to the last century, there is no doubt that the prevalence of rickets would have been greater and its form more severe. We know this both from older reports about people with dark skin in Great Britain (Harris, 1935; Bicknell and Prescott, 1946), and from the 25(OH)D concentrations reported for non-White children and adults in northern countries now (Meulmeester *et al.*, 1990; Koch and Burmeister, 1993; Gessner *et al.*, 1997; Lawson *et al.*, 1999). The natural history of untreated rickets is one of severe anatomical

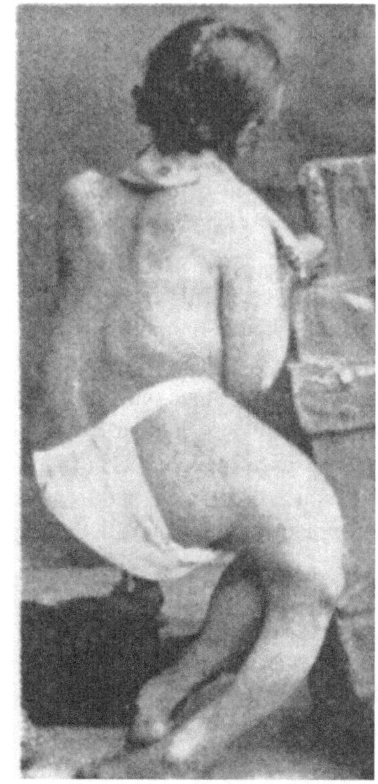

Figure 9.2. The consequence of vitamin D deficiency is rickets in the child, and osteomalacia in the adult. This is one of the numerous cases of osteomalacia seen in Central Europe after World War I, illustrating "marmalade legs." (Harris, 1935) © reprinted with permission of Cambridge University Press.

deformity (Figure 9.2). Normal childbirth would be impossible for women or girls with unresolved rickets, and for nutritionally marginal women delivery would have become progressively more difficult. More often than not, it was during pregnancy that asymptomatic vitamin D deficiency manifest itself in adulthood, as osteomalacia (Harris, 1935; Bicknell and Prescott, 1946). With poor vitamin D nutrition, pelvic deformity became worse with each pregnancy. The contracted pelvic opening made a vaginal delivery impossible (Figure 9.3).

The improved vitamin D nutrition facilitated by a whiter skin or diets of ocean fish (the only meaningful nutritional source of vitamin D) would have been essential for human reproduction at northern latitudes. However, depigmented skin by itself may not have been enough of an adaptation to prevent rickets at northern latitudes. It has been argued that high calcium intakes were needed. To achieve this, human populations in northern Europe adapted to permit consumption of milk into adulthood, by the process of natural selection favoring high intestinal lactase activity beyond childhood (Fuller, 2000).

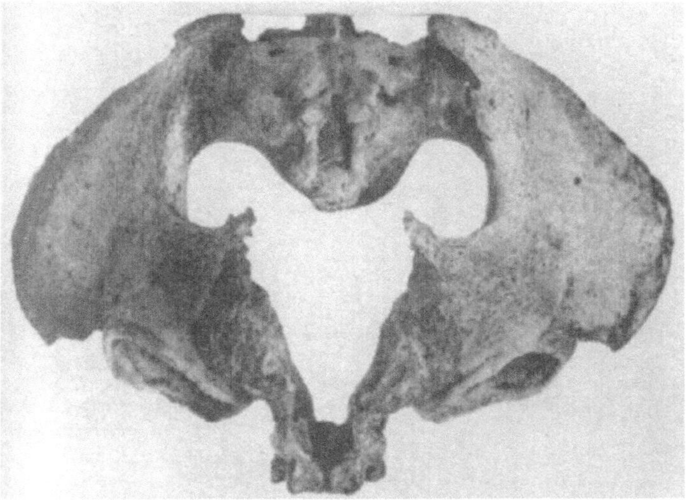

Figure 9.3. Women with osteomalacia exhibit a contracted pelvis, which is a progressive condition. It was said that the earliest symptom of vitamin D deficiency in younger women is pain and deformation around the pelvic area. The diminished size of the pelvic outlet made a vaginal delivery impossible, and older medical texts advised simply that these women be "forbidden" from becoming pregnant (Bicknell and Prescott, 1946) reprinted with permission ©.

7. Nutritional Implications of Vitamin D in Human Biology

Senile osteoporosis has long been thought to be a consequence of prolonged, mild vitamin D deficiency (Bicknell and Prescott, 1946; Parfitt, 1990; Heaney, 1999). In terms of severity of vitamin D deficiency, rickets is the most severe stage of the resulting bone disease. Less severe is the adult onset of osteomalacia during nutritionally stressed periods. The consequence for bone of still milder vitamin D insufficiency would be osteoporosis. This view is supported by the modern clinical evidence of fracture prevention with vitamin D in the elderly (Chapuy *et al.*, 1992; Dawson-Hughes *et al.*, 1997).

Osteoporosis and most of the other conditions listed in Table 9.1 are unlikely to have contributed to natural selection, because only rickets and osteomalacia would have affected reproductive capacity. Therefore, there is no reason to assume that natural selection for skin color and greater dietary calcium were sufficient to eliminate the predisposition to the other vitamin D deficiency related diseases listed in Table 9.1.

The amounts of vitamin D needed to bring about the kinds of 25(OH)D concentrations associated with abundant sunshine exposure exceed the current official safety limit of 50 μg/d (2,000 IU/day) (Standing Committee on the Scientific Evaluation of Dietary Reference Intakes, 1997; Vieth, 2001). Figure 9.4 compares circulating 25(OH)D concentrations as they would have been through primate and early human evolution, against levels that are now common for adults, and levels attained with vitamin D intakes far higher than current RDA's for the nutrient. In the broader context of this comparison, modern humans are relatively deprived of vitamin D, and even the most recently revised dietary

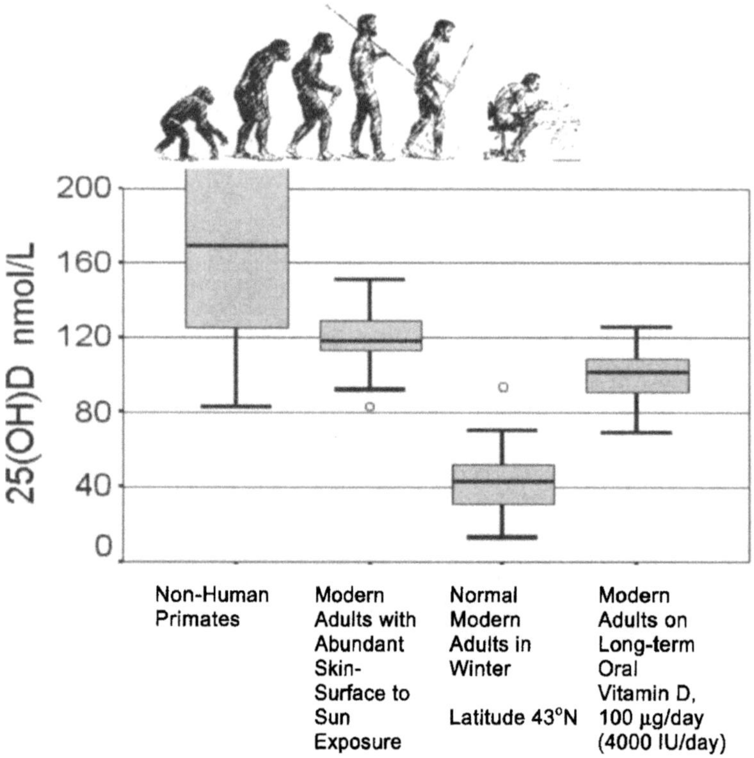

Figure 9.4. Summary of what is known about circulating 25(OH)D concentrations in non-human primates and in modern adults. The cartoon along the top serves only to provide symbolic reference points for the corresponding parts of the graph below. It is assumed here that since modern humans evolved in tropical regions and without clothing, early vitamin D nutrition was similar to that of modern humans living under similar conditions. Results for non-human primates and for sun-rich adults are from Table 9.2, with additional data for adults given artificial tanning sessions (Vieth, 1999). Data for modern adults in winter and their responses to vitamin D are from a recent study involving hospital workers in Toronto, Canada (Vieth, 2001). These plots include whiskers that show the lowest and highest values, the boxes show the range of the central 50% of the sample group, with a line indicating the median value of the group.

guidelines for this nutrient (Standing Committee on the Scientific Evaluation of Dietary Reference Intakes, 1997) are probably still woefully inadequate for adults.

The reason contemporary older adults require calcium intakes at levels attainable only with dairy foods or mineral supplements, may be because they are relatively vitamin D deprived. Because current nutrient recommendations provide far less vitamin D than is attainable through sunshine, modern medical thinking effectively maintains adults in a state of relative vitamin D insufficiency, compensated for by high requirements for calcium. In contrast, early humans living in sun-rich environments were relatively vitamin D rich—probably at least 100 µg/day (4,000 IU/day). Therefore, early humans may not have required as much calcium to prevent osteoporosis or rickets. Moreover, maintenance of higher vitamin D supplies may have optimized cellular control mechanisms that prevented many diseases that have not been classically associated with vitamin D nutrition.

References

Adams, J.E., Gacad, M.A., Baker, A.J., and Rude, R.K. (1985). Serum concentrations of 1,25-dihydroxyvitamin D_3 in Platyrrhini and Cathrrhini: A phylogenetic appraisal. *Am. J. Primatol.* **9**, 219–224.

Al Arabi, K.M., Elidrissy, A.W., and Sedrani, S.H. (1984). Is avoidance of sunlight a cause of fractures of the femoral neck in elderly Saudis? *Trop. Geogr. Med.* **36**, 273–279.

Alagol, F., Shihadeh, Y., Boztepe, H., Tanakol, R., Yarman, S., Azizlerli, H., and Sandalci, O. (2000). Sunlight exposure and vitamin D deficiency in Turkish women. *J. Endocrinol. Invest.* **23**, 173–177.

Better, O.S., Shabtai, M., Kedar, S., Melamud, A., Berenheim, J., and Chaimovitz, C. (1980). Increased incidence of nephrolithiasis in lifeguards in Isreal. In S.G. Massry, E. Ritz, and G. Jahreis (eds), *Phosphate and Minerals in Health and Disease*. Plenum Press, New York, pp. 467–472.

Bicknell, F. and Prescott, F. (1946). Vitamin D. The antirachitic or calcifying vitamin. In F. Bicknell and F. Prescott (eds), *Vitamins in Medicine*. Whitefriars Press, London, pp. 630–707.

Bikle, D.D. and Pillai, S. (1993). Vitamin D, calcium, and epidermal differentiation. *Endocr. Rev.* **14**, 3–19.

Blumberg, R.W, Forbes, G.B., Fraser, D., Hansen, A.E., Lowe, C.U., Smith, N.J., Sweeney, M.J., and Fomon, S.J. (1963). The prophylactic requirement and the toxicity of vitamin D. *Pediatrics* **31**, 512–525.

Carpenter, K.J. and Zhao, L. (1999). Forgotten mysteries in the early history of vitamin D. *J. Nutr.* **129**, 923–927.

Chan, T.Y. (2000). Vitamin D deficiency and susceptibility to tuberculosis. *Calcif. Tissue Int.* **66**, 476–478.

Chapuy, M.C., Arlot, M.E., Duboeuf, F., Brun, J., Crouzet, B., Arnaud, S., Delmas, P.D., and Meunier, P.J. (1992). Vitamin D_3 and calcium to prevent hip fractures in the elderly women. *N. Engl. J. Med.* **327**, 1637–1642.

Chel, V.G., Ooms, M.E., Popp-Snijders, C., Pavel, S., Schothorst, A.A., Meulemans, C.C., and Lips, P. (1998). Ultraviolet irradiation corrects vitamin D deficiency and suppresses secondary hyperparathyroidism in the elderly. *J. Bone Miner. Res.* **13**, 1238–1242.

Chesney, R.W., Hamstra, A.J., and DeLuca, H.F. (1981). Rickets of prematurity: Supranormal levels of serum 1,25-dihydroxyvitamin D. *Am. J. Dis. Child.* **135**, 34–37.

Davie, M.W., Lyawson, D.E., Emberson, C., Barnes, J.L., Roberts, G.E., and Barnes, N.D. (1982). Vitamin D from skin: Contribution to vitamin D status compared with oral vitamin D in normal and anticonvulsant-treated subjects. *Clin. Sci.* **63**, 461–472.

Dawson-Hughes, B., Dallal, G.E., Krall, E.A., Harris, S., Sokoll, L.J., and Falconer, G. (1991). Effect of vitamin D supplementation on wintertime and overall bone loss in healthy postmenopausal women. *Ann. Int. Med.* **115**, 505–512.

Dawson-Hughes, B., Harris, S.S., Krall, E.A., and Dallal, G.E. (1997). Effect of calcium and vitamin D supplementation on bone density in men and women 65 years of age or older. *N. Engl. J. Med.* **337**, 670–676.

Dent, C.E., Round, J.M., Rowe, D.J., and Stamp, T.C. (1973). Effect of chapattis and ultraviolet irradiation on nutritional rickets in an Indian immigrant. *Lancet* **1**, 1282–1284.

Douglas, A.S., Ali, S., and Bakhshi, S.S. (1998). Does vitamin D deficiency account for ethnic differences in tuberculosis seasonality in the UK? *Ethn. Health* **3**, 247–253.

Dusso, A., Finch, J., Delmez, J., Rapp, N., Lopez-Hilker, S., Brown, A., and Slatopolsky, E. (1990). Extrarenal production of calcitriol. *Kidney Int. Suppl.* **29**, S36–S40.

Eaton, S.B. and Nelson, D.A. (1991). Calcium in evolutionary perspective. *Am. J. Clin. Nutr.* **54**, 281S–287S.

Embry, A.F., Snowdon, L.R., and Vieth, R. (2000). Vitamin D and seasonal fluctuations of gadolinium-enhancing magnetic resonance imaging lesions in multiple sclerosis. *Ann. Neurol.* **48**, 271–272.

Eva, J.K. (1999). Vitamin D supplement in early childhood and risk for Type I (insulin-dependent) diabetes mellitus. The EURODIAB Substudy 2 Study Group. *Diabetologia* **42**, 51–54.

Falkenbach, A., Unkelbach, U., Boehm, B.O., Regeniter, A., Stein, J., Seiffert, U., and Wendt, T. (1993). Bone metabolism before and after irradiation with ultraviolet light. *Eur. J. Appl. Physiol.* **66**, 55–59.

Fiennes, R.N. (1974). Problems of rickets in monkeys and apes. *Proc. R. Soc. Med.* **67**, 309–314.

Fonseca, V., Tongia, R., el Hazmi, M., and Abu-Aisha, H. (1984). Exposure to sunlight and vitamin D deficiency in Saudi Arabian women. *Postgrad. Med. J.* **60**, 589–591.

Fraser, D.R. (1983). The physiological economy of vitamin D. *Lancet* **I**, 969–972.

Fuleihan, G.E. and Deeb, M. (1999). Hypovitaminosis D in a sunny country. *N. Engl. J. Med.* **340**, 1840–1841.

Fuller, K. (2000). Lactose, rickets, and the coevolution of genes and culture. *Hum. Ecol.* **28**, 471–477.

Gacad, M.A. and Adams, J.S. (1992). Specificity of steroid binding in New World primate B95-8 cells with a vitamin D-resistant phenotype. *Endocrinology* **131**, 2581–2587.

Garabedian, M., Bainsel, M., Mallet, E., Guillozo, H., Toppet, M., Grimberg, R., NGuen, T.M., and Balsan, S. (1983). Circulating vitamin D metabolite concentrations in children with nutritional rickets. *J. Pediatr.* **103**, 381–386.

Garland, C.F., Garland, F.C., and Gorham, E.D. (1999). Calcium and vitamin D. Their potential roles in colon and breast cancer prevention. *Ann. NY Acad. Sci.* **889**, 107–119.

Gessner, B.D., deSchweinitz, E., Petersen, K.M., and Lewandowski, C. (1997). Nutritional rickets among breast-fed black and Alaska Native children. *Alaska Med.* **39**, 72–74, 87.

Haddad, J.G. and Kyung, J.C. (1971). Competitive protein-binding radioassay for 25-hydroxycholecalciferol. *J. Clin. Endocrinol.* **33**, 992–995.

Haddad, J.G., Matsuoka, L.Y., Hollis, B.W., Hu, Y.Z., and Wortsman, J. (1993). Human plasma transport of vitamin D after its endogenous synthesis. *J. Clin. Invest.* **91**, 2552–2555.

Haddock, L., Corcino, J., and Vazquez, M.D. (1982). 25(OH)D serum levels in the normal Puerto Rican population and in subjects with tropical sprue and parathyroid disease. *P. R. Health Sci. J.* **1**, 85–91.

Harris, L.J. (1935). Vitamin D and rickets. In Anonymous. *Vitamins in Theory and Practice*. Cambridge University Press, Cambridge, pp. 107–150.

Harris, L.J. (1956). Vitamin D and Bone. In G.H. Bourne (ed.), *The Biochemistry and Physiology of Bone*. Academic Press, New York, pp. 581–622.

Hayes, C.E., Cantorna, M.T., and DeLuca, H.F. (1997). Vitamin D and multiple sclerosis. *Proc. Soc. Exp. Biol. Med.* **216**, 21–27.

Heaney, R.P. (1999). Lessons for nutritional science from vitamin D. *Am. J. Clin. Nutr.* **69**, 825–826.

Heikinheimo, R.J., Inkovaara, J.A., Harju, E.J., Haavisto, M.V., Kaarela, R.H., Kataja, J.M., Kokko, A.M., Kolho, L.A. *et al.* (1992). Annual injection of vitamin D and fractures of aged bones. *Calcif. Tissue Int.* **51**, 105–110.

Henry, H. and Norman, A.W. (1975). Presence of renal 25-hydroxyvitamin-D-1-hydroxylase in species of all vertebrate classes. *Comp. Biochem. Physiol.* **50B**, 431–434.

Hewison, M., Zehnder, D., Bland, R., and Stewart, P.M. (2000). 1Alpha-hydroxylase and the action of vitamin D. *J. Mol. Endocrinol.* **25**, 141–148.

Holick, M.F. (1992). Evolutionary biology and pathology of vitamin D. *J. Nutr. Sci. Vitaminol.* Spec No: 79–83.

Holick, M.F. (1995). Environmental factors that influence the cutaneous production of vitamin D. *Am. J. Clin. Nutr.* **61**, 638S–645S.

Holick, M.F., MacLaughlin, J.A., and Doppelt, S.H. (1981). Regulation of cutaneous previtamin D_3 photosynthesis in man: Skin pigment is not an essential regulator. *Science* **211**, 590–593.

Hsu, J.Y., Feldman, D., McNeal, J.E., and Peehl, D.M. (2001). Reduced 1alpha-hydroxylase activity in human prostate cancer cells correlates with decreased susceptibility to 25-hydroxyvitamin D_3-induced growth inhibition. *Cancer Res.* **61**, 2852–2856.

Jablonski, N.G. and Chaplin, G. (2000). The evolution of human skin coloration. *J. Hum. Evol.* **39**, 57–106.

Kewenig, S., Schneider, T., Hohloch, K., Lampe-Dreyer, K., Ullrich, R., Stolte, N., Stahl-Hennig, C., Kaup, F.J. *et al.* (1999). Rapid mucosal CD4(+) T-cell depletion and enteropathy in simian immunodeficiency virus-infected rhesus macaques. *Gastroenterology* **116**, 1115–1123.

Koch, H.C. and Burmeister, W. (1993). [Vitamin D status of children and adolescents of African and Asian diplomats in Germany]. [German]. *Klin. Padiatr.* **205**, 416–420.

Krause, R., Buhring, M., Hopfenmuller, W., Holick, M.F., and Sharma, A.M. (1998) Ultraviolet B and blood pressure. *Lancet* **352**, 709–710.

Lane, N.E., Gore, L.R., Cummings, S.R., Hochberg, M.C., Scott, J.C., Williams, E.N., and Nevitt, M.C. (1999). Serum vitamin D levels and incident changes of radiographic hip osteoarthritis: A longitudinal study. Study of Osteoporotic Fractures Research Group. *Arthritis Rheum.* **42**, 854–860.

Lawson, M., Thomas, M., and Hardiman, A. (1999). Dietary and lifestyle factors affecting plasma vitamin D levels in Asian children living in England. *Eur. J. Clin. Nutr.* **53**, 268–272.

Mahon, B.D., Bemiss, C., and Cantorna, M.T. (2001). Altered cytokine profile in patients with multiple sclerosis following vitamin D supplementation. *FASEB J.* **837**, 4.

Marx, S.J., Jones, G., Weinstein, R.S., Chrousos, G.P., and Renquist, D.M. (1989). Differences in mineral metabolism among nonhuman primates receiving diets with only vitamin D_3 or only vitamin D_2. *J. Clin. Endocrinol. Metab.* **69**, 1282–1289.

Matsuoka, L.Y., Wortsman, J., and Hollis, B.W. (1990). Suntanning and cutaneous synthesis of vitamin D_3. *J. Lab. Clin. Med.* **116**, 87–90.

Mawer, E.B., Berry, J.L., Sommer-Tsilenis, E., Beykirch, W., Kuhlwein, A., and Rohde, B.T. (1984). Ultraviolet irradiation increases serum 1,25-dihydroxyvitamin D in vitamin-D-replete adults. *Miner. Electrolyte Metab.* **10**, 117–121.

McAlindon, T.E., Felson, D.T., Zhang, Y., Hannan, M.T., Aliabadi, P., Weissman, B., Rush, D., Wilson, P.W., and Jacques, P. (1996). Relation of dietary intake and serum levels of vitamin D to progression of osteoarthritis of the knee among participants in the Framingham Study. *Ann. Intern. Med.* **125**, 353–359.

McGrath, J. (2001). Does "imprinting" with low prenatal vitamin D contribute to the risk of various adult disorders? *Med. Hypotheses* **56**, 367–371.

Meulmeester, J.F., van den Berg, H., Wedel, M., Boshuis, P.G., and Hulshof, K.F.L.R. (1990). Vitamin D status, parathyroid hormone and sunlight in Turkish, Moroccan and Caucasian children in The Netherlands. *Eur. J. Clin. Nutr.* **44**, 461–470.

Muhe, L., Lulseged, S., Mason, K.E., and Simoes, E.A. (1997). Case-control study of the role of nutritional rickets in the risk of developing pneumonia in Ethiopian children. *Lancet* **349**, 1801–1804.

Nestle, M. (2000). Paleolithic diets: A sceptical view. *BNF Nutrition Bulletin* **25**, 43–47.

Nykjaer, A., Dragun, D., Walther, D., Vorum, H., Jacobsen, C., Herz, J., Melsen, F., Christensen, E.I. *et al.* (1999). An endocytic pathway essential for renal uptake and activation of the steroid 25-(OH) vitamin D_3. *Cell* **96**, 507–515.

Ott, S.M., Lipkin, E.W., and Newell-Morris, L. (1999). Bone physiology during pregnancy and lactation in young macaques. *J. Bone Miner. Res.* **14**, 1779–1788.

Parfitt, A.M. (1990). Osteomalacia and related disorders. In Louis V. Arioli and Stephen M. Krane (ed.), *Metabolic Bone Disease and Clinically Related Disorders, 2nd edn.* W.B. Saunders, Philadelphia, pp. 329–396.

Pfeifer, M., Begerow, B., Minne, H.W., Abrams, C., Nachtigall, D., and Hansen, C. (2000). Effects of a short-term vitamin D and calcium supplementation on body sway and secondary hyperparathyroidism in elderly women. *J. Bone Miner. Res.* **15**, 1113–1118.

Relethford, J.H. (1997). Hemispheric difference in human skin color. *Am. J. Phys. Anthropol.* **104**, 449–457.

Rostand, S.G. (1997). Ultraviolet light may contribute to geographic and racial blood pressure differences. *Hypertension* **30**, 150–156.

Schwartz, G.G., Wang, M.H., Zang, M., Singh, R.K., and Siegal, G.P. (1997). 1 Alpha,25-dihydroxyvitamin D (calcitriol) inhibits the invasiveness of human prostate cancer cells. *Cancer Epidemiol. Biomarkers Prevent.* **6**, 727–732.

Schwartz, G.G., Whitlatch, L.W., Chen, T.C., Lokeshwar, B.L., and Holick, M.F. (1998). Human prostate cells synthesize 1,25-dihydroxyvitamin D_3 from 25-hydroxyvitamin D_3. *Cancer Epidemiol. Biomarkers Prevent.* **7**, 391–395.

Sedrani, S.H., Elidrissy, A.W., and El Arabi, K.M. (1983). Sunlight and vitamin D status in normal Saudi subjects. *Am. J. Clin. Nutr.* **38**, 129–132.

Stamp, T.C. (1975). Factors in human vitamin D nutrition and in the production and cure of classical rickets. *Proc. Nutr. Soc.* **34**, 119–130.

Stamp, T.C., Haddad, J.G., and Twigg, C.A. (1977). Comparison of oral 25-hydroxycholecalciferol, vitamin D, and ultraviolet light as determinants of circulating 25-hydroxyvitamin D. *Lancet* **1**, 1341–1343.

Standing Committee on the Scientific Evaluation of Dietary Reference Intakes. (1997). *Dietary Reference Intakes: Calcium, Phosphorus, Magnesium, Vitamin D, and Fluoride.* National Academy Press.

Stene, L.C., Ulriksen, J., Magnus, P., and Joner, G. (2000). Use of cod liver oil during pregnancy associated with lower risk of Type I diabetes in the offspring. *Diabetologia* **43**, 1093–1098.

Sturm, R.A., Box, N.F., and Ramsay, M. (1998). Human pigmentation genetics: The difference is only skin deep. *Bioessays* **20**, 712–721.

Trang, H., Cole, D.E., Rubin, L.A., Pierratos, A., Siu, S., and Vieth, R. (1998). Evidence that vitamin D_3 increases serum 25-hydroxyvitamin D more efficiently than does vitamin D_2. *Am. J. Clin. Nutr.* **68**, 854–848.

Varghese, M., Rodman, J.S., Williams, J.J., Brown, A., Carter, D.M., Zerwekh, J.E., and Pak, C.Y. (1989). The effect of ultraviolet B radiation treatments on calcium excretion and vitamin D metabolites in kidney stone formers. *Clin. Nephrol.* **31**, 225–231.

Vieth, R. (1994). Simple method for determining specific binding capacity of vitamin D-binding protein and its use to calculate the concentration of "free" 1,25-dihydroxyvitamin D. *Clin. Chem.* **40**, 435–441.

Vieth, R. (1999). Vitamin D supplementation, 25-hydroxyvitamin D concentrations, and safety. *Am. J. Clin. Nutr.* **69**, 842–856.

Vieth, R. (2001). Reply to J Hathcock and I Munro. *Am. J. Clin. Nutr.* **74**, 866–867.

Vieth, R., Kessler, M.J., and Pritzker, K.P. (1987). Serum concentrations of vitamin D metabolites in Cayo Santiago rhesus macaques. *J. Med. Primatol.* **16**, 349–357.

Vieth, R., McCarten, K., and Norwich, K.H. (1990). Role of 25-hydroxyvitamin D_3 dose in determining rat 1,25-dihydroxyvitamin D_3 production. *Am. J. Physiol.* **258**, E780–E789.

Walters, M.R., Kollenkirchen, U., and Fox, J. (1992). What is vitamin D deficiency? *Proc. Soc. Exp. Biol. Med.* **199**, 385–393.

Webb, A.R., DeCosta, B.R., and Holick, M.F. (1989). Sunlight regulates the cutaneous production of vitamin D_3 by causing its photodegradation. *J. Clin. Endocrinol. Metab.* **68**, 882–887.

Webb, A.R., Kline, L., and Holick, M.F. (1988). Influence of season and latitude on the cutaneous synthesis of vitamin D_3: Exposure to winter sunlight in Boston and Edmonton will not promote vitamin D_3 synthesis in human skin. *J. Clin. Endocrinol. Metab.* **67**, 373–378.

Part IV

Bone Loss and Osteoporosis in Past Populations

10

Techniques for the Investigation of Age-Related Bone Loss and Osteoporosis in Archaeological Bone

Megan B. Brickley and Sabrina C. Agarwal

1. Introduction

With increasing awareness of age-related bone loss and osteoporosis in modern Western populations, a growing number of studies have set out to investigate whether individuals in the past were similarly affected (Martin and Armelagos, 1979; Bennike and Bohr, 1990; Lees *et al.*, 1993; Agarwal and Grynpas, 1996; Brickley and Howell, 1999; Drusini *et al.*, 2000; Mays, 2000). Research has demonstrated that age-related bone loss and osteoporosis results in changes to cortical bone (Derisquebourg *et al.*, 1994), structural changes to trabecular bone (at a gross and microscopic level [Jayasinghe, 1994]), and bone mass and density (Cummings *et al.*, 1993). Bone turnover and age-related bone loss are highly complex processes (see Chapters 1 and 2, this volume). The interaction between bone loss in both cortical and trabecular bone throughout the skeleton allows a variety of possible approaches to the study of bone loss. A range of techniques have been developed, each of which allows assessment of a different aspect of bone loss. Although this area has generated a great deal of recent interest, the epidemiology of age-related bone loss and fragility fractures, both in clinical and archaeological contexts, is unclear. The history of the development of the disease is not yet fully understood and a range of possibilities is currently being explored. For example, Neese and Williams (1994) suggest that increasing bone loss may be an evolutionary trend (see also Chapter 8, this volume).

This chapter examines the range of possible techniques that can be applied to the assessment of bone loss and osteoporosis in archaeological bone. Each technique is reviewed and information provided on its advantages and disadvantages. The exact aspect of bone loss being measured along with any factors that should be taken into account when considering archaeological material will be discussed.

Megan B. Brickley • Institute of Archaeology and Antiquity, University of Birmingham.

Sabrina C. Agarwal • Department of Anthropology, University of Toronto.

Bone Loss and Osteoporosis: An Anthropological Perspective, edited by Sabrina C. Agarwal and Sam D. Stout. Kluwer Academic/Plenum Publishers, New York, 2003.

The chapter is divided into four broad sections according to the region of bone examined: visual examination of the complete bone, investigations of cortical bone, investigations of trabecular bone, and investigative techniques that assess both cortical and trabecular bone in combination.

1.1. Background

Osteoporosis has been defined as "a disease characterized by abnormalities in the amount and architectural arrangement of bone tissue that lead to impaired skeletal strength and undue susceptibility to fracture" (Melton *et al.*, 1992: 15). However, in earlier studies the term osteoporosis may have been applied to a different range of conditions than would be applied currently; the meaning of the term has changed since it was initially coined. As pointed out by Weaver (1998: 27–8) it is important that correct terminology be used. The term osteoporosis should only be used in cases of extreme osteopenia where natural bone loss has been exaggerated and the individual is liable to suffer from one of the associated fractures (Gallagher, 1990). The World Health Organization defines normal bone mineral content (BMC) or bone mineral density (BMD) as within one standard deviation of the young adult reference mean, osteopenia or low bone mass as between 1 and 2.5 SD below young adult mean, and osteoporosis or very low mass as greater than 2.5 SD below young adult mean (WHO Geneva, 1994). While this definition of osteoporosis does not address the change that can occur in bone quality independent of bone mass (see also Chapter 3, this volume), it provides an idea of the relative amounts of bone being talked about.

The most important characteristic given in the definition by Melton and coworkers is the susceptibility to fracture risk. Therefore, the best way to diagnose osteoporosis in archaeological bone is to examine for osteoporosis-related fractures (fragility fractures). Fragility fractures are commonly manifest as vertebral crush or wedge fractures, fractures of the distal radius (Colles' fractures), and hip fractures (fractures of the neck of the femur). The fracture most commonly reported from the archaeological record has been the vertebral crush fracture (Brickley, 2002b). Vertebral crush fracture and Colles' fracture are linked to Type I Osteoporosis or post-menopausal bone loss. This type of bone loss affects women immediately after menopause and is manifest in the loss of trabecular bone (Kanis, 1994). Type II Osteoporosis affects both men and women in older age categories (60+), and both cortical and trabecular bone is lost. This combined pattern of bone loss not only leads to fractures of the vertebral bodies but also predisposes individuals to hip fractures.

1.2. Problems with Diagenetic Change

Diagenesis is a term used to describe changes occurring in bone after death. It includes all processes that affect degradation and remineralization, both in and out of the ground, but excludes the effects of high temperature and pressure (Lapedes, 1978; Pate and Brown, 1985). Schultz (Chapter 11 this volume) discusses microscopic diagenetic change in greater detail, but there are a number of points that are worth mentioning briefly in the light of considerations of techniques for investigation of age-related bone loss and osteoporosis in archaeological bone.

Any non-invasive density determination technique that is applied to archaeological bone, which does not examine the mineral make up of the sample analyzed may produce erroneous results. An important consideration is that the presence of diagenetic changes may not be discernable from visual examination of bones. Indeed, bones that appear well preserved may have undergone considerable change (Stout and Simmons, 1979; Bell, 1990).

Investigation of age-related bone loss has demonstrated the presence of "foreign" minerals within the structure of archaeological bone (Farquharson and Brickley, 1997), in this case calcium carbonate. Brickley (1998) has demonstrated that soil infiltration is relatively common in archaeological bone. This fact is not very surprising, but what is more concerning is the demonstration that it is very difficult to detect such infiltration even from careful examination of radiographic images (Brickley, 1998; Agarwal, 2001). Clearly diagenetic change is an important consideration for any investigation of age-related bone loss and osteoporosis in archaeological bone.

2. Visual Examination of Complete Bones

There are a number of recent reported cases of fracture from archaeological bone assemblages that may be due to age-related bone loss (Roberts and Wakely, 1992; Foldes *et al.*, 1995; Frigo and Lang, 1995; Mays, 1996; Dequeker *et al.*, 1997). One such specimen, discovered during excavations at the Roman site of Pella in Jordan, exhibited a fracture characteristic of osteoporosis (Sambrook *et al.*, 1988). The bone, a lower thoracic vertebra of a mature (50–60 year old) male, displayed a wedged deformity typical of an osteoporotic fracture. Further illustrations and examples of the type of vertebral crush fractures that may be related to age-related bone loss are given in Aufderheide and Rodríguez-Martín (1998: 314–315).

While an example of hip fracture is illustrated in Roberts and Manchester (1995: 179), few fragility-related hip fractures have been reported from the archaeological record. A number of authors have discussed the seemingly low number of typical fragility fractures in the past (Agarwal and Grynpas, 1996; Weaver, 1998; Pfeiffer, 2000). There seems to be an *a priori* expectation that age-related fragility fractures would have occurred in most archaeological populations. However, as in modern human populations, there may simply have been population-specific conditions that contributed to a low prevalence of fragility fracture in some groups. There are, however, a number of explanations for the paucity of reported cases that must be considered when dealing with mortality samples. The lack of hip fracture in the past may reflect heterogeneity in archaeological samples, whereby those who did live to a greater age in the past could have been biologically fitter than elderly people today who have benefited from modern medicine. Further, on average, individuals would have had to live to a much greater age in order to sustain hip fractures as opposed to other types of fracture. Although in past societies there would have been a significant number of individuals who reached old age (examination of ancient texts, burial, and historical records [see Jackes, 2000] demonstrates this), the proportion of the population living into their seventies and eighties would have been much smaller than today. However, it should also be noted that in modern times fracture risk is not tied exclusively to life expectancy. Today, there is a secular trend whereby the increment in the population over the age of 80 has and will continue to rise exponentially as compared to the overall population growth (Kanis, 1994). However, the change in demographics does not account entirely for the present increased incidence of several types of fragility fracture. For example, Kanis (1994) notes that hip fracture incidence in Oxford, England doubled in the 27 years following the 1950s, and similar increases have been documented in other parts of the world. It is clear that life expectancy is not the only factor involved in the increasing incidence of osteoporosis.

Hip fractures are also associated with a high level of morbidity (Spector, 1991). They cause a significant shock to the system of an elderly individual and are very difficult to heal (Sneed and Van Bree, 1990). As such, many individuals in the past would have died from such a fracture and the bones may well have be un-united when they were buried (Brickley, 2002). There is great difficulty in determining if bones that are fractured when a skeleton is excavated are perimortem or postmortem (Pfeiffer, 2000). The difficulty is compounded as it is rare for an osteologist to be present throughout an excavation and so the individual compiling the report may not have been able to observe the bones *in situ*. Ortner and Putschar (1985) discuss the examination of perimortem or postmortem fractured bones. Simply feeling the weight of a bone to decide if it is very "light" is not sufficient to diagnose osteopenia or bone fragility. There are many taphonomic and diagenetic changes that could affect bone, making this type of investigation unsound.

In considering a differential diagnosis of age-related osteoporosis a number of factors will have to be considered, such as age and sex of the individual, location of fracture, and any other pathological changes present on the skeleton. There are a number of pathological conditions that can cause osteopenia and in severe cases can lead to a pathological fracture (e.g., leprosy and scurvy) (Brickley, 2000).

Further, although examination of fractures in bone may be the most direct way of looking at osteoporosis, there are limitations to this type of approach. The first problem is that it is impossible to be exactly sure when a fracture occurred in an individual's life (Roberts, 2000). Although an individual with typical fragility fracture may be an "old adult" it is possible that the injury occurred at a younger age and was not linked to age-related bone loss. Traumatic fractures can often be mistaken as fragility-related fractures.

3. Investigations of Cortical Bone

There are a number of ways in which cortical bone can be analyzed and these can involve both invasive and non-invasive techniques. Cortical bone loss is often directly assessed by measurement from cross-sections of bone that can yield estimates of the amount of bone present. However, as noted by Weaver (1998), these methods do not tell us about the density or quality of the bone measured.

3.1. Metacarpal Radiogrammetry

This technique is relatively straightforward and non-destructive in that a calculation of the amount of cortical bone present in a metacarpal is determined from measurements obtained from standard radiographs. The equipment and technical knowledge required are simple. A number of studies have been carried out on archaeological bone (Ekenman *et al.*, 1995; Mays, 1996, 2000, 2001; Ives, 2002). One important advantage of this technique is that prior to widespread use of techniques such as Dual Energy X-ray Absorptiometry (DEXA), metacarpal radiogrammetry was commonly used in clinical investigations and so data from modern individuals are available.

Typically the second metacarpal has been selected for analysis in both clinical (Virtama and Helelä, 1969; Meema and Meema, 1987) and paleopathological investigations. In studies of archaeological bone it has been noted that the shape of the second metacarpal allows positioning of the bone on the film to simulate positioning in living subjects (Mays, 1996: 145). Measurements are taken from the images obtained and used to calculate the cortical thickness and cortical index. The measurements required are the total length, total width, and medullary width. The formula used to calculate the cortical index is:

$$\text{Cortical index} = \frac{\text{Total width} - \text{Medullarywidth}}{\text{Total width}} \times 100$$

The cortical index gives the percentage of bone width taken up by the cortex.

Bones that have been weathered should not be included in this type of analysis, but most forms of diagenetic change will have little effect on the technique. However, there are exceptions, for example heavy soil infiltration may make bones unsuitable for study. Bones should be unbroken so that the midpoint can accurately be calculated. Information on film type and settings to be used can be found in a number of reports (Mays, 1996; Ives, 2002) but advice should always be sought from a radiographer.

While this technique is easy to apply to archaeological bone, criticisms identified in the clinical literature should be considered. As only cortical bone is measured, no information on important losses in the trabecular tissue are made, and it does not measure bone loss at an area of the skeleton typically affected by fragility-related fractures (Derisquebourg *et al.*, 1994). However, interesting results have been obtained and the technique does have a role to play in investigations of age-related bone loss in archaeological bone.

3.2. Cortical Histomorphometry

While general microscopic bone loss or porosity can be examined in archaeological bone with histology (see Chapter 11, this volume), histomorphometry offers a quantitative examination of morphological changes at the tissue and cellular level. Histomorphometry is the measurement of microscopic bone features based on the fact that bone is constantly remodeling. As the resorption and formation of bone work together in what is termed a basic multicellular unit (BMU), and are generally coupled, any change or loss reflects a disruption of this balance (see also Chapter 2, this volume). Histomorphometry can help identify if this balance has been disrupted by metabolic conditions, such as osteoporosis. Most examinations of cortical bone microstructure utilize thin sections and light microscopy, although backscattered electron microscopy or microradiography can give suitable images for static histomorphometry. Cortical histomorphometry is commonly used as an aging technique in archaeological bone, but can be used to examine bone remodeling and bone loss in past populations (for more extensive review see Chapters 12 and 13, this volume). A number of studies have examined bone loss and cortical remodeling in archaeological populations from various geographic regions (e.g., Laughlin *et al.*, 1979; Martin and Armelagos, 1979, 1985; Richman *et al.*, 1979; Ericksen, 1980; Thompson and Gunness-Hey, 1981; Stout, 1983; Burr *et al.*, 1990; Stout and Lueck, 1995), and the femur and rib are sites that have been most commonly examined. For histological thin sections, some technical experience is required to embed, grind, and section specimens (for discussion on preparation of archaeological samples consult Pfeiffer, 2000 or Stout, 1989). Histomorphometric measurements can then be made with the aid of microscope eyepiece reticules or more recently with the use of automated image analysis systems and software. The static histomorphological structures usually studied are the number and size of secondary osteons and associated canals, and from these several derived measurements such as osteonal population density (OPD), mean wall thickness (MWT), and porosity can be calculated, as well as estimates of activation frequency and bone turnover rate (see Chapter 13, this volume).

Some issues need to be considered when examining histomorphological changes in archaeological samples. Most importantly, it is often difficult to separate the various factors that can affect bone remodeling. Age, metabolic disturbances, and biomechanical loading can all affect histomorphological features. The histological examination of bone from various skeletal sites, and/or in conjunction with trabecular tissue could aid in the interpretation of histomorphometric data. Further, histomorphometric measurements in archaeological bone are limited to static indices, and derived measurements such as activation frequency rely on accurate assignment of chronological age to skeletal remains. Researchers should also follow parameters and standardized nomenclature set forth by Parfitt *et al.* (1987).

As histological methods are invasive, curators are often unwilling to sacrifice skeletal elements to be sectioned. As Pfeiffer (2000) notes, the use of smaller skeletal elements such as the rib or metacarpal can offer a compromise between the preservation of valuable archaeological samples and the need for microscopic research. With the confounding effects of diagenesis in non-invasive measurements of bone density in archaeological samples, histomorphometry offers a valuable tool to examine bone remodeling and loss.

4. Investigations of Trabecular Bone

Trabecular bone makes up approximately 20% of the skeletal mass (Woolf and St John Dixon, 1988) and forms the main component of the vertebral bodies and epiphyses of the long bones. There are also small amounts of trabecular bone at other skeletal sites. The trabeculae form a semi-rigid framework of bony struts, arranged so as to provide support to the structure of the bone in relation to the forces placed upon it. Trabecular bone has a high surface area and for this reason is generally assumed to be more metabolically active than cortical bone (Dargent and Breart, 1993). The importance of trabecular bone in the occurrence of osteoporosis-related fractures is indicated by the occurrence of fractures in skeletal regions with high trabecular bone content and the number of investigations that have focused on this type of bone. A number of studies utilizing a variety of methods have confirmed post-menopausal and age-related changes in the vertebral trabecular architecture, and have further demonstrated that architecture does play a role, independent of mass, in bone strength (Kleerekoper *et al.*, 1985; Garrahan *et al.*, 1986; Mosekilde, 1988, 1989, 1993; Mellish *et al.*, 1991; Vesterby *et al.*, 1991; Parfitt, 1992; Compston, 1994; Jayasinghe *et al.*, 1994).

4.1. Visual Examination of Trabecular Bone Structure

Visual examination of the trabecular bone present can give an indication of bone loss and bone quality. At a gross scale it may be possible to observe phenomena such as trabecular bone loss and cortical thinning. At a slightly more detailed level it may be possible to observe features such as free-ending trabecular struts and micro-callus formation in association with architectural change to trabecular bone. These features of micro-architectural deterioration have been noted in studies of archaeological bone (Roberts and Wakely, 1992;

Brickley, 1998). However, if a meaningful analysis is to be undertaken there needs to be some method by which such changes can be quantified. Simple visual examination with no standard method of recording that could be applied by subsequent workers is of little value in comparisons of spatial and temporal changes in age-related bone loss and osteoporosis.

4.2. Singh Index

Simple radiographic images of bone can be examined in order to determine the amount and pattern of bone present. The simplest technique involving visual examination of radiographic images is the Singh index (Singh *et al.*, 1970), as it does not require complex equipment, just the scoring of the pattern of trabecular bone. Standard radiographs of the region of the proximal femur known as Ward's Triangle are examined visually and compared to written descriptions of the pattern of the trabecular bone within this region (six stages are described). Mielke *et al.* (1972) conducted an early study of trabecular patterning in a Nubian archaeological sample. However, testing of this technique on archaeological bone demonstrated that there were a number of problems in applying the technique (Brickley, 1998). One point noted is the difficulty in obtaining repeatable scores. It would be hard for two individuals working independently to consistently award the same score. Middle scores were the least consistent; consistency was greatest at either extreme. This result indicates that six stages may be too many. However, the extremes are relatively easy to determine and scores at the top and bottom of the range could be used as a way of expressing complete trabecular bone preservation or loss of structural integrity of trabecular elements in this region. In studies of modern individuals it is not clear how useful the Singh index is in determining bone loss and predicting fracture (Hadberg and Nilsson, 1977). Although some studies have identified a link between scores awarded for the Singh index and other measures of bone loss, the studies by Kawashima and Uhtoff (1991) and Brickley (1998) found only moderate correlations between the Singh index and other measures of bone loss.

4.3. Image Analysis of Trabecular Architecture

The quantitative examination of trabecular tissue has been used to investigate metabolic disease in case studies of archaeological skeletons (Weinstein *et al.*, 1981; Cook *et al.*, 1988). More recently, it has been demonstrated that age- and sex-related change in trabecular architecture can be successfully quantitatively examined in archaeological bone with the use of image analysis (Agarwal *et al.*, in press; Agarwal, 2001). Using X-rays of thick bone sections this method can provide a relatively simple assessment of age-related change in trabecular microstructure (Agarwal *et al.*, in press; Agarwal, 2001). This can be used to examine changes in trabecular bone microstructure as well as connectivity. Image analysis has been used extensively in clinical research to examine age-related changes in trabecular bone microstructure from samples that have been processed as thin sections (Garrahan *et al.*, 1986; Compston *et al.*, 1987; Vesterby, 1990; Amling *et al.*, 1996; Croucher *et al.*, 1996; Lundon *et al.*, 1997; Thomsen *et al.*, 2000), photographs of thick sections (Twomey *et al.*, 1983; Bergot *et al.*, 1988), and computed tomography (CT) images (Gordon *et al.*, 1998; Banse *et al.*, 2001). Although the different methods of obtaining images are not directly comparable, the different images provide similar information on trabecular structure and each offer different advantages. Digital image analysis of X-rays of trabecular bone architecture has been used in previous studies (Geraets *et al.*, 1990, 1993; Grynpas *et al.*, 1992, 1994), and the reliability of the technique is well established (Korstjens *et al.*, 1997). Radiographic images also capture trabecular structure throughout the entire section, and it has been demonstrated that radiographic properties of trabecular bone architecture significantly correlate to biomechanical characteristics (Korstjens *et al.*, 1998). Further, entire sections of large bones (e.g., sections of the vertebral body) are not easily processed to obtain thin sections. 3-D imaging instruments such as CT can obtain good images of the trabecular structure, although, these instruments are not often readily available for study with archaeological specimens. There are concerns with microstructural analysis using 2-D images. 2-D images are not an exact representation of the 3-D structure of the trabecular bone, but certainly are highly related to 3-D structure.

Images of trabecular microstructure can be analyzed with standard image analysis tools. Images are generally first scanned to obtain image files that can be accessed by an automated image processing and analysis system. Usually a masked area is used on the image to include only the trabecular tissue of the entire section, excluding the surrounding cortical bone. After thresholding the gray level images, binary images are obtained from which a further pruned version of the binary trabeculae is created. From this binary image mathematical morphology and standard image analysis tools can provide quantitative information on the connectivity of the trabecular architecture using strut analysis (Serra, 1982; Mellish *et al.*, 1991), and can also give information on structural histomorphometric parameters such as trabecular bone volume, average trabecular thickness, trabecular number, and trabecular separation as calculated by Parfitt *et al.* (1987). As with cortical histomorphometry, this method allows the examination of changes in bone remodeling at the tissue level without the concern for chemical diagenesis. More importantly, the examination of trabecular connectivity gives some idea of the bone quality.

The major disadvantage with the method is that most anthropological departments do not routinely use image analysis instruments and software, and some degree of technical experience is required with the image manipulation software. However, the equipment is becoming more readily available, and when used with newer CT imaging methods would provide an ideal non-invasive method to examine and quantify trabecular bone loss and architecture in archaeological populations.

4.4. Stereometry

Stereometry is a simple approach that allows the analysis of three dimensional trabecular structure. In a stereometric study of bone from modern individuals Jayasinghe (1991) found that there is a significant decrease in horizontal and vertical trabeculae with age. More importantly, there is highly significant decrease in horizontally oriented trabeculae with age, while the length of the remaining trabeculae increases with age, findings that were backed up by Brickley and Howell (1999). With complicated structures, such as the network formed by trabecular bone, stereo-measurement techniques are important for the correct interpretation of spatial relationships.

The technique is destructive in that it requires a 5 mm plane-parallel slice of bone to be cut to allow analysis of the trabecular architecture. In order for measurements to be made, stereo-pair photographs are taken and a stereocomparator is required to allow visual examination of the sample and measurements to take place. In the studies by Jayasinghe (1991) and Brickley and Howell (1999) the equipment used was an SFS-3 stereocomparator (Ross Instruments Ltd. Morgansvale Road, Redlynch, Salisbury, Wiltshire, UK) (Ross, 1986). Both the studies undertaken demonstrated a clear link between changes in trabecular architecture and age. However, there are a number of drawbacks to the technique. First the technique is invasive and second the equipment required to view and record the trabecular bone is not widely available.

4.5. Energy Dispersive Low Angle X-ray Scattering (EDLAXS)

Energy Dispersive Low Angle X-ray Scattering (EDLAXS) is an energy dispersive diffraction technique. This is just one of the newer techniques that have been investigated with a view to providing clinicians with a more reliable tool than DEXA. However, results obtained to date indicate that the radiation dose may be too high for the technique to be used clinically. Although the radiation dose is not problematic for investigations of archaeological bone the fact that the technique is not likely to be used in a clinical setting means that such an apparatus will not be widely available, but confined to a relatively small number of laboratory setups. The limited availability has clear implications for the potential of the technique to contribute to future understanding of age-related bone loss in past populations.

The system uses a polyenergetic beam of X-rays produced in an X-ray tube. An energy sensitive detector is placed so as to detect the scattered photons from an object at a fixed angle (Farquharson and Brickley, 1997). Only certain wavelengths (and hence photon energies) will satisfy the Bragg condition for constructive interference from the scattering planes to occur. The energies at which diffraction takes place are detected and an intensity versus energy spectrum can be measured. A plot of the relative intensity of the scattering spectra is produced, and from this a plot of different minerals can be recognized and their quantities can be calculated. The measurement area can be adjusted and it is possible to measure the trabecular bone alone or both trabecular and some cortical bone. The results of the measurements using EDLAXS are expressed in counts of photons. EDLAXS measurements on bone have the potential to reveal all the mineral components present in the tissue. As a result techniques such as EDLAXS have the potential to detect the type of minerals present as well as the "density" of a bone (Farquharson, 1996; Farquharson and Brickley, 1997). Studies by Brickley in which the measurement area was configured to measure only trabecular bone (1998) demonstrated that the technique produced accurate results. The main limitation of this technique is its accessibility, rather than its accuracy.

5. Investigative Techniques that Measure Whole Bone

The diagnosis of bone loss and assessment of risk of fracture in the clinical setting is routinely made with the non-invasive *in vivo* measurement of bone density. There are a variety of non-invasive densitometry methods, including recent methods such as quantitative CT and ultrasound (Grampp *et al.*, 1993; Jergas and Genant, 1993; Genant *et al.*, 1996). However, bone mass is routinely examined with the use of absorptiometric methods that are based on the differential absorption of radiation by bone and soft tissues. While the key advantage of the application of these methods to archaeological bone is that they are non-invasive, each of the methods have some concerns that are addressed below.

5.1. Optical/Photo Densitometry

One method to examine bone density in the whole bone is optical or photo densitometry. In this technique a relative measure of bone density is calculated from radiographs. Clinically, the wrist and hand are the most commonly used sites (Kruse and Kuhlencordt, 1983; Bland *et al.*, 1989). An object of known density, or more frequently a scaled marker such as a step wedge made of aluminum, is placed on the X-ray film next to the area to be radiographed. The steps of the step wedge allow a range of known optical densities to be obtained. Densities can be read from the film using an optical densitometer. The film is placed between a light source and a photoelectric cell, the output of which has been calibrated. A calibration curve may be constructed using these standards, allowing a density figure to be given to any part of the picture on film. In clinical studies a water bath may be used to eliminate soft tissue differences around bone (Barnett and Nordin, 1960). A number of measurements should be taken from the region of interest and the average calculated. If a whole bone is radiographed then trabecular as well as cortical bone will be included in the measurement.

The results obtained from applying this technique to archaeological bone will not be comparable to those obtained in clinical studies. The presence of soft tissue will influence the results of a clinical study, hence the need to use a water bath in some clinical investigations. However, the results obtained from an investigation using archaeological bone have been found to be accurate and the technique is therefore suitable for studies that seek to look at differences in the density of bone between individuals from an archaeological collection (Brickley, 1998). One serious concern that exists with the technique is the possible influence of diagenetic change. Although the radiographic image obtained will allow some diagenetic changes to be observed, many changes taking place in archaeological bone are difficult to detect through simple visual analysis of a radiographic image. Therefore, before any large-scale study involving the technique is used careful testing of the mineral make up of the bones to be investigated should be carried out. This could be done with a technique such as X-ray powder diffraction that requires relatively small samples. Although the equipment used is widely available and the technique simple to use and inexpensive, these limitations of non-invasive density assessment must be considered.

5.2. Dual Energy X-ray Absorptiometry (DEXA)

DEXA was developed for clinical use and is a widely used aid to identify individuals at risk of fracture (Thompson, 1991; Peel and Eastell, 1995). It has been utilized in a number of recent studies investigating archaeological material (Bennike and Bohr, 1990; Lees *et al.*, 1993; Ekenman *et al.*, 1995; Mays *et al.*, 1998; Poulsen *et al.*, 2001). Absorptiometric methods are tempting to use in the case of archeological specimens as they offer non-invasive diagnosis and are generally accepted as the gold standard for the assessment of bone loss in the clinical setting.

Unlike earlier absorptiometric methods, DEXA utilizes a stable X-ray source for the measurement of mineral content. The area of interest is scanned using two energies of radiation that are absorbed by the soft tissue and bone. Computer analysis of the absorption patterns allows the measurement of bone mineral content and density. The way in which absorption patterns are analyzed means that the bone mineral density is expressed as grams of hydroxyapatite per cm^2. DEXA equipment and software used in the clinical setting are designed based on a number of assumptions. For example, it is assumed soft tissue is present and that all mineral encountered is hydroxyapatite.

There are a number of ways in which the problems related to lack of soft tissue can be approached. One approach is to use the forearm option available with machines such as the Lunar DPX-L (GE Lunar Corp, Madison, WI). Scans using this setting can be performed in air providing the tissue equivalent platform made of delrin is included in the scan. Delrin (Acetal/Celcon) is a homopolymer material. Alternatively a water bath, rice, or other substitute material can be used. Using a "slow" scan mode with DPX-L scans and the manual analysis option to define the region of interest help increase accuracy, but there are still problems associated with the technique (Brickley, 1998). In each case error will be introduced to the calculations due to the fact that in almost all clinical DEXA scans soft tissue is taken into consideration in calculations, and the body index of the "patient" is required. Another alternative is to use the specialized small animal software that is available for most scanners. This software is specifically designed for use in small animals samples without soft tissue. However, again some type of plastic or polystyrene container is needed to simulate the soft tissue. The use of specialized peripheral densitometers has also been recently used to effectively examine age-related changes in bone mineral density in thick sections of archaeological bones (Agarwal, 2001). Specialized peripheral densitometers, such as the GE Lunar Piximus densitometer are primarily used for small animal analyses, but also utilize dedicated software designed for small excised bones without soft tissue. Further, the instrument has the advantage of short scan time (with the use of cone beam energy), as well as good precision and spatial resolution, making it ideal to examine thick sections of archeological bones (Agarwal, 2001). However, due to its small maximum scan area, only small bones or sections of bones can be scanned. Further, the instrument is not readily available, although peripheral research instruments may allow more accurate measurements of bone mineral density in archeological samples in the future.

It should be noted that, since DEXA measurements are projectional, measured bone density is not a true volumetric density but an areal density. The normalization by the projected area reduces the effect of body size, but can be problematic, for example, in the case of true volume of a whole vertebra (Ott *et al.*, 1997; Nelson and Koo, 1999). With a constant volumetric density a larger vertebrae would give higher areal BMD results as compared to a smaller vertebrae (Genant *et al.*, 1996; Ebbesen *et al.*, 1998; Nelson and Koo, 1999). There have been attempts to estimate true volumetric bone density from DEXA scans (Carter *et al.*, 1992; Compston, 1995; Jergas *et al.*, 1995; Ott *et al.*, 1997), however, while these estimates more accurately determine true volumetric density, they do not improve predictions of fracture risk (Genant *et al.*, 1996; Ott *et al.*, 1997). The difference between volumetric and areal BMD is certainly important when studying BMD in children during growth or longitudinal studies, and when comparing vertebrae of very different sizes (Agarwal, 2001).

However, the most serious concerns with absorptiometric methods in dry archaeological bone is diagenesis. A number of investigators have questioned the reliability of BMD measurements in archaeological bone (Kneissel *et al.*, 1994; Agarwal and Grynpas,

1996; Mays, 1996; Brickley and Waldron, 1998). Although radiographic assessment of bone specimens prior to scanning can help exclude samples with obvious inclusions, it is essentially impossible to determine the extent of diagenetic alteration without invasive or chemical methods.

6. Conclusions

Postmenopausal and age-related bone loss is a complex process with a multifactorial etiology. While bone loss in archaeological bone can be studied at the gross and microscopic level with various methodologies, it should be noted that these techniques offer insight into different aspects of bone remodeling and maintenance. More importantly, these methods are not directly comparable. While there is a push to apply methods that are routinely used in the clinical setting to archaeological remains, these methods are not always applicable due to the confounding effects of diagenesis or the lack of soft tissue. Also, effort needs to be made to develop and maintain current standards with any of the methods and nomenclature used to facilitate better comparison of results by different researchers.

In order to gain a more complete picture of bone loss in the past, loss at different skeletal sites composed of differing tissues (cortical and trabecular) must be considered within samples. Similarly, as Agarwal and Grynpas (1996) have emphasized, the role of bone quality (such as bone material or architecture) must be considered alongside the role of bone mass or density. The success of examining age-related bone loss in the past also relies heavily on the accuracy of age estimations of archaeological skeletons. As such, there also needs to be continued effort to examine bone loss and fragility in historical known age at death collections.

It is evident that the growing number of methodologies used to examine bone loss and its complex etiology, combined with the unique issues surrounding the study of archaeological bone, make the study of bone loss in the past difficult. However, what makes the picture of bone loss and fragility so complex also makes it so compelling and interesting to examine in past populations.

References

Agarwal, S.C. (2001). The influence of age and sex on trabecular architecture and bone mineral density in three British historical populations. Doctoral thesis, University of Toronto, Toronto.

Agarwal, S.C. and Grynpas, M.D. (1996). Bone quantity and quality in past population. *Anat. Rec.* **249**, 423–432.

Agarwal, S.C., Dimitriu, M., and Grynpas, M.D. (in press). Medieval trabecular bone architecture: The influence of age, sex and lifestyle. *Am. J. Phys. Anthropol.*

Amling, M., Herden, S., Pösl, M., Hahn, M., Ritzel, H., and Delling, G. (1996). Heterogeneity of the skeleton: Comparison of the trabecular microarchitecture of the spine, the iliac crest, the femur, and the calcaneus. *J. Bone Miner. Res.* **11**, 36–45.

Aufderheide, A.C. and Rodríguez-Martín, C. (1998). *The Cambridge Encyclopedia of Human Paleopathology*. Cambridge University Press, Cambridge.

Banse, X., Devogelaer, J.P., Munting, E., Delloye, C., Cornu, O., and Grynpas, M. (2001). Inhomogeneity of human vertebral cancellous bone: Systematic density and structure patterns inside the vertebral body. *Bone* **28**, 563–571.

Barnett, E. and Nordin, B.E.C. (1960). The radiological diagnosis of osteoporosis: A new approach. *Clin. Radiol.* **11**, 166–174.

Bell, L.S. (1990). Palaeopathology and diagenesis: An evaluation of structural changes using backscattered electron imaging. *J. Arch. Sci.* **17**, 85–102.

Bennike, P. and Bohr, H. (1990). Bone mineral content in the past and present. In C. Christiansen and K. Overgaard (eds) *Third International Symposium on Osteoporosis*. Osteopress, Copenhagen, pp. 89–91.

Bergot, C., Laval-Jeantet, A.M., Preteux, F., and Meunier, A. (1988). Measurement of anisotropic vertebral trabecular bone loss during aging by quantitative image analysis. *Calcif. Tissue Int.* **43**, 143–149.

Bland, J.S., Brooks, D.H., Kent, D.J., and Fisher, W.H. (1989). Evaluation of the clinical significance of appendicular skeletal assessment by radiographic photodensitometry. *J. Manipulative Physiol. Ther.* **12**, 113–119.

Brickley, M. (1998). Age-related bone loss and osteoporosis in archaeological bone: A study of two London collections, Redcross Way and Farringdon Street. Doctoral thesis, University of London, London.

Brickley, M. (2000). The diagnosis of metabolic bone disease in archaeological bone. In M. Cox and S. Mays (eds) *Human Osteology in Archaeology and Forensic Science*. Greenwich Medical Media, London, pp. 183–198.

Brickley, M. (2002). Recognition and understanding of age-related bone loss and osteoporosis-related fractures in the eighteenth and nineteenth centuries. In R. Arnott (ed.) *The Archaeology of Medicine*. British Archaeological Reports, British Series, Oxford, pp. 141–146.

Brickley, M. (2002b). An investigation of historical and archaeological evidence for age-related bone loss and osteoporosis. *Int. J. Osteoarchaeol.* **12**, 364–371.

Brickley, M. and Howell, P.G.T. (1999). Measurement of changes in trabecular bone structure with age in an archaeological population. *J. Arch. Sci.* **26**, 151–157.

Brickley, M. and Waldron, T. (1998). Relationship between bone density and osteoarthritis in a skeletal population from London. *Bone* **22**(3), 279–283.

Burr, D.B., Ruff, C.B., and Thompson, D.D. (1990). Patterns of skeletal histological change through time: Comparison of an archaic native American population with modern populations. *Anat. Rec.* **26**, 307–313.

Carter, D.R., Bouxsein, M.L., and Marcus, R. (1992). New approaches for interpreting projected bone densitometry data. *J. Bone Miner. Res.* **7**, 137–145.

Compston, J.E. (1994). Connectivity of cancellous bone: Assessment and mechanical implications. *Bone* **15**, 463–466.

Compston, J.E. (1995). Bone density: BMC, BMD, or corrected BMD? *Bone* **16**, 5–7.

Compston, J.E., Mellish, R.W., and Garrahan, N.J. (1987). Age-related changes in iliac crest trabecular microanatomic bone structure in man. *Bone* **8**, 289–292.

Cook, M., Molto, E., and Anderson, C. (1988). Possible case of hyperparathyroidism in a Roman period skeleton from the Dakhleh Oasis, Egypt, diagnosed using bone histomorphometry. *Am. J. Phys. Anthropol.* **75**, 23–30.

Croucher, P.I., Garrahan, N.J., and Compston, J.E. (1996). Assessment of cancellous bone structure: Comparison of strut analysis, trabecular bone pattern factor, and marrow space star volume. *J. Bone Miner. Res.* **11**, 955–961.

Cummings, S.R., Black, D.M., Nevitt, M.C., Browner, W., Cauley, J., Ensrud, J., Genant, H.K., Palermo, L. *et al.* (1993). Bone density at various sites for prediction of hip fractures. *Lancet* **341**, 72–75.

Dargent, P. and Breart, G. (1993). Epidemiology and risk factors of osteoporosis. *Curr. Opin. Rheumatol.* **5**, 339–345.

Dequeker, J., Ortner, D.J., Stix, A.I., Cheng, X., Brys, P., and Boonen, S. (1997). Hip fracture and osteoporosis in a XIIth dynasty female skeleton from Lisht, Upper Egypt. *J. Bone Miner. Res.* **12**, 881–888.

Derisquebourg, T., Dubois, P., Devogelaer, J., Duquesnoy, B., Nagent de Deuxchaisnes, C., Delcambre, B., and Marchandis, X. (1994). Automated computerized radiogrammetry of the second metacarpal and its correlation with absorptiometry of forearm and spine. *Calcif. Tissue Int.* **54**, 461–465.

Drusini, A.G., Bredaroil, S., Carrara, N., and Bonati, M. (2000). Cortical bone dynamics and age-related osteopenia in a Longobard archaeological sample from three graveyards of the Veneto Region (Northeast Italy). *Int. J. Osteoarchaeol.* **10**, 268–279.

Ebbesen, E.N., Thomsen, J.S., Beck-Nielsen, H., Nepper-Rasmussen, H.J., and Mosekilde, L. (1998). Vertebral bone density evaluated by dual energy X-ray absorptiometry and quantitative computed tomography *in vitro*. *Bone* **23**, 283–290.

Ekenman, I., Eriksson, A., and Lindgren, J. (1995). Bone density in Medieval skeletons. *Calcif. Tissue Int.* **56**, 355–358.

Ericksen, M.F. (1980). Patterns of microscopic bone remodelling in three aboriginal American populations. In D.L. Brownman (ed.) *Early Native Americans: Prehistoric Demography, Economy, and Technology*. Houton, The Hague, pp. 239–270.

Farquharson, M.J. (1996). *Characterisation of Bone Tissue Using Coherently Scattered X-ray Photons*. Doctoral thesis, University of London, London.

Farquharson, M.J. and Brickley, M. (1997). Determination of mineral composition of archaeological bone using energy-dipersive low-angle X-ray scattering. *Int. J. Osteoarchaeol.* **7**, 95–99.

Foldes, A.J., Moscovici, A., Popovtzer, M.M., Mogle, P., Urman, D., and Zias, J. (1995). Extreme osteoporosis in a sixth century skeleton from the Negev desert. *Int. J. Osteoarchaeol.* **5**, 157–162.

Frigo, P. and Lang, C. (1995). Osteoporosis in a woman of the Early Bronze Age. *N. Engl. J. Med.* **333**, 1468.

Gallagher, J.C. (1990). The pathogenesis of osteoporosis. *Bone Miner.* **9**, 215–227.

Garrahan, N.J., Mellish, R.W., and Compston, J.E. (1986). A new method for the two-dimensional analysis of bone structure in human iliac crest biopsies. *J. Microsc.* **142**, 341–349.

Genant, H.K., Engelke, K., Fuerst, T., Gluer, C.C., Grampp, S., Harris, S.T., Jergas, M., Lang, T. *et al.* (1996). Noninvasive assessment of bone mineral and structure: State of the art. *J. Bone. Miner. Res.* **11**, 707–730.

Geraets, W.G., Van der Stelt, P.F., and Elders, P.J. (1993). The radiographic trabecular bone pattern during menopause. *Bone* **14**, 859–864.

Gordon, C.L., Lang, T.F., Augat, P., and Genant, H.K. (1998). Image-based assessment of spinal trabecular bone structure from high-resolution CT images. *Osteoporos. Int.* **8**, 317–325.

Grampp, S., Jergas, M., Gluer, C.C., Lang, P., and Genant, H.K. (1993). Radiologic diagnosis of osteoporosis. Current methods and perspectives. *Radiol. Clin. North Am.* **31**, 1133–1145.

Grynpas, M.D., Acito, A., Dimitriu, M., Mertz, B.P., and Very, J.M. (1992). Changes in bone mineralization, architecture and mechanical properties due to long-term (1 year) administration of pamidronate (APD) to adult dogs. *Osteoporos. Int.* **2**, 74–81.

Grynpas, M.D., Kasra, M., Dumitriu, M., Nespeca, R., Very, J.M., and Mertz, B.P. (1994). Recovery from pamidronate (APD): A two-year study in the dog. *Calcif. Tissue Int.* **55**, 288–294.

Hadberg, L. and Nilsson, B.E. (1977). Can fracture of the femoral neck be predicted? *Geriatrics* **32**, 55–61.

Ives, R.A. (2002). An investigation of metacarpal radiogrammetry and age-related cortical bone loss in Post-Medieval London Collections. M.Phil. thesis, The University of Birmingham, Birmingham, UK.

Jackes, M. (2000). Building the bases for paleodemographic analysis: Adult age determination. In M.A. Katzenberg and S.R. Saunders (eds) *Biological Anthropology of the Human Skeleton*. Wiley-Liss, New York, pp. 417–466.

Jayasinghe, J.A.P. (1991). *A study of change in human trabecular bone structure with age and during osteoporosis*. Doctoral thesis, University of London, London.

Jayasinghe, J.A.P., Jones, S.J., and Boyde, A. (1994). Three-dimensional photographic study of cancellous bone in human fourth lumbar vertebral bodies. *Anat. & Embryol. (Berl.)* **189**, 259–274.

Jergas, M., Breitsenseher, M., Gluer, C.C., Yu, W., and Genant, H.K. (1995). Estimates of volumetric bone density from projectional measurements improve the discriminatory capability of dual X-ray absorptiometry. *J. Bone Miner. Res.* **10**, 1101–1110.

Jergas, M. and Genant, H.K. (1993). Current methods and recent advances in the diagnosis of osteoporosis. *Arthritis Rheum.* **36**, 1649–1662.

Kanis, J.A. (1994). *Osteoporosis*. Blackwell Scientific Publications, Oxford.

Kawashima, T. and Uhthoff, H.K. (1991). Pattern of bone loss of the proximal femur: A radiologic, densitometric and histomorphometric study. *J. Orthop. Res.* **9**, 634–640.

Kleerekoper, M., Villanueva, A.R., Staneiu, J., Sudhaker Rao, D., and Parfitt, A.M. (1985). The role of three-dimensional trabecular mico-structure in the pathogenesis of vertebral compression fractures. *Calcif. Tissue Int.* **37**, 594–597.

Kneissel, M., Boyde, A., Hahn, M., Treschler-Nicola, M., Kalchhauser, G., Plenk, H., Jr. (1994). Age- and sex-dependent cancellous bone changes in a 4000y BP population. *Bone* **15**, 539–545.

Korstjens, C.M., Spruijt, R.J., Geraets, W.G., Mosekilde, L., and Van der Stelt, P.F. (1997). Reliability of an image analysis system for quantifying the radiographic trabecular pattern [letter]. *IEEE Trans. Med. Imaging* **16**, 230–234.

Korstjens, C.M., Spruijt, R.J., Mosekilde, L., Geraets, W.G., and Van der Stelt, P.F. (1998). Agreement between radiographic and photographic trabecular patterns. *Acta. Radiol.* **39**, 625–631.

Kruse, H.I.P. and Kuhlencordt, F. (1983). Studies in primary osteoporosis. In A. St John Dixon, R.G.G. Russell, and T.C.B. Stamp (eds) *Osteoporosis, A Multi-Disciplinary Problem*. Academic Press, London, pp. 149–152.

Lapedes, D.N. (ed.) (1978). *Mc Graw-Hill Encyclopaedia of the Geological Sciences*. Mc Graw-Hill Inc, New York, pp. 153–155.

Laughlin, W.S., Harper, A.B., and Thompson, D.D. (1979). New approaches to the pre- and post-contact history of Arctic peoples. *Am. J. Phys. Anthropol.* **51**, 579–587.

Lees, B., Molleson, T., Arnett, T.R., and Stevenson, J.C. (1993). Differences in proximal femur bone density over two centuries. *Lancet* **341**, 673–675.

Lundon, K., Dumitriu, M., and Grynpas, M.D. (1997). Supraphysiologic levels of testosterone affect cancellous and cortical bone in young female cynomolgus monkey. *Calcif. Tissue Int.* **60**, 54–62.

Martin, D.L. and Armelagos, G.J. (1979). Morphometrics of compact bone: An example from Sudanese Nubia. *Am. J. Phys. Anthropol.* **51**, 571–578.

Martin, D.L. and Armelagos, G.J. (1985). Skeletal remodeling and mineralisation as indicators of health: An example from prehistoric Sudanese Nubia. *J. Hum. Evol.* **14**(5), 527–537.

Mays, S.A. (1996). Age-dependent cortical bone loss in a Medieval population. *Int. J. Osteoarchaeol.* **6**, 144–154.

Mays, S. (2000). Age dependent cortical bone loss in women from 18th and early 19th century London. *Am. J. Phys. Anthropol.* **112**(3), 349–362.

Mays, S. (2001). Effects of age and occupation on cortical bone in a group of 18th–19th century British Men. *Am. J. Phys. Anthropol.* **116**, 34–44.

Mays, S., Lees, B., and Stevenson, J. (1998). Age-dependent bone loss in the femur in a medieval population. *Int. J. Osteoarchaeol.* **8**, 97–106.

Meema, H.E. and Meema, S. (1987). Postmenopausal osteoporosis: Simple screening method for diagnosis before structural failure. *Radiology* **164**, 405–410.

Mellish, R.W.E., Ferguson-Pell, M.W., Cochran, G.V.B., Lindsay, R., and Dempster, D.W. (1991). A new manual method for assessing two-dimensional cancellous bone structure: Comparison between iliac crest and lumbar vertebra. *J. Bone Miner. Res.* **6**, 689–696.

Melton, J.L., **III**, Chrischilles, E.A., Cooper, C., Lane, A.W., and Riggs, L.B. (1992). Perspective, how many women have osteoporosis. *J. Bone Miner. Res.* **7**, 1005–1010.

Mielke, J.H., Armelagos, G.J., and Van Gerven, D.P. (1972). Trabecular involution in femoral heads of a prehistoric (X-Group) population from Sudanese Nubia. *Am. J. Phys. Anthropol.* **36**(1), 39–44.

Mosekilde, L. (1988). Age-related changes in vertebral trabecular bone architecture, assessed by a new method. *Bone* **9**, 247–250.

Mosekilde, L. (1989). Sex differences in age-related loss of vertebral trabecular mass and structure—biomechanical consequences. *Bone* **10**, 425–432.

Mosekilde, L. (1993). Vertebral structure and strength *in vivo* and *in vitro*. *Calcif. Tissue. Int.* **53** (Suppl 1), S121–S125.

Neese, R.M. and Williams, G.C. (1994). *Why We Get Sick*. Times Books, New York.

Nelson, D.A. and Koo, W.W.K. (1999). Interpretation of absorptiometric bone mass measurements in the growing skeleton: Issues and limitations. *Calcif. Tissue Int.* **65**, 1–3.

Ortner, D.J. and Putschar, W.G.J. (1985). *Identification of Pathological Conditions in Human Skeletal Remains* (2nd edn.). Smithsonian Institution Press, Washington.

Ott, S.M., O'Hanlan, M., Lipkin, E.W., and Newell-Morris, L. (1997). Evaluation of vertebral volumetric vs. aerial bone mineral density during growth. *Bone* **20**, 553–556.

Parfitt, A.M. (1992). Implications of architecture for the pathogenesis and prevention of vertebral fracture. *Bone* **13** (Suppl 2), S41–S47.

Parfitt, A.M., Drezner, M.K., Glorieux, F.H., Kanis, J.A., Malluche, H., Meunier, P.J., Ott, S.M., and Recker, R.R. (1987). Bone histomorphometry: Standardization of nomenclature, symbols, and units. Report of the ASBMR Histomorphometry Nomenclature Committee. *J. Bone Miner. Res.* **2**, 595–610.

Pate, F.D. and Brown, K.A. (1985). The stability of bone strontium in the geochemical environment. *J. Hum. Evol.* **14**, 483–491.

Peel, N. and Eastell, R. (1995). ABC of rheumatology: Osteoporosis. *Brit. Med. J.* **15**, 310 (6985), 989–992.

Pfeiffer, S. (2000). Paleohistology: Health and disease. In A. Katzenberg and S. Saunders (eds) *Biological Anthropology of the Human Skeleton*. Wilry-Liss, New York, pp. 287–302.

Poulsen, L.W., Qvesel, D., Brixen, K., Vesterby, A., and Boldsen, J.L. (2001). Low bone mineral density in the femoral neck of medieval women: A result of multiparity? *Bone* **28**, 454–458.

Richman, E.A., Ortner, D.J., and Schulter-Ellis, F.P. (1979). Differences in intracortical bone remodeling in three aboriginal American populations: Possible dietary factors. *Calcif. Tissue Int.* **28**, 209–214.

Roberts, C. (2000). Trauma in biocultural perspective: Past, present and future work in Britain. In M. Cox and S. Mays (eds) *Human Osteology in Archaeology and Forensic Science*. Greenwich Medical Media, London, pp. 337–356.

Roberts, C. and Manchester, K. (1995). *The Archaeology of Disease* 2nd edn. Cornell University press, New York.

Roberts, C. and Wakely, J. (1992). Microscopical findings associated with the diagnosis of osteoporosis in palaeopathology. *Int. J. Osteoarchaeol.* **2**, 23–30.

Ross, H.F. (1986). A new comparator for SEM Stereophotogrammetry. *Scanning* **8**, 216–220.

Sambrook, P.N., Browne, C.D., Eisman, J.A., and Bourke, S.J. (1988). A case of crush fracture osteoporosis from late Roman Pella in Jordan. *OSSA* **13**, 167–171.

Serra, J. (1982). *Image Analysis and Mathematical Morphology*. Academic Press, London.

Singh, M., Nagrath, A.R., and Maini, P.S. (1970). Changes in the trabecular pattern of the upper end of the femur as an index of osteoporosis. *J. Bone Joint Surg. Br.* **52**a, 457–467.

Sneed, N.V. and Van Bree, K.M. (1990). Treating ununited fractures with electricity: Nursing implications. *J. Gerentol. Nursing* **16**, 26–31.

Stout, S.D. (1983). The application of histomorphometric analysis to ancient skeletal remains. *Anthropos* (Greece), **10**, 60–71.

Stout, S.D. (1989). Histomorphometric analysis of human skeletal remains. In M. Iscan and K. Kennedy (eds) *Reconstruction of Life from the Skeleton*. Alan R Liss, New York, pp. 41–52.

Stout, S.D. and Lueck, R. (1995). Bone remodeling rates and skeletal maturation in three archaeological skeletal populations. *Am. J. Phys. Anthropol.* **93**, 123–129.

Stout, S. and Simmons, D.J. (1979). Use of histology in ancient bone research. *Yearbook of Phys. Anthropol.* pp. 228–249.

Spector, T.D. (1991). The epidemiology of osteoporosis. In J.C. Stevenson (ed.) *Osteoporosis*. Reed Healthcare, Guildford, pp. 7–9.

Thompson, D.D. and Gunness-Hey, M.E. (1981). Bone mineral-osteon analysis of Yupik-Inupiaq skeletons. *Am. J. Phys. Anthropol.* **55**(1), 1–7.

Thompson, P.W. (1991). Assessment of the skeleton. In J.C. Stevenson (ed.) *Osteoporosis*. Reed Healthcare, Guildford, pp. 19–22.

Thomsen, J.S., Ebbesen, E.N., and Mosekilde, L. (2000). A new method of comprehensive static histomorphometry applied on human lumbar vertebral cancellous bone. *Bone* **27**, 129–138.

Twomey, L., Taylor, J., and Furniss, B. (1983). Age changes in the bone density and structure of the lumbar vertebral column. *J. Anat.* **136**, 15–25.

Weaver, D. (1998). Osteoporosis in the bioarchaeology of women. In A.L. Grauer and P. Stuart-Macadam (eds) *Sex and Gender in Paleopathological Perspective*. Cambridge University Press, Cambridge, pp. 27–44.

Weinstein, R.S., Simmons, D.J., and Lovejoy, C.O. (1981). Ancient bone disease in a peruvian mummy revealed by quantitative skeletal histomorphometry. *Am. J. Phys. Anthropol.* **54**, 321–326.

Woolf, A.D. and St John Dixon, A. (1988). *Osteoporosis a Clinical Guide*. M. Dunitz, London.

World Health Organisation. (1994). *Assessment of Fracture Risk and its Application to Screening for Postmenopausal Osteoporosis*. Report of a WHO study group, WHO technical report series **843**. WHO, Geneva.

Vesterby, A. (1990). Star volume of marrow space and trabeculae in iliac crest: Sampling procedure and correlation to star volume of first lumbar vertebra. *Bone* **11**, 149–155.

Vesterby, A., Mosekilde, L., Gundersen, H.J., Melsen, F., Mosekilde, L., Holme, K., and Sorensen, S. (1991). Biologically meaningful determinants of the *in vitro* strength of lumbar vertebrae. *Bone* **12**, 219–224.

Virtama, P. and Helelä, T. (1969). Radiographic measures of cortical bone. Variations in a normal population between 1 and 90 years of age. *Acta Radiol. Suppl.* **293**.

11

Differential Diagnoses of Intravitam and Postmortem Bone Loss at the Micro-Level

Michael Schultz

1. Introduction

In paleopathology and forensic anthropology the examination of bone frequently reveals difficulties in the interpretation of porotic bone structures (Schultz, 2001a). Most notably, it is not always easy to differentiate between intravitam and postmortem bone loss in macerated, that is dry bones, through macroscopic examination. Therefore, in paleopathology, forensic anthropology, or legal medicine as well as in prehistoric or historic archaeology, microscopic research is necessary to establish reliable diagnoses. The causes of intravitam changes that lead to porosity are relatively well known (e.g., osteoporosis due to inactivity or old age; osteoclastic processes such as malignant tumors, tuberculosis, and other inflammatory processes; insufficient blood supply or hemorrhage). The nature and the causes of postmortem factors of decomposition and diagenesis are still not completely understood (Schultz, 1997, 2001a). The most important factors of diagenesis causing bone loss in dry bones are, for instance, soil and water, plant roots, fungi, algae, bacteria, protozoa, and arthropods and their larvae (Schultz, 1986, 1997, 2001a, b). This chapter makes a contribution to the differential diagnoses of intravitam and postmortem bone loss and shows the microscopic examination of thin ground sections of samples taken from dry bones to be the method of choice.

2. Methods and Techniques Used in Histological Research of Macerated Bone Specimens

As a rule, in paleopathology and prehistoric or historic anthropology, the skeletal remains from which samples for microscopic research were taken are relatively brittle and frequently poorly preserved, whereas the materials examined in forensic anthropology or

---

Michael Schultz • Zentrum Anatomie, University of Göttingen, Germany.

Bone Loss and Osteoporosis: An Anthropological Perspective, edited by Sabrina C. Agarwal and Sam D. Stout. Kluwer Academic/Plenum Publishers, New York, 2003.

legal medicine are much better preserved. Archaeological skeletal remains no longer have the quality of fresh bone. Thus, archaeological undecalcified bone samples, embedded or not, should never be cut by microtome. Otherwise, microfractures may occur which can cause serious artifacts leading to false diagnoses. Of course, decalcified bone is easier to cut, however, if a poorly preserved bone sample is decalcified, nothing much remains worth analyzing. Therefore, for archaeological or sometimes even forensic specimens, the technique of choice is the preparation of undecalcified thin ground sections (Schultz and Drommer, 1983; Schultz, 1988, 2001b) using modified already existing techniques (Hackett, 1976; Stout, 1992).

To prepare sufficiently good thin ground sections for the histological examination in the author's laboratory, a special technique was developed based upon the method of plastination established by Hagens (1979), but modified for histological purposes by M. Schultz and M. Brandt (Schultz, 1988, 2001b, 2003). The embedding medium is a special epoxy resin. Before the embedding procedure, the samples are dehydrated in an ascending ethanol series (e.g., solutions of 40, 50, 60, 75, 80, 85, 90, and 95% of ethanol). Lastly, the sample is in methyl chloride as an intermediate solution for the exchange of substances after which they are ready to be embedded. The most suitable embedding substance for such bone samples is the epoxy resin Biodur®, developed by Gunther von Hagens (1979). Biodur® is much easier to handle than methyl methacrylate during the embedding procedure, which takes place under a relative vacuum preserved by a motor vacuum pump. Biodur® is highly suitable for organic materials which might still contain minimal vestiges of moisture. The embedded samples are mounted on a glass slide and cut with a special circular saw (e.g., Dr Steeg and Reuter, Frankfurt am Main). Using the same saw fitted with a special circular disk the samples are ground down to final thicknesses of 100, 70, and 50 μm for unstained thin ground sections to be examined in plane or polarized light, or 15 μm for stained thin ground sections that are to be examined for cells, collagen bundles, and special soft tissue structures in plane light. The polished ground sections are labeled and protected by a thin glass cover. Specimens prepared by this procedure, even from brittle or rotted bone, can usually be examined satisfactorily.

3. Intravitam Changes

When paleopathologists examine the vestiges of ancient diseases in archaeological bones, as a rule, none of the soft tissues or cells, which play an important role in diagnosing pathological conditions in recent materials, are preserved. Therefore, soft tissue histology and cytological examinations cannot be carried out. A similar situation exists when forensic anthropologists use light microscopy to study skeletal remains that are preserved over several decades in the ground. Thus, the options for diagnosing diseases from dry bones are limited.

Because of the limited diagnostics and the large number of diseases that lead to bone loss, paleopathologists should first try to understand the mechanisms of pathophysiology, before diagnosing diseases (Schultz, 2001b, 2003). (For discussions relating to mechanisms of bone loss, see Chapter 1, 2, and 8, this volume.) Therefore, selected examples of intravitam bone loss are presented in this contribution. Abnormal intravitam bone loss is often described by the term osteoporosis.

3.1. Primary Osteoporosis

Three types of primary osteoporosis are known: (a) idiopathic osteoporosis, (b) postmenopausal osteoporosis (type I osteoporosis), and (c) senile or involutional osteoporosis (type II osteoporosis). All three types can be observed in archaeological skeletal remains and can be studied by microscopic techniques.

3.1.1. Idiopathic Osteoporosis

This kind of osteoporosis is rare and occurs in children and young adults with normal gonadal function. Up to now, no archaeological case has been described.

3.1.2. Postmenopausal Osteoporosis

These days, postmenopausal osteoporosis is frequently seen and occurs in individuals between the ages of 50 and 75 years. The frequency in females is six times greater than in males (Kuhlencordt, 1992; Bätge and Renz-Polster, 2000). In females, the decrease in the production of estrogen, and in males the decrease in production of testosterone leads to rarefaction of the cancellous bone trabeculae and the cortical and compact bone substances. This phenomenon causes bone fractures, such as crush fractures of the vertebral bodies and Colles' fractures (fracture in the distal shaft of the radius). Up to now, we have only uncertain information from the archaeological record.

3.1.3. Senile Osteoporosis

Senile osteoporosis, which usually occurs in modern populations in individuals older than 60 years, is associated with the normal process of aging that is characterized by a gradual decrease of the number of osteoblasts. As a rule, the number of osteoclasts is not necessarily enlarged. Further, senile osteoporosis is a more or less multifactorial process, since in old age not only the gonadal function (postmenopausal osteoporosis) but also the functions of all other metabolic processes are reduced. Typical fractures are found in the femoral neck, vertebral bodies, proximal shaft of the humerus, proximal shaft of the tibia, and the pelvis.

There are many papers dealing with this type of osteoporosis in archaeological skeletal remains. However, there are only a few which focus on the problem of aging techniques of archaeological specimens (e.g., Kerley, 1965, 1969; Ahlquist and Damsten, 1969; Stout, 1976, 1992; Kerley and Ubelaker, 1978; Martin and Armelagos, 1979; Uytterschaut, 1985; Wolf, 1999) and on paleodemographic problems in the diagnosis of osteoporosis in ancient populations (e.g., Agarwal and Grynpas, 1996; Beilner, 2001) using histological techniques.

The microscopic examination of thin ground sections taken from the compact bone substance of the diaphysis of long bones shows a characteristic morphological pattern in the transverse section using low power microscopy (Figure 11.1). By viewing thin ground sections demonstrating severely developed age-related osteoporosis, the typical changes, such as decrease in the relative number and the size of Haversian systems and increase in the diameter of the Haversian canals, can be observed (Figure 11.2).

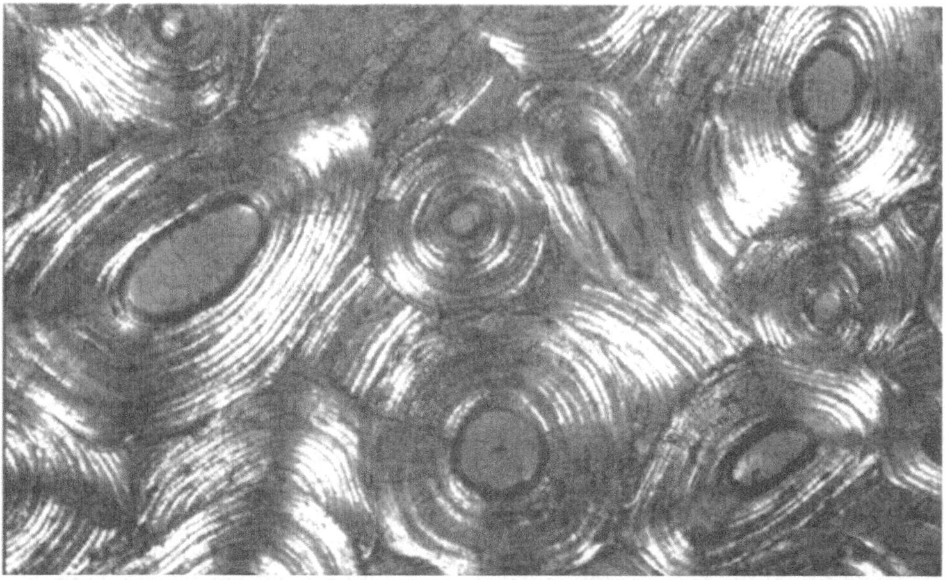

Figure 11.1. Lamellar bone consisting of Haversian systems and interstitial lamellae representing the characteristic bone formation of the compact bone substance of the shaft of long bones (femur). Adult individual from the Iron Age (Celtic) settlement of Manching (southern Germany). Undecalcified thin ground section (50 μm) viewed through the microscope in polarized light using a hilfsobject red 1st order (quartz) as compensator. Magnification 100×.

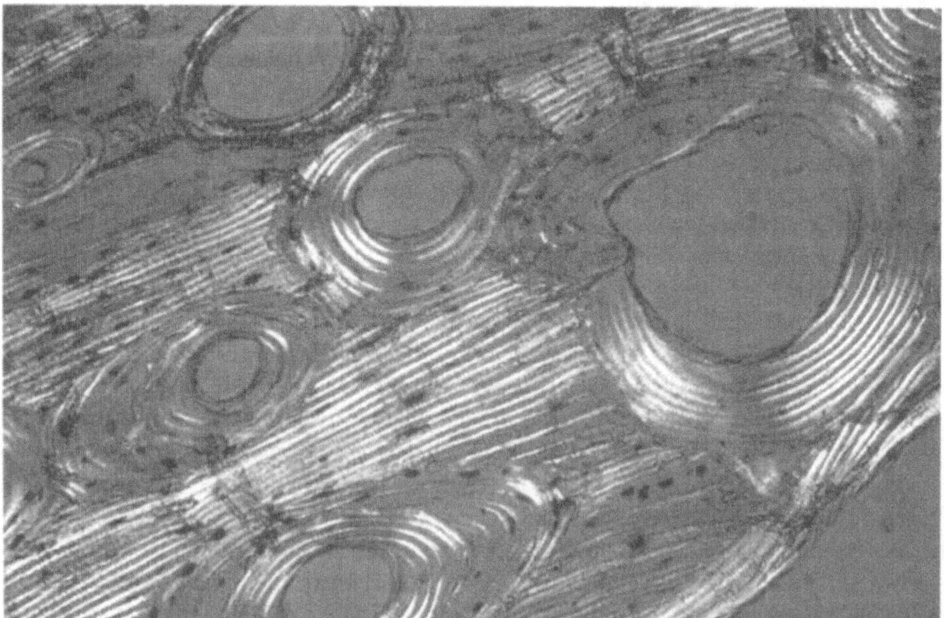

Figure 11.2. Old-age osteoporosis in the cross section of the shaft of the femur of a senile male from an Eneolithic cemetery of central Ukraine (Baštečki). Undecalcified thin ground section (50 μm) viewed through the microscope in polarized light using a hilfsobject red 1st order (quartz) as compensator. Magnification 100×.

3.2. Secondary Osteoporosis

Secondary osteoporosis accounts for less than 5% of all osteoporosis cases. Most of these osteoporosis types still cannot be reliably diagnosed in archaeological skeletal remains (e.g., endocrine, metabolic: Cushing's disease, hyperthyroidism, hypogonadism, diabetes mellitus, homocystinuria; para-infectious, immunogen: rheumatoid arthritis, Crohn's enteritis syndrome; hereditary collagenoses: Ehlers-Danlos' syndrome; complex osteopathy: chronic renal failure, and chronic intestinal syndromes). This means that, of course, bone loss can be diagnosed, but not the exact cause of the osteoporosis. However, some types of secondary osteoporosis can be diagnosed in archaeological specimens using macroscopic and microscopic techniques (e.g., endocrine, metabolic: hyperparathyroidism, acromegalia; hereditary collagenoses: Marfan's syndrome and osteogenesis imperfecta [brittle bone disease]). Some other types, which are also diagnosable using macroscopic and microscopic techniques, will now be discussed.

3.2.1. Osteoporosis due to Inactivity and Immobilization

Microscopic investigations of thin ground sections can detect osteoporotic changes that result from chronic inactivity and immobilization caused by disability or paralysis, such as long-term bed rest, paraplegia, hemiplegia, and paralysis after poliomyelitis (Schultz, 1997, 2001b, 2003). Sometimes, these lesions are not clearly observable macroscopically (Schultz, 2001a).

An interesting example is the Neanderthal individual whose skeletal remains were found in 1856 in the "Kleine Feldhofer Grotte," 13 km east of Düsseldorf (Germany). This skeleton of a young mature male was the first representative of a Neanderthal individual to be described. His left ulna had been fractured during his lifetime. The microscopic investigation of thin ground sections prepared from a sample taken from this bone reveals enlarged Haversian canals and an increase of cancellous bone in the endosteal area of the primarily compact bone substance (Figure 11.3). Thus, the traumatically affected ulna shows evidence of osteoporosis. Because of the young mature age of this male, this osteoporotic structure cannot be the result of age-dependent bone involution. The bone substance of the right ulna shows a regular structure characteristic of the compact bone of a mature individual and no vestiges of osteoporosis (Figure 11.4). These results are striking and can be interpreted as follows. This man suffered from a fracture of his left ulna, which healed relatively well during his lifetime, however, leaving a disability. In comparison to his right ulna (Figure 11.4), which, in the microscopic record, presents a regular bone structure, there is severe osteoporosis in the fractured left ulna (Figure 11.3), due to inactivity atrophy. This means that after the accidental trauma broke the bone, this individual could not use his left arm in the same way as his right arm for the rest of his life. He was unable to carry out the physically hard work of every day life in a normal way. As he survived for many years after this accident, there was likely some kind of social care, which means that other individuals of his group helped him to lead his life, particularly in situations in which the strength of both arms would have been needed (Schultz, 1999). Severe inactivity atrophy caused by extensive loss of myokinetic and skeletal activity is characterized not only by osteoporosis but also by a relative decrease in the number of Haversian systems and the development of tangential lamellae that are situated within the compact bone substance and replace osteonal structures (Knese *et al.*, 1954; Schultz, 1986, 1997,

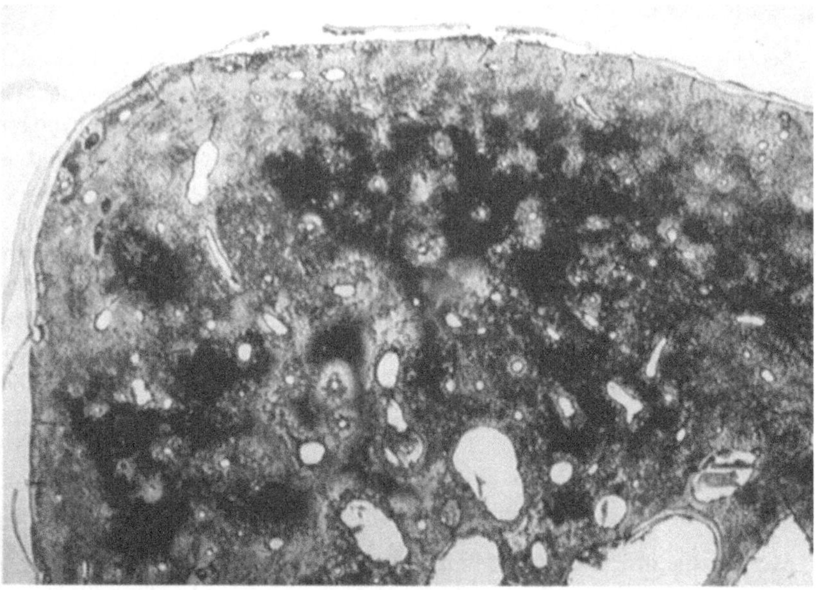

Figure 11.3. Neanderthal man from the Neander Valley. Mature male. Transverse section through left fractured ulna. Compact bone demonstrating osteoporosis by large resorption holes. Undecalcified thin ground section (50 μm) viewed through the microscope in plane (normal) light. Magnification 25×.

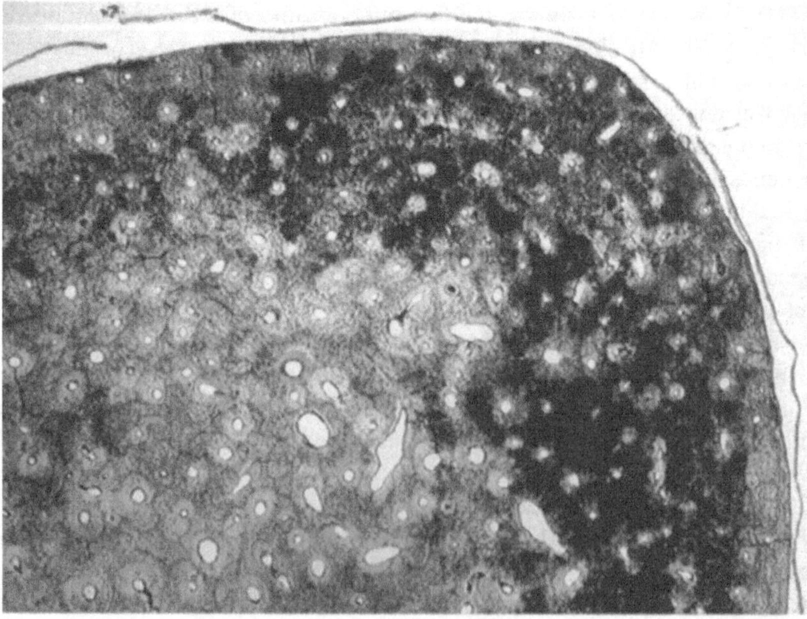

Figure 11.4. Neanderthal man from the Neander Valley. Mature male. Transverse section through right ulna. Compact bone showing no pathological changes. Thin ground section (50 μm) viewed through the microscope in plane (normal) light. Magnification 25×.

2001b, 2003). Tangential lamellae and a significant reduction in the number of the Haversian systems was not observed in the compact substance of the left ulna of this Neanderthal male, it seems evident that he still used his crippled left lower arm to some extent.

3.2.2. Bone Loss Caused by Inflammatory Processes

In macerated bones demonstrating vestiges of inflammatory processes, not only products of proliferative (Schultz, 2001b, 2003), but also of osteolytic (osteoclastic) processes can be observed (Figure 11.5). These osteolytic changes represent typical intravitam bone loss that is characterized by Howship's lacunae. The number and distribution of Howship's lacunae give a relevant impression of the nature of an osteolytic process. Thus, the frequency of Howship's lacunae observed in a thin ground section representing an inflammatory osteolytic process is a good indicator of the intensity (e.g., speed of spread, virulence of pathological agent, immune system of patient) of the disease process. As these relatively small, primary areas of intravitam bone loss can flow together; an osteolytic pattern can originate which looks similar to what is seen in primary osteoporosis. Therefore, occasionally, the inexperienced investigator can confuse these changes.

3.2.3. Bone Loss Caused by Tumorous Processes

Tumorous diseases, particularly metastasizing carcinomas, frequently produce severe bone loss. In macerated skeletal remains, especially in archaeological specimens, these lesions can easily be overlooked because they are mistaken for the vestiges of postmortem destruction (see below). If a tumorous osteoclastic resorption is relatively regular (Figure 11.6), the changes can falsely be diagnosed by paleopathologists as lesions caused by primary osteoporosis. Occasionally, the nature of osteoclastic resorption

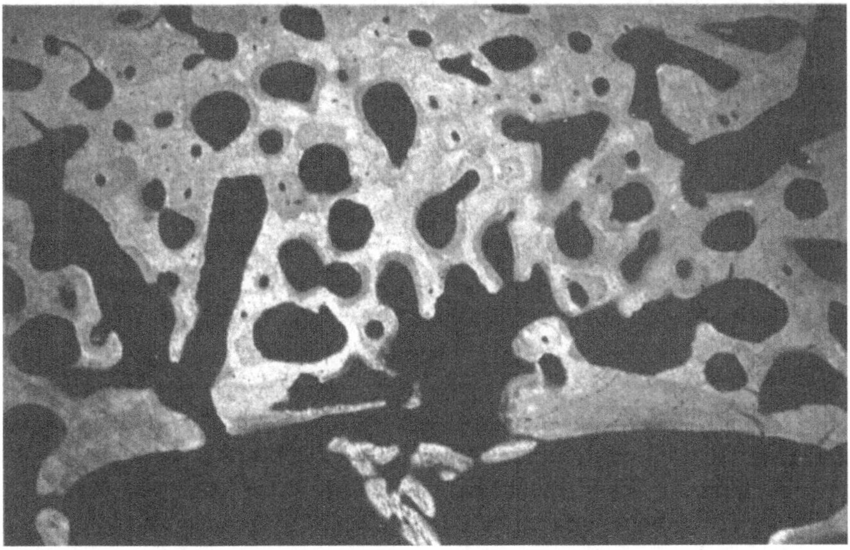

Figure 11.5. Microradiographic image of a cross section of a femur fragment of an adult individual from the Smoky Bear Ruin (Arizona). Osteolytic changes caused by a severe inflammatory process. Magnification 25×.

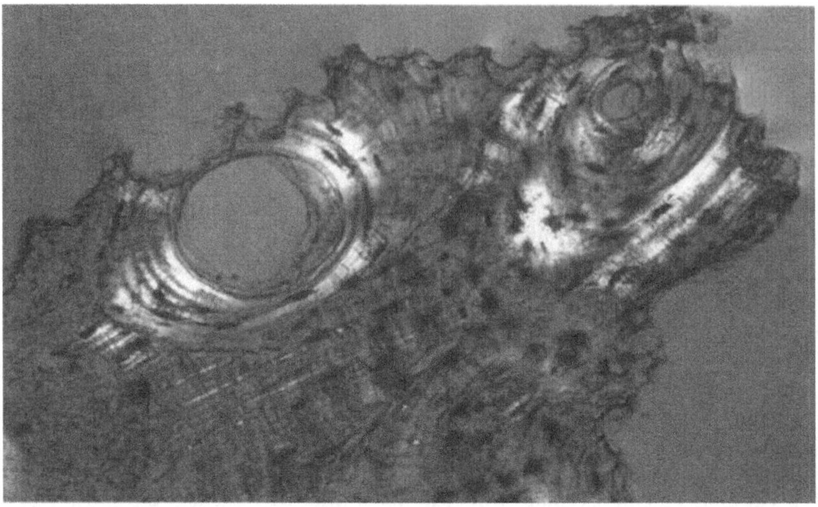

Figure 11.6. Section through a fragment of the skull vault of a 35–45 year-old female from Sayala (Egyptian Nubia). Metastasizing carcinoma. Coptic Period (Early Middle Ages), individual K-68/2. Masses of Howship's lacunae have demarcated a small piece of dead bone (sequester) which can relatively frequently be found with a similar appearance in chronic inflammatory bone processes (osteomyelitis). Undecalcified thin ground section (50 μm) viewed through the microscope in polarized light using a hilfsobject red 1st order (quartz) as compensator. Magnification 100×.

(e.g., growth direction of metastases from the periosteal bone area [Figure 11.7], from the endosteal bone area, or from the Haversian canals [Figure 11.8]) can contribute to the classification of a tumor (Schultz, 1993, 1997). Similarly, as already described in the paragraph dealing with bone loss caused by inflammatory processes, the frequency of Howship's lacunae is a good indicator of the intensity of, for example, metastasizing processes (Figure 11.9).

4. Causes of Postmortem Bone Loss

As most of the changes of postmortem bone loss are primarily only visible at the micro-level, the degree of diagenesis has to be more advanced to produce changes that are macroscopically observable. These vestiges of postmortem damage can falsely be diagnosed by paleopathologists as lesions caused intravitam by diseases (pseudopathology). Many of these changes cannot be differentiated by macroscopic or radiological analysis, but are easily diagnosable by microscopic techniques (Schultz, 1986, 2001b, 2003).

4.1. Soil and Water

It is relatively easy to differentiate changes caused by soil and water from intravitam changes. However, sometimes, the correct diagnosis is difficult when dry soil remains, such as earth, sinter, or other deposits that cannot be removed without destroying brittle bone structures, cover bone surfaces and fill the modules of the red bone marrow. In such a case, histological examination can exclude postmortem changes due to soil and water erosion (Figure 11.10). Severe damage can also be caused by humic acids that can dissolve bony tissues.

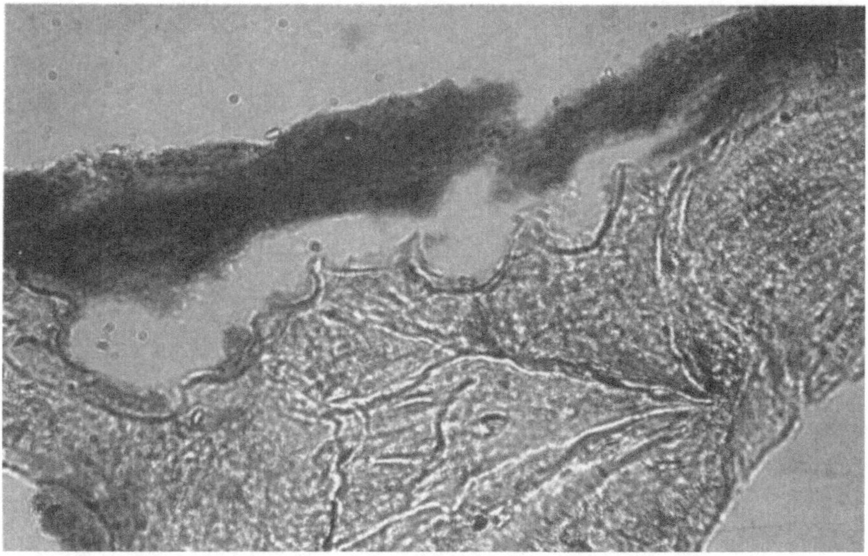

Figure 11.7. Surface of occipito-lateral wall of left maxillary sinus of a 35–45 year-old male from Sayala (Egyptian Nubia). Coptic Period (Early Middle Ages), individual I-3. Vestiges of primary tumor represented by Howship's lacunae covered by mummified remains of soft tissue. The process was spreading from the submucosal periosteal area. Undecalcified thin ground section (50 μm) viewed through the microscope in plane (normal) light. Magnification 250×.

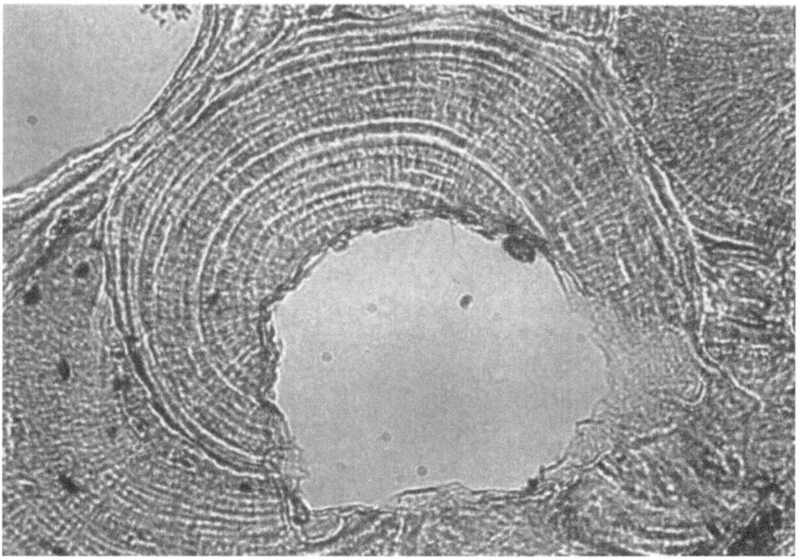

Figure 11.8. Osteoclastic resorption by Howship's lacunae spreading from a Haversian canal in the cross section of the shaft of the left tibia of a 35–55 year-old female from the Late Roman cemetery of Linz (Austria). Undecalcified thin ground section (50 μm) viewed through the microscope in plane (normal) light. Magnification 160×. The bone sample was given to the author by Prof Dr Maria Teschler-Nicola, Museum of Natural History, Vienna (Austria).

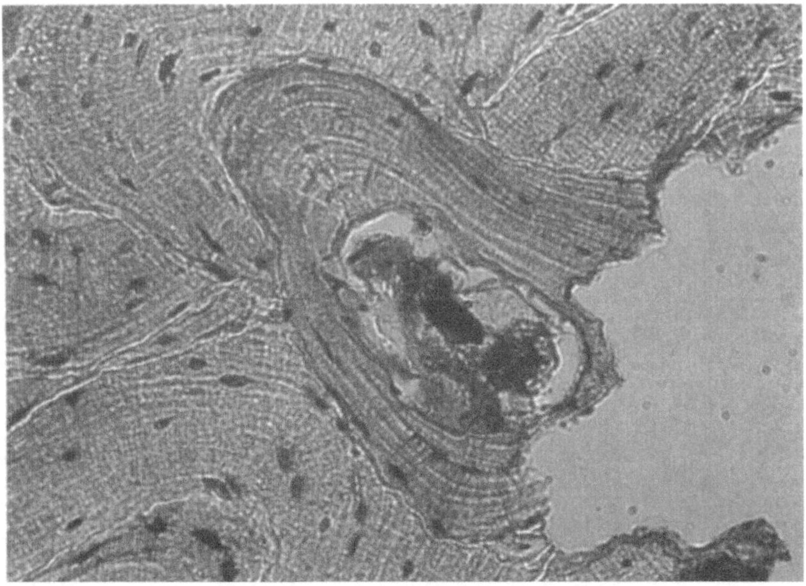

Figure 11.9. Section through the shaft of the left clavicle of a 35–45 year-old female from Sayala (Egyptian Nubia). Metastasizing carcinoma. Coptic Period (Early Middle Ages), individual K-68/2. Masses of Howship's lacunae characterize a marked, very intensive osteoclastic process. Undecalcified thin ground section (50 μm) viewed through the microscope in plane (normal) light. Magnification 160×.

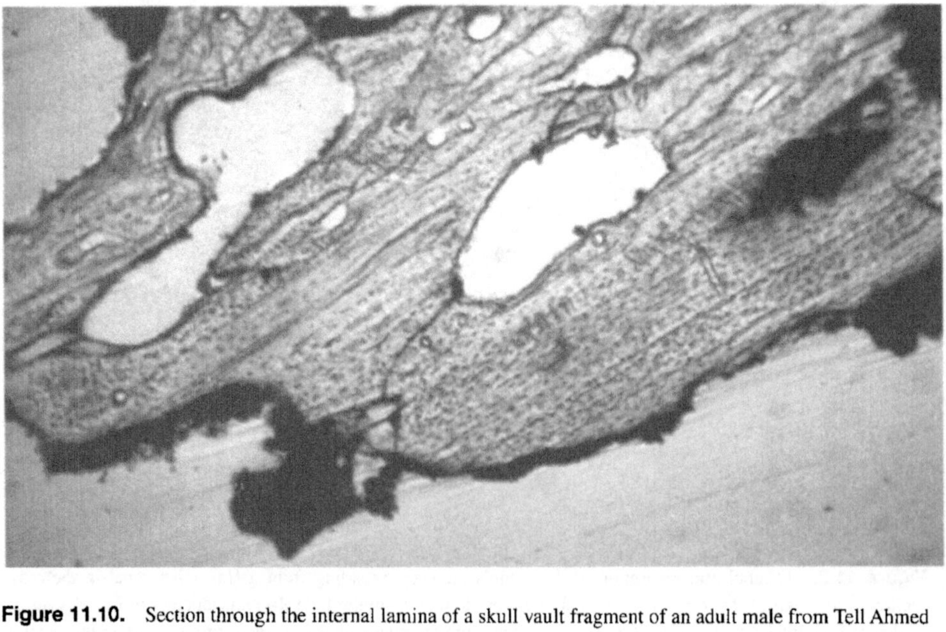

Figure 11.10. Section through the internal lamina of a skull vault fragment of an adult male from Tell Ahmed al-Hattu (Iraq). Early Dynastic Period, individual 7. Destruction caused by soil and water erosion. Undecalcified thin ground section (50 μm) viewed through the microscope in plane (normal) light. Magnification 160×.

4.2. Plant Roots

The growth traces of plant roots causing bone loss by tunneling through the bony tissue are characterized by holes. These changes can easily be differentiated by macroscopic investigation. However, if several different factors, such as soil and water, come together and affect a bone, the typical lesion due to plant roots cannot clearly be differentiated. Very small, hair-like roots are able to destroy the compact bone substance. As a rule, the destruction zone of these fine roots is found at and along the external bone surfaces.

4.3. Fungi, Algae, Bacteria, and Protozoa

Compact bone, in particular, can be destroyed by characteristic tunnel-like canals caused by the postmortem growth of fungi or algae (Wedl, 1864; Hackett, 1981). These tunnels can flow together and produce relatively large destruction holes (Figure 11.11), which, macroscopically, resemble intravitam osteoporosis or vestiges of a metastasizing tumor (Schultz, 2003). As a rule, the tunnels produced by algae are smaller than those

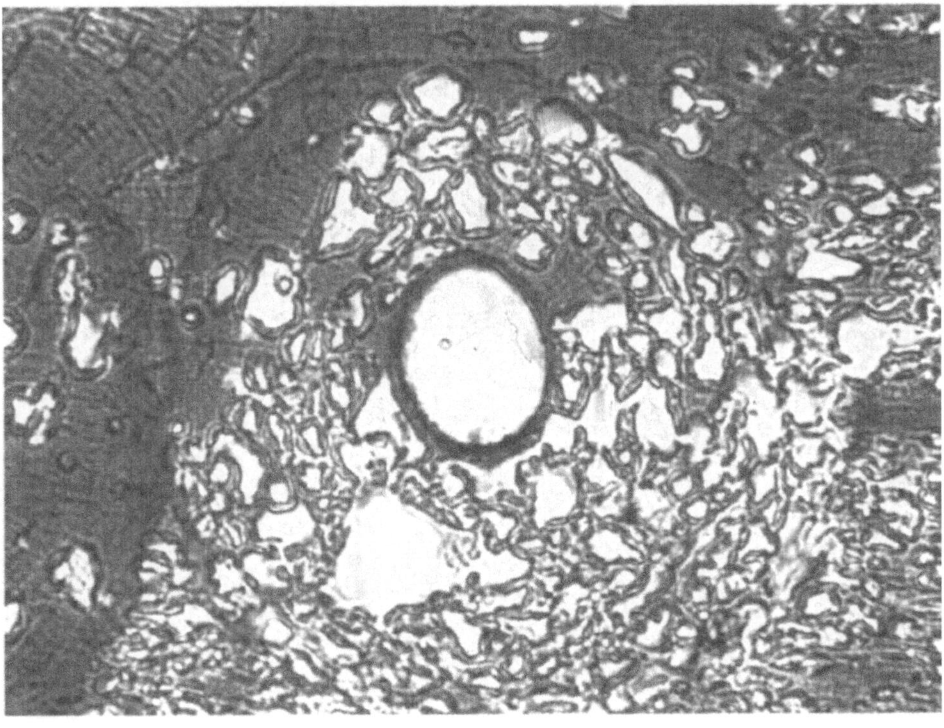

Figure 11.11. Cross section through long bone fragment of an adult individual from Künzing (southern Germany), Late Roman Period. Tunnel-like canals mainly caused by fungi have destroyed compact bone substance of a Haversian system. Undecalcified thin ground section (25 μm) stained with fuchsin viewed through the microscope in plane (normal) light. Magnification 25×.

built up by fungi (Bertozzi, 1982). Destruction holes caused by bacteria are difficult to diagnose in thin ground sections using light microscopy. They are characterized by their irregular shape and patch-like distribution. Using scanning electron microscopy, these defects can be detected more efficiently (Figure 11.12). Relatively rare are vestiges caused by the growth of *actinomycetes* which are small bacteria growing like mycelia. These changes cannot be reliably diagnosed alone by viewing thin ground sections with a light microscope using plane transmission light. However, in scanning electron microscopy, the characteristic size and pattern of these changes are relatively easy to detect (Figure 11.13).

Up to now, no vestiges characteristic of protozoa have been observed. However, there is no doubt that during diagenesis protozoa can also destroy the bony tissues.

4.4. Arthropods and their Larvae

Changes due to arthropods, for example insects and their larvae, are mainly found in spongy bone, but as a rule, not in the compact cortical bone substance. Large holes caused by arthropods can be mistaken for the product of plant roots. These vestiges can be diagnosed well in scanning electron microscopy (Figure 11.14). Particularly, smaller holes

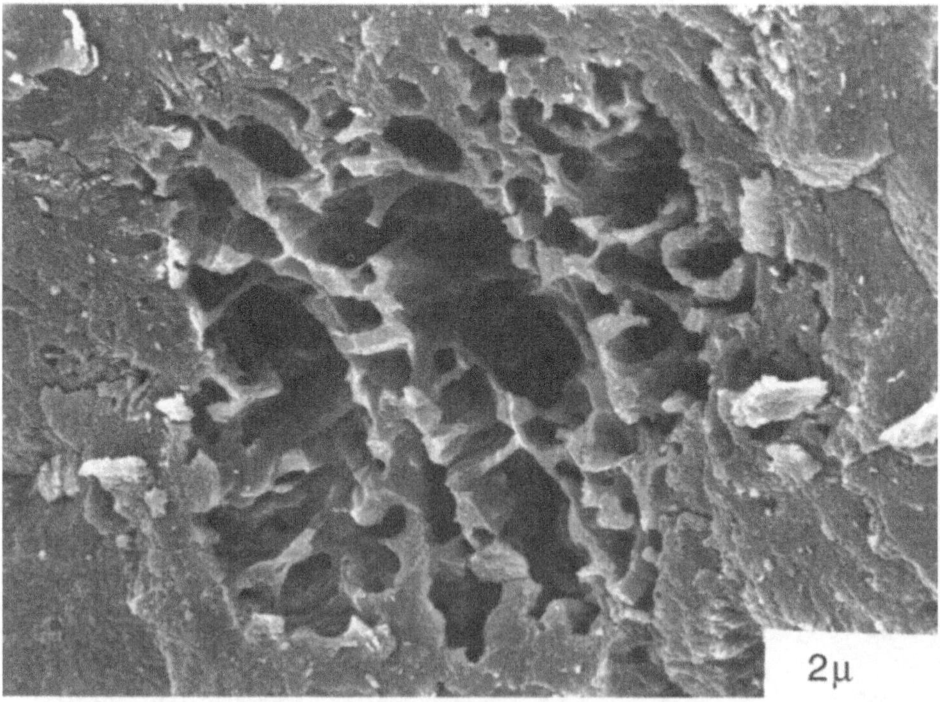

Figure 11.12. Scanning-electron microscopic image of a long bone fragment from the pre-Classi site of Tetelpan (Mexico). Destruction holes caused by actinomycetes. Probably due to bacteria. Magnification: bar = 1 μm. The bone fragment was given to the author by Dr Carmen M. Pijoan Aguade, National Museum of Anthropology, INAH (Mexico).

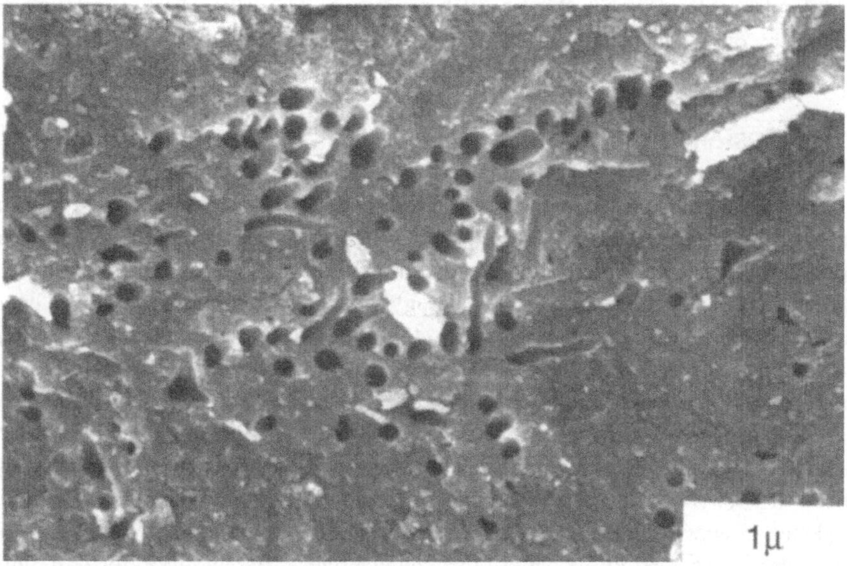

Figure 11.13. Scanning-electron microscopic image of a long bone fragment from the pre-Classic site of Tetelpan (Mexico). Destruction holes caused by actinomycetes. Magnification: bar = 1 µm. The bone fragment was given to the author by Dr Carmen M. Pijoan Aguade, National Museum of Anthropology, INAH (Mexico).

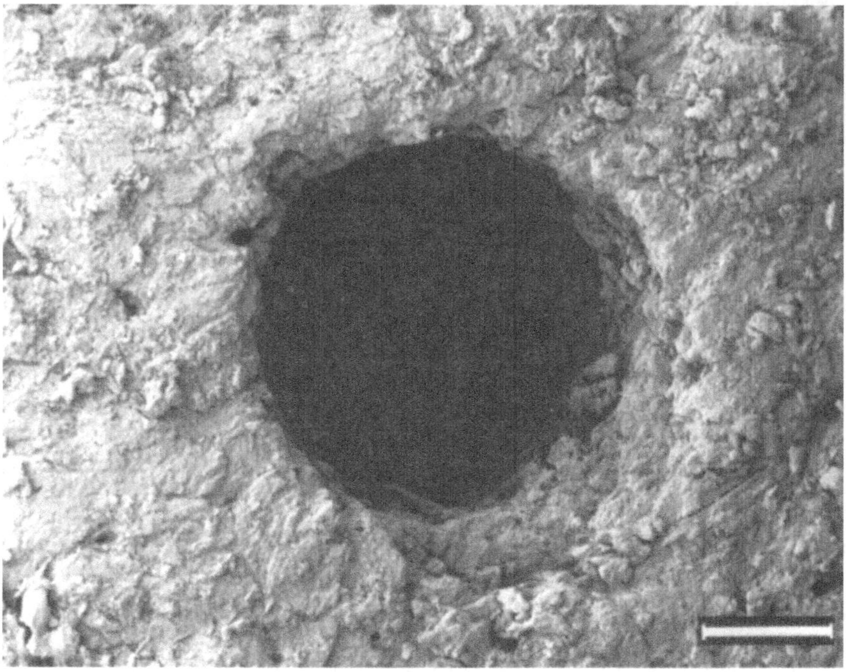

Figure 11.14. Scanning-electron microscopic image. Skull of a 35–45 year-old male from Sayala (Egyptian Nubia). Coptic Period (Early Middle Ages), individual J-1/6. Hole made by insects. Magnification: bar = 1 mm.

are difficult to diagnose in thin ground sections because they look similar to holes produced by other agents, such as those described above.

5. Conclusions and Summary

The study of intra vitam and postmortem bone loss in macerated skeletal remains represents an interdisciplinary research field in which various methods such as macroscopic, radiological, and microscopic techniques are all required. A good working knowledge of the microscopic structure, physiology, histogenesis and the growth of bone, as well as the influences of diagenesis can help to differentiate between the various factors of intravitam and postmortem bone loss. The method of choice is the microscopic examination of macerated bone specimens by thin ground sections.

Various degrees of intravitam bone loss reflect specific pathological bone behavior, which is expressed by the extent of osteoclastic activity. This activity is represented by the number of Howship's lacunae and other histomorphological indicators of an altered remodeling process. Thus, according to these features at the micro-level, osteolytic changes can be grouped into a pattern that characterizes different processes (e.g., inflammatory, tumorous). However, there are also other factors that influence the nature of osteolytic activity (e.g., speed of spreading of inflammatory or tumorous processes). These include, for example, age and condition of the immune system of the patient, general living conditions (e.g., nutrition, housing, working, sanitary, hygienic) and the virulence of disease-causing agents.

In this contribution, it has been demonstrated that the histological examination of archaeological skeletal remains provides greater reliability in diagnosing the various causes of bone loss. The patterns of changes observed in archaeological skeletal remains, particularly in the compact cortical bone structures, provide significant insight into the various mechanisms of bone loss. In macerated skeletal remains we can differentiate at the microscopic level between morphological features that are produced intravitam (e.g., Howship's lacunae) or postmortem (e.g., growth traces of plant roots or fungi).

6. Acknowledgments

The author wishes to thank Michael Brandt and Ingrid Hettwer-Steeger (Department of Anatomy, University of Göttingen, Germany) for preparing the ground sections used to create the illustrations in this chapter, and Cyrilla Maelicke (Department of Histology, University of Göttingen, Germany) for reading and editing the English text.

References

Ahlquist, J. and Damsten, O. (1969). A modification of Kerley's method for the microscopic determination of age in human bone. *J. For. Sci.* **14**, 205–212.

Agarwal, S.C. and Grynpas, M.D. (1996). Bone quantity and quality in past populations. *Anat. Rec.* 1031, **246**, 423–432.

Bätge, B. and Renz-Polster, H. (2000). Kalziotrope Hormone und metobolische Knochenerkrankungen. In H. Renz-Polster and J. Braun (eds) *Basislehrbuch Innere Medizin*. Urban-Fischer, München/Jena, pp. 720–734.

Beilner, T. (2001). Histomorphometrische Untersuchungen zur Osteoporoseprädisposition in frühmittelalterlichen Bevölkerungen. In M. Schultz (ed.) Beiträge zur Paläopathologie, Vol. 5. Cuvillier Verlag, Göttingen, pp. 1–146.

Bertozzi, B. (1982). Doctoral dissertation, Department of Anatomy, University of Göttingen, Germany.

Hackett, C.J. (1976). Diagnostic criteria of syphilis, yaws and treponarid (treponematoses) and some other diseases in dry bones. *Sitzber. Heidelb. Akad. Wiss.* **4**, 1–124.

Hackett, C.J. (1981). Microscopical focal destruction (tunnels) in exhumed human bones. *Med. Sci. Law* **21**, 234–265.

Hagens, V.G. (1979). Impregnation of soft biological specimens with thermostetting resins and elastomers. *Anat. Rec.* **194**, 247–255.

Kerley, E.R. (1965). The microscopic determination of age in human bone. *Am. J. Phys. Anthropol.* **23**, 149–163.

Kerley, E.R. and Ubelaker, D.H. (1978). Revision in the microscopic method of estimating age at death in human cortical bone. *Am. J. Phys. Anthropol.* **49**, 545–546.

Knese, K.-H., Voges, D., and Ritschl, I. (1954). Untersuchungen über die Osteon- und Lamellenformen im Extremitätenskelett des Erwachsenen. *Z. Zellforsch.* **40**, 323–360.

Kuhlencordt, F. (1992). Osteoporose. In H. Hornbostel, W. Kaufmann, and W. Siegenthaler (eds) *Innere Medizin in Praxis und Klinik.* Georg Thieme Verlag, Stuttgart/New York, pp. 9.25–9.37.

Martin, D.L. and Armelagos, G.J. (1979). Morphometrics of compact bone: An example of Sudanese Nubia. *Am. J. Phys. Anthropol.* **51**, 571–578.

Schultz, M. (1986). Die mikroskopische Untersuchung prähistorischer Skeletfunde. Anwendung und Aussagemöglichkeiten der differentialdiagnostischen Untersuchung in der Paläopathologie. Archäologie und Museum, Vol. 6. Kanton Baselland, Liestal, pp. 5–140.

Schultz, M. (1988). Methoden der Licht- und Elektronenmikroskopie. In R. Knussmann (ed) *Anthropologie. Handbuch der vergleichenden Biologie des Menschen*, Vol. 1. G. Fischer, Stuttgart/New York, pp. 698–730.

Schultz, M. (1993). Microscopic investigation on tumorous lesions from Christian Sayala (Egyptian Nubia). *Anthrop. Anz.* **51**, 117–121.

Schultz, M. (1997). Microscopic investigation of excavated skeletal remains: A contribution to paleopathology and forensic medicine. In W.D. Haglund and M.H. Sorg (eds) *Forensic Taphonomy. The Postmortem Fate of Human Remains.* CRC, Boca Raton/New York/London/Tokyo, pp. 201–222.

Schultz, M. (1999). Microscopic investigation in fossil Hominoidea. A clue to taxonomy, functional anatomy and the history of diseases? *Anat. Record.* (New Anat.) **257**, 225–232.

Schultz, M. (2001a). Mikroskopische Identifikation von Krankheiten an mazerierten Skelettfunden.—Identification of diseases in macerated skeletal remains. In M. Oehmichen and G. Geserick (eds) *Osteologische Identifikation und Altersschätzung*. Schmidt-Römhild, Lübeck, pp. 197–220. [Osteological Identification and Estimation of Age.]

Schultz, M. (2001b). Paleohistopathology of bone. A new approach to the study of ancient diseases. *Yearb. Phys. Anthropol.* **44**, 106–147.

Schultz, M. (2003). Light microscopic analysis in skeletal paleopathology. In D.J. Ortner (ed.) *Identification of Pathological Conditions in Human Skeletal Remains.* 2nd edn. Academic Press/Elsevier Science, London/New York, pp. 73–108.

Schultz, M. and Drommer, R. (1983). Möglichkeiten der Präparateherstellung aus dem Gesichtsschädelbereich für die makroskopische und mikroskopische Untersuchung unter Verwendung neuer Kunststofftechniken. In W.G. Hoppe (ed.) Fortschritte der Kiefer- und Gesichts-Chirurgie 28. Experimentelle Mund-Kiefer-Gesichts-Chirurgie. Mikrochirurgische Eingriffe. G. Thieme, Stuttgart/New York, pp. 95–97.

Stout, S.D. (1976). Histomorphometric analysis of archaeological bone. Doctoral dissertation, Department of Anthropology, Washington University, St. Louis.

Stout, S.D. (1992). Methods of determining age at death using bone microstructure. In S.R. Saunders and M.A. Katzenberg (eds) *Skeletal Biology of Past Peoples. Research Methods.* New York: Wiley-Liss, pp. 21–35.

Uytterschaut, H. (1985). Determination of skeletal age by histological methods. *Z. Morph. Anthrop.* **75**, 331–340.

Wedl, C. (1864). Über einen im Zahnbein und Knochen keimenden Pilz. Sitzber. *Kais. Akad. Wiss. Wien, Math. Nat. Cl. Abt.*1, **50**, 171–193.

Wolf, M. (1999). Ergebnisse makro- und mikroskopischer Untersuchungen an den römischen Brandgräbern von Rheinzabern (Rheinland-Pfalz). In M. Schultz (ed.) Beiträge zur Paläopathologie, Vol. 3. Cuvillier Verlag, Göttingen, pp. 1–171.

12

Histomorphology, Geometry, and Mechanical Loading in Past Populations

Alexander G. Robling and Sam D. Stout

1. Introduction

A common goal of most anthropological research is to gain some understanding of the diversity among human groups, whether it is related to biology, behavior, or beliefs. Physical anthropology is concerned primarily with the first of these three endeavors, though behavior (or environmental conditions in more general terms) is intimately intertwined with the biology. A prime example of this union is the effects of physical activity on skeletal dimensions, proportions, and morphology. There is clear genetic control of skeletal size and shape, but the genetically specified phenotype is modified by local mechanical loads endured by the bones during ontogeny, and less so, during adulthood.

Variation in physical activity levels has also attracted the attention of the medical community in recent years in light of the observed population-level differences in age-associated bone fragility and exercise (Schnitzler, 1993; Dougherty and Al-Marzouk, 2001). Bone loss, to the degree found in some modern sedentary populations, appears to be a relatively recent phenomenon. In addition, evidence of osteoporotic fracture is relatively rare in past populations (Agarwal and Grynpas, 1996). Although the etiology of bone loss in past and present populations is almost certainly multifactorial, physical activity has been invoked as a significant determinant in the accrual and maintenance of bone mass. Past human populations practiced a wide range of subsistence economies, with consequently different types and levels of mechanical loading endured by the skeleton. Studying skeletal remains from populations that practiced differing subsistence strategies can shed insight onto the role of physical activity in modulating bone mass and structure in humans, and can reveal the long-term skeletal outcomes that can be expected from certain lifestyles.

Below, we summarize the results from a biomechanical and histological analysis of a series of skeletons recovered from Paloma, a prehistoric archaeological site located on the central coast of Peru. The skeletons originated from three distinct and contiguous layers of sediment, dating to 5800–2600 BC. The faunal and floral specimens recovered from the site

Alexander G. Robling • Department of Anatomy & Cell Biology, Indiana University School of Medicine.
Sam D. Stout • Department of Anthropology, The Ohio State University.

Bone Loss and Osteoporosis: An Anthropological Perspective, edited by Sabrina C. Agarwal and Sam D. Stout. Kluwer Academic/Plenum Publishers, New York, 2003.

reveal a shift in subsistence economies through time, beginning with almost an exclusive hunting and gathering lifestyle which led the inhabitants across the steep foothills of the Andes. Toward the end of the occupation, a more local, sedentary maritime economy had been adopted. The skeletal remains offer a rare opportunity to study the effects of a shift in subsistence and consequent physical activity on skeletal morphology and histomorphology.

2. Mechanobiology Methods for Preserved Skeletal Remains

2.1. Interpreting Preserved Evidence of Mechanical Loading History from Bone Geometry

The structure and composition of mammalian bone presents an interpretable record of the organism's life history and developmental environment. The *in vivo* adaptive nature of bone to extrinsic physical forces, coupled with its *ex vivo* durability and excellent preservational qualities, allow the skeletal paleobiologist to make behavioral inferences from the skeletons of populations long extinct. Understanding physical activity levels in past populations requires extracting information on the mechanical loading history encoded in the preserved hard tissues. Fortunately, principles founded in modern bone biology can be used to characterize the *in vivo* loading environment from preserved bone morphology.

Most biomechanical analyses of skeletal remains are based on Wolff's Law which, simply stated, asserts that bone mass and architecture are tuned to match the loads borne by the skeleton. Greater than 80% of the strains produced in long bone cortices are caused by bending moments (Rubin *et al.*, 1990). Long bone cortices must be adapted primarily to withstand bending loads if functional competence is to be maintained. Comparisons of limb bones from exercised and nonexercised animals illustrate this point clearly; cortices experiencing vigorous mechanical usage are usually more resistant to bending than cortices from less active individuals (Woo *et al.*, 1981; Jee *et al.*, 1991; Lieberman, 1996). The established role of mechanical usage in determining the bending rigidity of a long bone provides a useful model for deducing mechanical loading history from an estimated bending rigidity.

The bending (and torsional) rigidity of a long bone can be estimated using beam theory—a principle used in mechanical engineering to calculate a beam's capacity to resist bending and torsion. The long, tubular morphology of the typical long bone diaphysis enables it to be modeled as a hollow beam (Huiskes, 1982), and its capacity to resist bending and torsional moments can be estimated from cross sections taken normal to it's long (z) axis. The properties of a section most relevant to evaluating the bending and torsional rigidity of the shaft from which it came are the second moments of area (SMA), also known as the area moments of inertia. Beams with greater SMAs exhibit greater resistance to bending than beams with lesser SMAs, all other things (e.g., material properties) being equal (van der Meulen *et al.*, 2001).

The SMA considers two properties of a section—its cross-sectional area and the distribution of that area about the neutral axis of bending. It is derived by dividing the section into a series of small areas, and multiplying each area (dA) by its squared distance from the neutral bending axis (y^2). This procedure is integrated over the entire cross section and is expressed in mm^4:

$$I = \int_A y^2 dA$$

The SMA can be calculated about any axis that passes through the section's center of mass. Conventionally, the SMA calculated about the neutral axis parallel to the mediolateral plane of a bone is denoted I_X. Thus, I_X estimates the bone's rigidity when bent in an anteroposterior plane. Bending rigidity in about the anteroposterior axis (mediolateral bending) is conventionally denoted I_Y. The plane of greatest bending rigidity is known as the major axis, and the SMA along that axis is denoted I_{MAX}. The plane of least bending rigidity is known as the minor axis, and the SMA along that axis is denoted I_{MIN}.

The polar SMA (J) is another informative geometric property; it represents the beam's potential to resist twisting (torsion). It can be calculated using the equation shown above, except that the squared distance from the centroid (radius of gyration or r) replaces the squared distance from the neutral axis. The polar SMA is equivalent to the sum of any two perpendicular bending moments from the same section.

Several factors bear on the SMA of lower limb bones, as illustrated in Figure 12.1. Body mass has a significant effect on the SMA. In humans, heavier individuals typically have a greater SMA in the lower limb bones than lighter individuals. To avoid interpreting a structurally rigid cortex (e.g., femur) from a heavy individual as evidence for greater

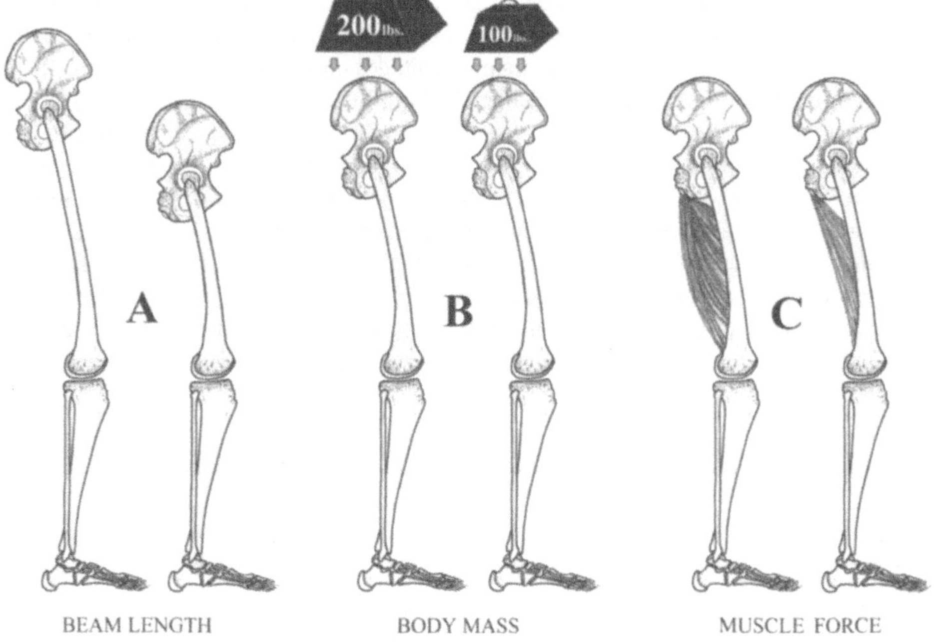

Figure 12.1. Factors affecting the bending rigidity of the femur. (A) A longer femur will generate stress and strain than a shorter femur for the same load. Consequently, the femur on the left (the longer one) will exhibit a greater second moment of area (SMA), even though the same loads (equal physical activity) were applied to each femur. (B) Greater body mass will generate greater stress and strain in the femur than lesser body mass. Consequently, the femur on the left (from a heavier individual) will exhibit a greater SMA, even though the vigor of mechanical use may have been equal. (C) The greater force generated by stronger muscles will deform the femur more than forces generated from weaker muscles. The femur on the left should exhibit a greater SMA than the femur on the right. A biomechanical interpretation of long bone cross-sectional geometry should remove the effects of A and B to reveal the effects of C.

physical activity, the effects of body mass on the section properties should be removed. Second, the length of a bone has a significant effect on the SMA. During loading, the amount of force generated at the root (e.g., hip joint) of a cantilever beam increases as the moment arm (femur length) increases. To avoid interpreting a structurally rigid femoral cortex from a taller individual as evidence for greater physical activity, the effects of bone length should be removed.

Skeletal remains do not offer direct information on body mass and stature, but these properties can be estimated from the skeletal dimensions and used to standardize geometric properties. Body mass can be estimated reliably from the bi-iliac breadth or from femoral head dimensions. Bone length can be directly measured and corrected with a constant to yield the biomechanical length, which is a more germane measurement for evaluating the moment arm of a bone.

2.2. Bone Microstructure and Mechanical Loading History

The effects of mechanical loading on intracortical remodeling dynamics also provide a useful model for studying mechanical loading history from cortical bone microstructure. Frost (1987a, 1990b) has summarized the relationship between mechanical loading and remodeling in his "mechanostat" model of skeletal mechanobiology (see also Chapter 2, this volume). The mechanostat is based on a set of strain thresholds that control the rate of remodeling within the cortex. If peak strain magnitudes do not surpass a *m*inimum *e*ffective *s*train required to suppress *r*emodeling (MES_R), the remodeling rate is accelerated. When peak strains exceed the MES_R, which appears to exist at about 100–150 $\mu\varepsilon$, the remodeling rate becomes suppressed (Figure 12.2A). However, in the suprathreshold range of strains (> 150 $\mu\varepsilon$), the remodeling rate is affected by an additional factor—microdamage. When bone is loaded repetitively, as occurs *in vivo*, small flaws and phase interfaces in the bone matrix develop into microscopically detectable cracks in the bone. The fatigue-damaged moieties of bone attract teams of osteoclasts and osteoblasts (called basic multicellular units, or BMUs), which ultimately replace the damaged bone with younger, more structurally competent bone (Mori and Burr, 1993). Because microdamage (MDx)

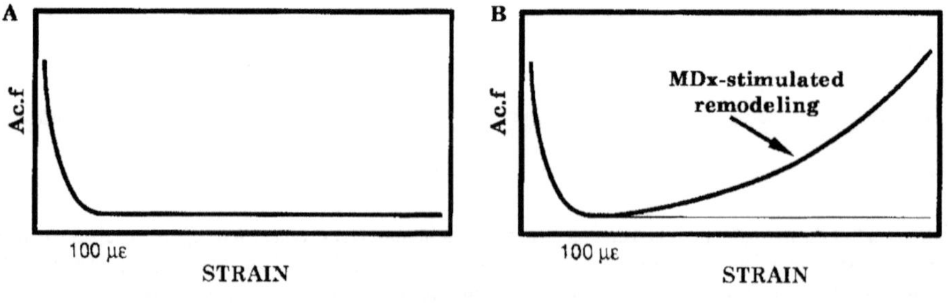

Figure 12.2. Frost's mechanostat. (A) Peak strains below 100 $\mu\varepsilon$ result in the "disuse state" wherein remodeling is increased. Peak strains greater than 100 $\mu\varepsilon$ depress remodeling. The effect of microdamage is not considered in graph A. (B) When the effect of microdamage (MDx) is added, the activation frequency in the post MES_R range increases with strain. Mechanical loading history can be inferred from the number of remodeling events in skeletal remains if only those individuals in the post MES_R range are considered. Modified from Frost (1987a, 1990b).

production in bone is a function of the vigor (e.g., strain magnitude, strain rate) with which the bone is loaded and/or the duration of loading (number of cycles), individuals engaged in more physically active lifestyles should create more damage in their skeletons, and consequently, exhibit a greater rate of BMU activation. Frost perhaps summarized this relation best:

> Because microscopic fatigue damage does occur even in normal bone and remodeling BMUs almost certainly usually repair it, yet complete fractures of intact bones rarely occur in healthy people, one may infer that Nature does proportion our annual remodeling activity to our annual MDx production. Otherwise, fatigue fractures of intact bones would occur far more often than they do. (Frost 1989: 380)

Increased remodeling in vigorously loaded bone is well established experimentally (Hert *et al.*, 1972; Lanyon and Baggot, 1976; Bouvier and Hylander, 1981, 1997; Burr *et al.*, 1995; Lieberman, 1997; Lieberman and Crompton, 1998). Thus the complete picture of cortical remodeling as a function of mechanical loading *in vivo* resembles Figure 12.2B. Beyond the disuse window, a positive association exists between BMU activation (remodeling) and mechanical stimulation. This relation can be used to interpret mechanical loading history (physical activity levels) from quantified bone remodeling parameters in preserved skeletons, provided that individual limb bones were not in a disuse state. Bone remodeling rates can be estimated from static histomorphometric parameters, readily measurable in thick sections from preserved cortical bone.

As a cortical BSU remodels bone, a secondary osteon is left in its wake. Thus the number of osteons (and osteon fragments—remnants of osteons that have been partially re-remodeled) counted in a cross section of cortical bone represents the number of BSUs that were activated over the lifespan of the tissue (Figure 12.3). If the age of the tissue is known, a mean activation frequency (# of BSUs created per year) can be estimated by dividing the osteon counts (called osteon population density or OPD) by mean tissue age. Further, if osteon size (On.Ar) is measured, then a mean annual volumetric bone remodeling rate can be calculated by multiplying mean osteon size by activation frequency. A few caveats apply to the preceding computations. First, as osteons accumulate with age, an increasing proportion of older osteons and fragments are obliterated by newer osteons, leaving no trace of the former's existence. Frost (1987d) developed an algorithm to account for these "missing" systems and to estimate total accumulated osteon creations (AOC) based on the visible OPD:

$$\mathrm{AOC} = \mathrm{OPD} \cdot (1 - \alpha^{3.5})^{-1}$$

where α is the observed OPD normalized to its asymptotic value. Alpha is calculated using the following formula:

$$\alpha = \mathrm{OPD} \cdot k\,(\mathrm{On.Ar} \cdot 4\pi^{-1})^{-1}$$

where k is a fragment packing operator that accounts for the overlapping distribution of osteons and fragments in a typical unit area of cortical bone. Several factors influence k, including cortical thickness, osteon geometry, and the ratio of intact to fragmentary osteons. Consequently, different bones are associated with different values of k:

$$k = \mathrm{OPD\ asymptote} \cdot \mathrm{On.Dm}^2$$

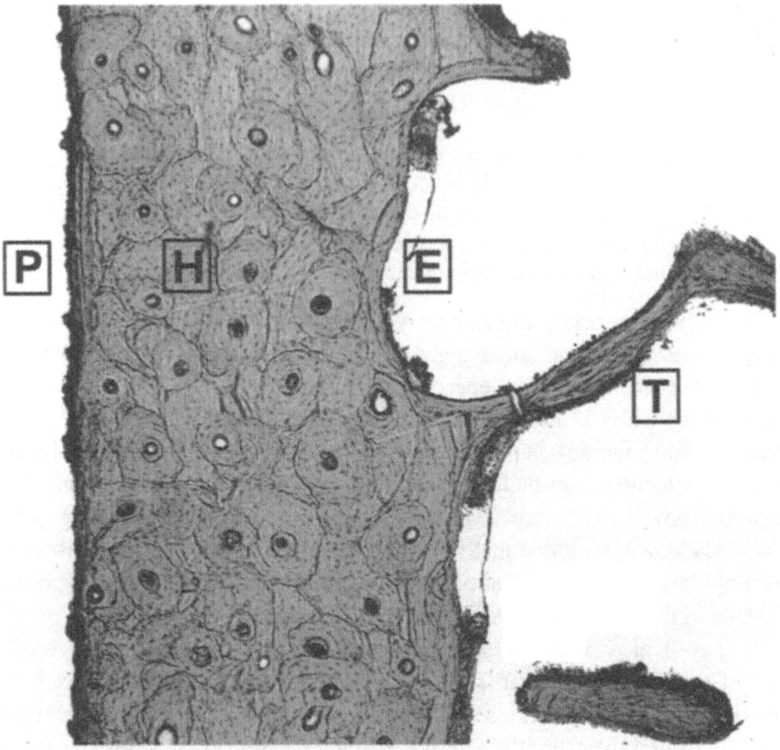

Figure 12.3. Photomicrograph of a heavily remodeled rib cortex from a ~45-year-old woman excavated at Paloma, Peru. The periosteal (P), endocortical (E), Haversian (H), and trabecular (T) surfaces are visible. Osteons and osteon fragments are visible throughout the cortex. Note the excellent microstructural preservation at Paloma.

where the OPD asymptote represents the point at which further creations of new osteons removes evidence of preexisting ones (Figure 12.4). The asymptote is usually calculated from an independent sample. On.Dm^2 is the squared diameter of the average osteon, and can be calculated from On.Ar by multiplying by 1.27 (assuming a circular osteon). A second consideration in the algorithm is that the mean tissue age is not the same as the chronological age of the individual. Mean age of the rib compacta, for example, is always less than chronological age because of modeling drifts that occur during ontogeny. In fact, none of the cortex in the adult rib is present before age 10, that is, it is all deposited during the second decade of life. Thus, any osteons present in the rib cortex of a 25-year-old man have had, at the most, 15 years to accumulate instead of the 25 years corresponding to his age. Most osteons will have had less time to accumulate than that, however, because the adult rib cortex only *begins* forming at age 10. Half of the cortex present in the adult rib is formed between ages 10 and 12.5, and the remaining half is formed between ages 12.5 and ~17.5 years (Frost and Wu, 1967; Wu *et al.*, 1970). The effective "birth" of adult compacta in the middle third of the sixth rib occurs at a mean age of 12.5 years. Thus, the mean age of the rib compacta in a 35-year-old man, in whom rapid modeling had essentially ceased, would be 22.5 years. The mean tissue age of the rib compacta in any normal adult can be estimated by subtracting 12.5 years from his or her chronological age.

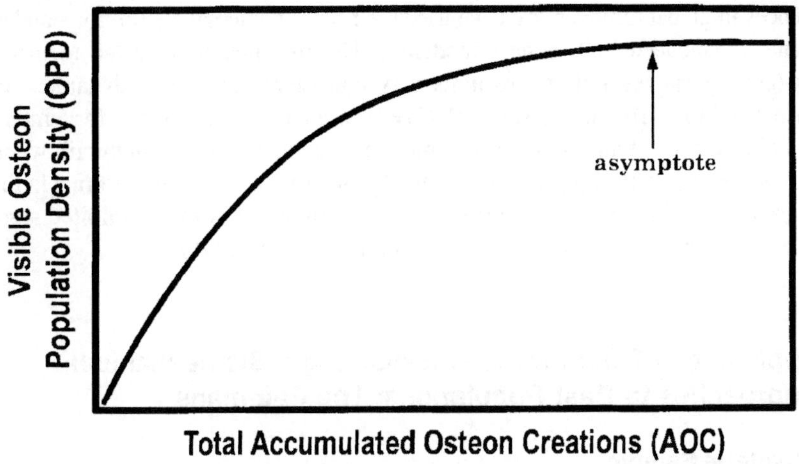

Figure 12.4. As osteons accumulate within the cortex of a long bone, evidence of preexisting osteons becomes obliterated. Initially, there is a 1 : 1 relation between visible and total accumulated osteons. As the amount of unremodeled circumferential bone diminishes, there is a greater probability that new BMUs will tunnel into preexisting osteons. This probability is represented by the curve, which eventually reaches asymptote, that is, any new osteon creations will come at the partial or total expense of older osteons. Frost (1987d) developed an algorithm to account for missing osteons.

The lack of modeling rate data in human bone other than the rib provides us with a less complete understanding of tissue age estimates in other skeletal elements, but most human cortical sampling sites are probably within ±3 years of the rib (Frost and Wu, 1967).

Like the cross-sectional geometric properties, interpretations of intracortical remodeling should be standardized for nonmechanical factors that might contribute considerable variation or bias to the interpretation. Specifically, there are a number of systemic influences such as endogenous hormones, serum levels of mineral ions, dietary intake, and other factors that affect cortical bone turnover. These "global" factors determine the number of remodeling events in all cortices of the skeleton, but are modified locally by the mechanical loading environment of each individual bone (Lanyon, 1984). Thus an observed microstructure (e.g., OPD) is the result of local biomechanical influences on bone remodeling superimposed onto those incurred by global (e.g., hormonal, biochemical) influences. Given that the global turnover rates exhibit substantial variation from individual to individual (Frost and Villanueva, 1961; Frost, 1963; Stout, 1986; Bouvier and Hylander, 1997) and from population to population (Stout, 1983; Schnitzler, 1993; Stout and Lueck, 1995), the effect of systemic influences on osteon counts in a loaded bone should be controlled for. For example, a heavily remodeled cortex (e.g., femur) from an individual with a greater systemic remodeling rate could be interpreted erroneously as evidence for greater physical activity if the effects of systemic turnover are not taken into account. Such standardization involves quantifying bone remodeling at an additional skeletal site that (a) is less affected by loading of the limb bones, that is, remote from the appendicular skeleton, and (b) when loaded *in vivo*, is done so in a similar manner from individual to individual; this criterion allows one to assume that the remodeling occurring in the control bone, though partly influenced by mechanical loading, receives the same contribution from mechanical forces across individuals, thereby manifesting relative differences in global turnover. We have used the rib as an internal control for standardizing mechanically induced limb bone remodeling. The rib, though subjected to mechanical forces (chiefly via respiration), exhibits very consistent remodeling dynamics, even in exercise conditions. Tommerup *et al.* (1993) exercised pigs on a treadmill for 5 months and found no difference in any static or dynamic remodeling parameters in the rib when compared to sedentary control pigs, despite a nearly threefold increase in heart rate in the exercised group. The limb bones (femora) from these animals, however, exhibited significant increases in Haversian remodeling parameters (Raab *et al.*, 1991).

3. Application of Geometric and Histologic Biomechanical Approaches to Past Populations: The Palomans

3.1. Skeletal Sample

The materials used in this study comprise rib and femur tissue samples from human skeletal remains excavated at Paloma, a prehistoric village on Peru's central coast. Paloma is located at the northern extent of the Chilca Valley, approximately 65 km south of Lima. Much of the Peruvian coast exhibits some of the driest and most inhospitable desert conditions in the world. There are, however, seasonally-moist, vegetation-rich "fog oases" along most of the desert coast, called *lomas*. Vegetation in the *lomas* flourishes during the Austral winter, when fog from the sea condenses on the trees and grasses of the *lomas*. At various times in the past, the stands of trees and bushes in the *lomas* were large enough to prevent evaporation and allow year-round growth (Quilter, 1989). Today, the northern edge of a *lomas* borders the site of Paloma (Engel, 1980).

Three major strata have been recognized at Paloma—levels 400, 300, and 200, and their ages have been established using radiocarbon dating (Benfer, 1990). The occupation of Paloma predates the appearance of agriculture on the central coast. The oldest layer containing human remains (L400) dates from 6,500 to 5,300 radiocarbon years BP. The middle layer and upper layers (L300 and L200) date from 5,300–5,100 and 5,100–4,700 radiocarbon years BP, respectively.

A number of analyses of the Paloma artifacts and ecofacts indicate that the subsistence economy was not uniform over time. It appears that the earlier inhabitants of the site (L400 and L300) practiced a more terrestrial hunter–gatherer mode of subsistence, exploiting small terrestrial animals and plants found in the scattered *lomas*. The later inhabitants (L200) appear to have focused their subsistence efforts almost exclusively on the nearby maritime resources, relying primarily on shellfish and anchovies (Benfer, 1990).

Concurrent with the observed shift in subsistence strategy at Paloma was a change in the types of activities practiced by the Palomans. The maritime subsistence economy of L200 appears to be associated with a more sedentary lifestyle compared to the earlier periods. Based on the faunal and floral remains at the site, Benfer (1990:304) noted that Paloma's occupation witnessed a "shift in activity toward more sedentism and fishing in place of extensive walking and carrying of plants and small animals." The change in activity levels, however, appears to be sex-specific. Preliminary data from muscle attachment rugosity and external diameters of the long bones suggest that males exhibited decreased physical activity

Table 12.1. Composition of Paloma Study Sample

		Males			Females			Pooled sex		
Level	Times span (BP)	*n*	Age range	Mean age	*n*	Age range	Mean age	*n*	Age range	Mean age
200	5100–4700	8	25–50	34.3	6	21–45	33.8	14	21–50	34.1
300	5300–5100	10	17–47	31.1	9	20–45	31.8	19	17–47	31.4
400	6500–5300	7	23–47	30.7	8	25–50	33.5	15	23–50	32.2
Total	6500–4700	25	17–50	32.0	23	20–50	32.9	48	17–50	32.4

through time, whereas the females exhibit evidence for increased physical activity through time. The Paloma skeletal sample used in our analysis is presented in Table 12.1.

3.2. Methods and Findings

From each skeleton, a section from the midshaft left or right femur and middle third of the fourth, fifth, or sixth rib was removed, embedded in plastic, sectioned (~60 μm) on a metallurgic wafering saw, and mounted on microscope slides. The femur sections were scanned on a flatbed scanner and imported into an image analysis program (NIH Image), where the maximum, minimum, and polar SMA were calculated from the periosteal and endocortical surfaces. The same femur sections used for geometric analysis were read on a compound microscope at 100× magnification. Using the point count technique (Parfitt, 1983), the number of intact and fragmentary osteons per mm^2 (OPD) was counted in eight 1 mm wide strips spanning from periosteum to endocortex (Figure 12.5A) (Iwaniec, 1997). For the rib sections, OPD was measured in every other microscopic field (Figure 12.5B).

We standardized the femoral geometric properties using the product of body mass and femur biomechanical length (Trinkaus *et al.*, 1998). Body mass was estimated from the maximum diameter of the femoral head using the regression formula presented in Ruff *et al.* (1997), which was found to produce a correlation coefficient of 0.98 between estimated body mass and actual body mass in a large, diverse modern human sample:

$$\text{body mass} = (2.268 \cdot \text{femoral head diameter}) - 36.5$$

The biomechanical length of the femur (length) was calculated by subtracting 5% of the maximum femur length (Ruff, 1994). Once a body size standard was calculated for each individual, their geometric variables (I_{MAX}, I_{MIN}, J) were logged and regressed onto log body size using reduced major axis regression (Ricker, 1973; Hofman, 1988). From these regressions, residual scores (^{R}) were calculated for each individual, which reflect the structural rigidity of the femur not accounted for by body size (Figure 12.6). This residual score is thus a size-independent measure of estimated bending rigidity. The assertion that body size has actually been removed by residual scores is illustrated in Figure 12.7, which shows that size standardization using the commonly used ratio of estimated bending rigidity (e.g., I_{MAX}) to body mass still exhibits a significant, positive correlation to body mass,

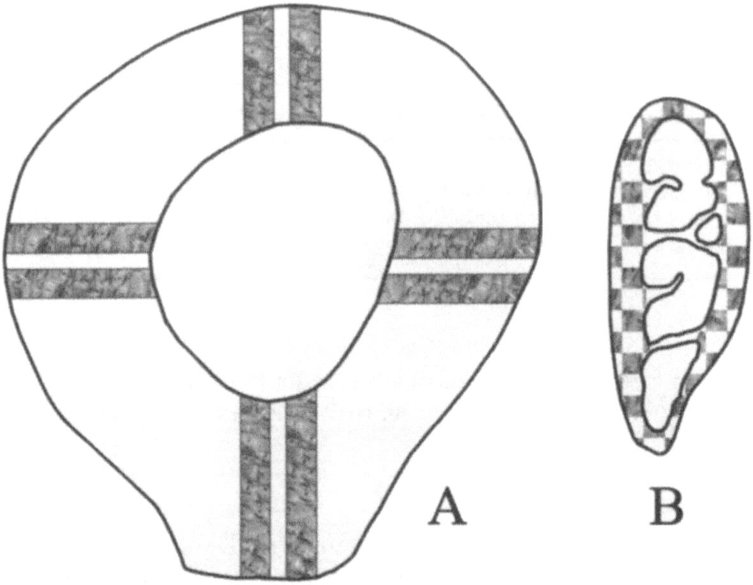

Figure 12.5. Topographic sampling method for static histomorphometry in the femur (A) and rib (B). The femur sampling strategy, which collects measurements from two 1 mm wide columns spanning from periosteum to endocortex in each of the four anatomical quadrants, was developed by Iwaniec (1997). The rib sampling strategy, which collects measurements in every other field (checkerboard), was developed by Stout (1986).

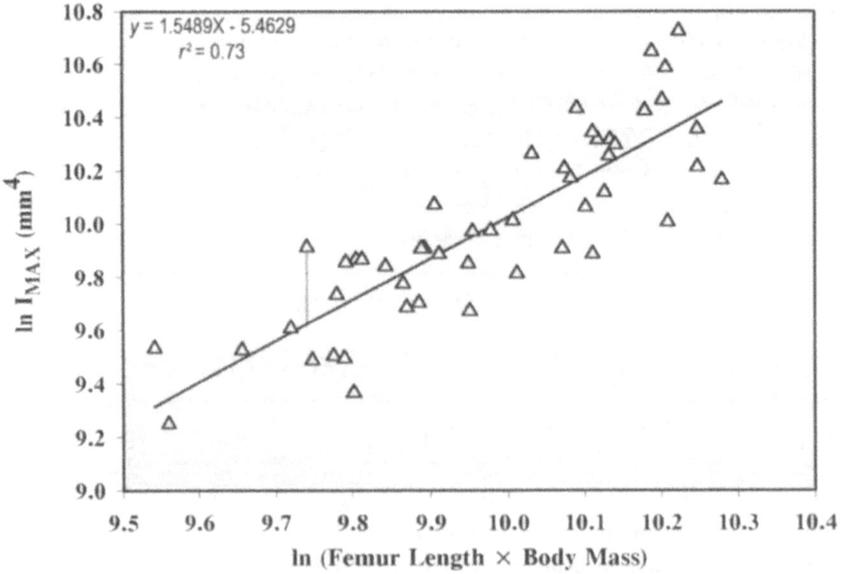

Figure 12.6. The maximum second moment of area (I_{MAX}) is tightly correlated with body size. However, much of the variance in this relation can be explained by mechanical loading history. The length of the gray vertical line, extending from the slope to one of the points, represents a residual score for that individual. The residual score indicates the degree and direction (+ or −) of deviation from an expected I_{MAX} value based on body size.

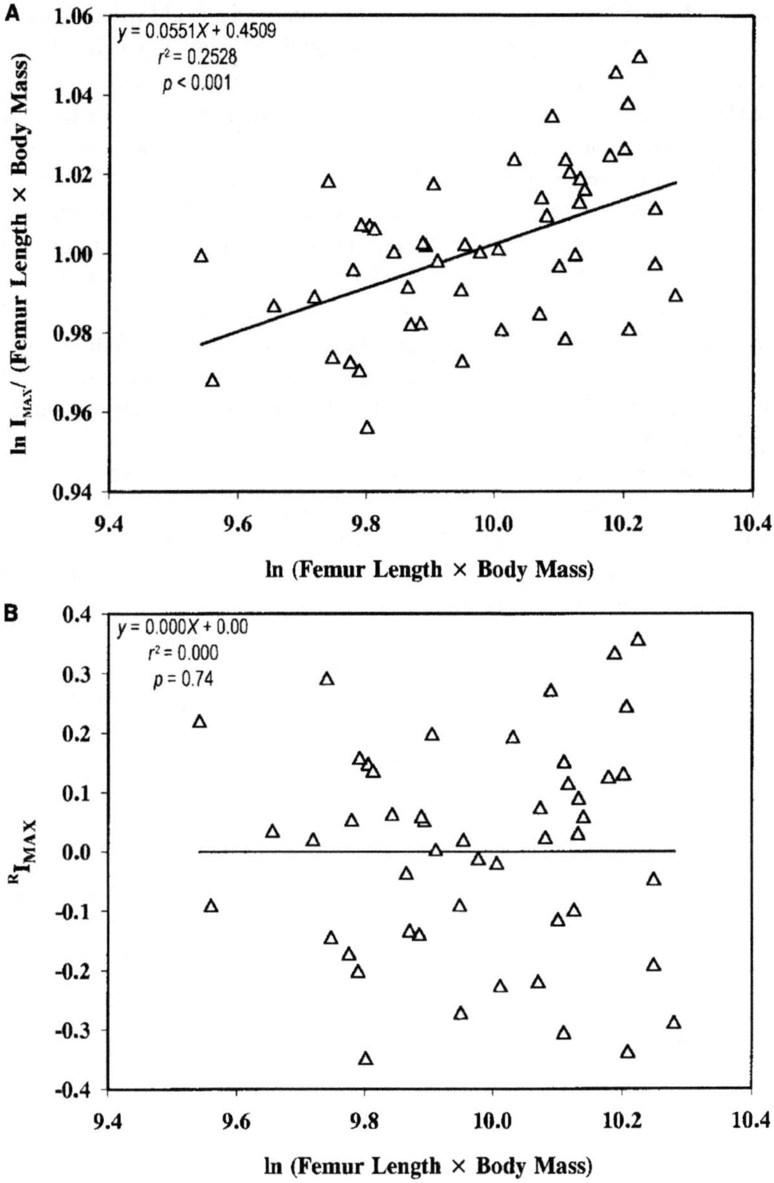

Figure 12.7. (A) Standardization of I_{MAX} for body size using the ratio of I_{MAX} to body size in the Paloma sample results in a significant ($p < 0.001$) correlation between the standardized variable and body size. Body size has not been removed from I_{MAX} using this technique. (B) Standardization of I_{MAX} for body size using residual scores in the Paloma sample results in a zero (ns) correlation between the standardized variable ($^{R}I_{MAX}$) and body size.

yet size standardization using the residual score of the same measure ($^{R}I_{MAX}$) regressed onto body mass shows no association (by definition of the technique) with body mass.

The residual I_{MAX} scores show that some individuals exhibited more, and others less, adaptation in the femur than would be predicted from body size alone. A biomechanical interpretation of these data would invoke differences in mechanical loading levels (physical activity levels) among individuals, with those exhibiting large positive $^{R}I_{MAX}$ scores probably having been more active than those with large negative scores.

We standardized intracortical remodeling in the femur with intracortical remodeling in the rib using the same statistical techniques as described for the geometric analysis. OPD in the femur was regressed onto OPD in the rib using the reduced major axis. From this regression, residual scores were calculated for each individual, which reflect remodeling in the femur not accounted for by remodeling in the rib (a surrogate for global turnover). The residual OPD scores for the femur ($^{R}OPD_F$) show that some individuals exhibited more, and others less, remodeling in the femur than would be predicted from the rib turnover alone. A biomechanical interpretation of these data would invoke differences in mechanical loading levels (physical activity levels) among individuals, with those exhibiting large positive $^{R}OPD_F$ scores probably having been more active than those with large negative scores.

To test these proposals, we subjected the residual geometric and histologic scores to correlation analysis. A strong, statistically significant association ($r = 0.56$, $p < 0.001$) was found between $^{R}I_{MAX}$ and $^{R}OPD_F$ (Figure 12.8). This relation was similar in males ($r = 0.59$, $p < 0.01$) and females ($r = 0.54$, $p < 0.01$). The relation between ^{R}J and $^{R}OPD_F$ was similarly strong (pooled sex $r = 0.51$, $p < 0.001$; males $r = 0.58$, $p < 0.01$; females $r = 0.46$, $p < 0.05$). $^{R}I_{MIN}$ exhibited a strong association with $^{R}OPD_F$ among females ($r = 0.54$, $p < 0.01$), but there was no association among males ($r = 0.16$, *ns*). Such a great sex difference in the relation between those two variables is interesting, and probably is a function of sexual dimorphism in the bony pelvis and its consequence on sex-related loading differences in the femur. Relative to body size, the female pelvis exhibits hip joints that are mediolaterally farther apart from the center of gravity than is exhibited in the male pelvis. This

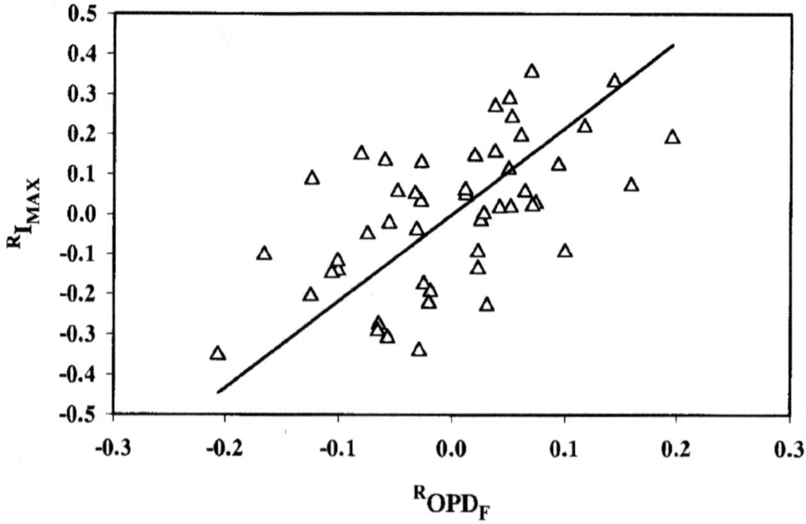

Figure 12.8. Residual I_{MAX} scores, which represent maximum bending rigidity not accounted for by body size, exhibit a significant, positive correlation with residual OPD scores in the midshaft femur (OPD in the femur not accounted from by OPD in the rib). The reduced major axis is shown.

difference has been linked to obstetric requirements in the female pelvic outlet. As a result of comparatively wider hip spacing, there is a relatively greater moment arm acting in the mediolateral plane of the femur than in the male hip and thigh (Lovejoy, 1988). Consequently, a relatively greater mediolateral bending moment is incurred on the proximal and mid-diaphyseal sections of the femur than would theoretically occur in males. It is difficult to say whether the orientation of I_{MIN} is aligned roughly with the mediolateral axis, but such an orientation would explain the stronger association between I_{MIN} and bone remodeling among females.

The geometric and remodeling data are consistent with the predictions of the mechanostat, in both the modeling and remodeling components. Under vigorous mechanical usage, the limb bones increase their modeling rate, resulting in a larger cross section that is better able to withstand bending and perhaps torsion. Concurrent with this adaptation at the periosteal and endocortical surfaces, the intracortical bone undergoes increased remodeling activity to keep pace with the microdamage burden that is accumulating as a result of the vigorous loading environment. Other studies of human skeletons have reached similar conclusions regarding the relation between bone geometry and remodeling, but the relation appears to be weaker if body size and global turnover are not taken into account (Lazenby, 1986; Walker *et al.*, 1994).

There still remains some unexplained variation between the geometric and histologic scores, and an explanation for this variance could be related to differences in the timing and duration of the adaptive response on the different bone envelopes. Bone modeling is retarded in the adult skeleton, particularly on the periosteal envelope. Because the gross rigidity of a diaphyseal cross section is influenced much more by periosteal bone apposition than by endosteal apposition, the rigidity of the femoral midshaft is largely determined by the time skeletal maturity is reached. Rubin *et al.* (1992) failed to find a significant alteration in bone mass or geometry in the ulnae of older (~3 years of age) turkeys after subjecting them to high (3000 $\mu\varepsilon$) strains. The same regimen applied to the ulnae of 1-year-old turkeys resulted in a 30% increase in cross-sectional area, the majority of which occurred on the periosteal surface. Therefore, cross-sectional geometric properties of the Paloma sample might more accurately reflect the mechanical loading environment prior to skeletal maturity and/or the age at which physically demanding (adult) activities began, as has been suggested by Knüsel (1993) for other archaeological samples. Haversian remodeling, on the other hand, is active throughout life, and is potentially sensitive to loading up to and including old age. Burr *et al.* (1995) demonstrated that the intracortical activation frequency in the humeral and femoral cortices of old (~12 years of age), treadmill-exercised dogs was from 2 to 4 times greater than that in the same bones from age-matched controls. Lieberman and Crompton (1998) have demonstrated the same phenomenon in the limb bones of young pigs. Thus, unlike the periosteal envelope, remodeling dynamics on the Haversian envelope appear to be sensitive to mechanical loading throughout life. Considering that Paloma sample used in this analysis comprised individuals in the adult age range only, some of the unexplained variance in the geometry–histology relations might be attributable to individual (or stratigraphic level) differences in the timing of supra-threshold physical activities endured over the lifetime.

3.3. Changes through Time at Paloma

When the data are partitioned by stratigraphic level, clear changes in physical activity levels emerge over time. Inhabitants of the earliest level (L400) exhibit the greatest

${}^{R}I_{MAX}$, ${}^{R}I_{MIN}$, and ${}^{R}J$. ${}^{R}OPD_F$ shows similar trends to those exhibited by the geometric measures (Figure 12.9), but statistical significance was not reached among groups. Taken together, the data show a rapid decrease in femoral geometry and remodeling from the early time period (L400) to the middle time period. The changes in bone geometry and remodeling were, however, sex-specific. Males exhibited a steady decline in geometric properties and intracortical remodeling in the femur, whereas females appear to have

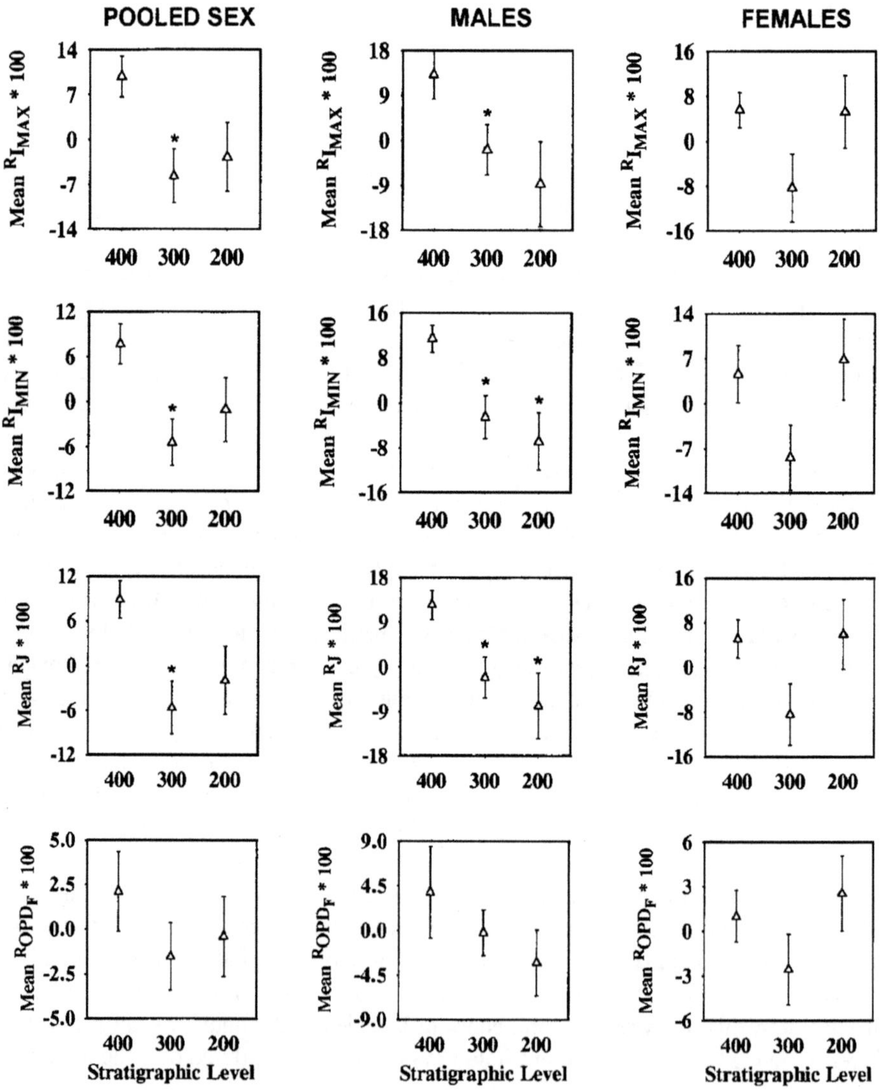

Figure 12.9. Residual maximum, minimum, and polar moments of inertia, and residual OPD in the femur, grouped by stratigraphic level. Note the similarity in trend between geometric and histologic residual scores by level. Activity levels appear to have decreased over time at Paloma, but the sex-specific plots show that this is true only for males. Females exhibited a decrease, followed by an increase, in geometric properties and remodeling activity over time. * = significantly different from L400 score.

exhibited a decrease followed by an increase that occurred between the middle and late periods. These differences in geometric properties among the three time periods were not significantly different for females. These results are consistent with Benfer's (1990) muscle marking scores, which showed that the rugosity of muscle attachment sites (using upper and lower limb bones) decreased in males but increased in females over time, resulting in decreased sexual dimorphism from L400 to L200.

4. Conclusions

The physical lifestyles of past populations were almost certainly more demanding than those of modern industrial populations, though the range of activity type, duration, and level was undoubtedly great. Nevertheless, it is curious to note that the shift to sedentary lifestyles among modern populations occurred concurrently with a decline in bone quantity, quality, and fracture resistance. Biomechanical analyses of skeletal remains from individuals that lived prior to modernization offer insight into the etiology and severity of the problem in modern times. Analysis of skeletal changes occurring over a period of time that spans a shift in daily activities (e.g., subsistence economy) can reveal the effects of physical activity changes on skeletal health at the population level. Approaches to studying physical activity levels in skeletal remains evolve as our understanding of bone mechanotransduction expands. Two skeletal attributes known to respond to mechanical loading are geometric adaptation of the cortex and intracortical remodeling within the bone. Histologic analysis is sometimes precluded because microscopic preservation of the cortical bone can be too severely affected by diagenesis. Conversely, geometric analysis is sometimes precluded because bone cortices are often fragmentary, and periosteal–endosteal tracings are not possible. The Paloma sample is perhaps a rare example, in that the skeletons were in pristine condition after several thousand years (in some cases, hair, eyes, and skin were well preserved). Consequently, geometric and histologic analyses were possible on the same specimens. However, the strong relation agreement of geometrically derived and histologically derived assessments of mechanical loading history suggest that both approaches are useful, and that the type of biomechanical approach to a particular specimen can be adapted to meet the condition of the sample when preservation conditions are not so ideal.

The remains from Paloma show a decrease in geometric properties and remodeling in the midshaft femur. These changes in skeletal morphology suggest that physical activity levels decreased through time at the site, concordant with a transition towards a less physically demanding subsistence economy. These findings have implications for the excessive bone loss observed in many sedentary modern populations, suggesting that reduced physical activity levels might contribute to the high incidence rates of osteoporotic fracture in those populations.

References

Agarwal, S.C. and Grynpas, M.D. (1996). Bone quantity and quality in past populations. *Anat. Rec.* **246**, 423–432.

Benfer, R.A. (1990). The Preceramic site of Paloma, Peru: Bioindications of improving adaptation to sedentism. *Latin Am. Antiq.* **1**, 284–318.

Bouvier, M. and Hylander, W.L. (1981). Effect of bone strain on cortical bone structure in macaques (*Macaca mulatta*). *J. Morphol.* **167**, 1–12.

Bouvier, M. and Hylander, W.L. (1997). The mechanical or metabolic function of secondary osteonal bone in the monkey *Macaca fascicularis*. *Arch. Oral Biol.* **41**, 941–950.

Burr, D.B., Yoshikawa, T., and Ruff, C.B. (1995). Moderate exercise increases intracortical activation frequency in old dogs. *Trans. Orthop. Res. Soc.* **20**, 204.

Dougherty, G. and Al-Marzouk, N. (2001). Bone density measured by dual-energy X-ray absorptiometry in healthy Kuwaiti women. *Calcif. Tissue Int.* **68**, 225–229.

Engel, F.A. (1980). Paloma village 613: A 6,000 year old "fog oasis" village in the lower central Andes of Peru. F.A. Engel (ed.) *Prehistoric Andean Ecology*. Humanities Press, New York, pp. 103–116.

Frost, H.M. (1963). *Bone Remodeling Dynamics*. Charles C. Thomas, IL.

Frost, H.M. (1987a). Bone "mass" and the "mechanostat": A proposal. *Anat. Rec.* **219**, 1–9.

Frost, H.M. (1987d). Secondary osteon populations: An algorithm for estimating the missing osteons. *Yearbk. Phys. Anthropol.* **30**, 239–254.

Frost, H.M. (1989). Transient-steady state phenomena in microdamage physiology: A proposed algorithm for lamellar bone. *Calcif. Tissue Int.* **44**, 367–381.

Frost, H.M. (1990b). Skeletal structural adaptations to mechanical usage (SATMU): 2. Redefining Wolff's Law: The remodeling problem. *Anat. Rec.* **226**, 414–422.

Frost, H.M. and Villanueva, A.R. (1961). Human osteoblastic activity-Part I. A comparative method of measurement with some results. *Henry Ford Hosp. Med. Bull.* **9**, 76–86.

Frost, H.M. and Wu, K. (1967). Histological measurement of bone formation rates in unlabelled contemporary, archeological, and paleontological compact bone. In William D. Wade (ed.) *Miscellaneous Papers in Paleopathology*. Museum of Northern Arizona, AZ, pp. 9–22.

Hert, J., Pribylova, E., and Liskova, M. (1972). Reaction of bone to mechanical stimuli. Part 3: Microstructure of compact bone of rabbit tibia after intermittent loading. *Acta. Anat.* **82**, 218–230.

Hofman, M.A. (1988). Allometric scaling in palaeontology: A critical survey. *Hum. Evol.* **3**, 177–188.

Huiskes, R. (1982). On the modeling of long bones in structural analyses. *J. Biomech.* **15**, 65–69.

Iwaniec, U.T. (1997). Effects of acidity on cortical bone remodeling: A histomorphometric assessment. Doctoral Dissertation, University of Wisconsin-Madison, WI.

Jee, W.S.S., Li, X.J., and Schaffler, M.B. (1991). Adaptation of diaphyseal structure with aging and increased mechanical usage in the adult rat: A histomorphometrical and biomechanical study. *Anat. Rec.* **230**, 332–338.

Knüsel, C.J. (1993). On the biomechanical and osteoarthritic differences between hunter–gatherers and agriculturalists. *Am. J. Phys. Anthropol.* **91**, 523–527.

Lanyon, L.E. (1984). Functional strain as a determinant for bone remodeling. *Calcif. Tissue Int.* **36**(Suppl), S56–S61.

Lanyon, L.E. and Baggott, D.G. (1976). Mechanical function as an influence on the structure and form of bone. *J. Bone Joint Surg.* **58B**, 436–443.

Lazenby, R.A. (1986). Porosity–geometry interaction in the conservation of bone strength. *J. Biomech.* **19**, 257–258.

Lieberman, D.L. (1996). How and why humans grow thick skulls: Experimental evidence for systemic cortical robusticity. *Am. J. Phys. Anthropol.* **101**, 217–236.

Lieberman, D.L. (1997). Making behavioral and phylogenetic inferences from hominid fossils: Considering the developmental influences of mechanical forces. *Annual Rev. Anthropol.* **26**, 185–210.

Lieberman, D.L. and Crompton, A.W. (1998). Responses of bone to stress: Constraints on symmorphosis. In E. Weibel, C.R. Taylor, and L. Bolis (eds) *Principles of Animal Design: The Optimization and Symmorphosis Debate*. Cambridge University Press, UK.

Lovejoy, C.O. (1988). Evolution of human walking. *Sci. Am.* (Nov.) 118–125.

Mori, S. and Burr, D.B. (1993). Increased intracortical remodelling following fatigue damage. *Bone* **14**, 103–109.

Parfitt, A.M. (1983). The physiologic and clinical significance of bone histomorphometric data. In R.R. Recker (ed.) *Bone Histomorphometry: Techniques and Interpretation*. CRC Press, FL, pp. 143–223.

Quilter, J. (1989). *Life and Death at Paloma*. University of Iowa Press, IA.

Raab, D.M., Crenshaw, T.D., Kimmel, D.B., and Smith, E.L. (1991). A histomorphometric study of cortical bone activity during increased weight-bearing exercise. *J. Bone Miner. Res.* **6**, 741–749.

Ricker, W.E. (1973). Linear regressions in fishery research. *J. Fish Res. Board Can.* **30**, 409–434.

Rubin, C.T., Bain, S.D., and McLeod, K.J. (1992). Supression of the osteogenic response in the aging skeleton. *Calcif. Tissue Int.* **50**, 306–313.

Rubin, C.T., McLeod, K.J., and Bain, S.D. (1990). Functional strains and cortical bone adaptation: Epigenetic assurance of skeletal integrity. *J. Biomech.* **23**(Suppl), 43–54.

Ruff, C.B. (1994). Biomechanical analysis of Northern and Southern plains femora: Behavioral implications. In D.W. Owsley and R.L. Jantz (eds) *Skeletal Biology in the Great Plains*: Migration, Warfare, Health, and Subsistence. Smithsonian Institution Press: Washington, D.C., pp. 235–245.

Ruff, C.B., Trinkaus, E., and Holliday, T.W. (1997). Body mass and encephalization in Pleistocene Homo. *Nature* **387**, 173–176.

Schnitzler, C.M. (1993). Bone quality: A determinant for certain risk factors for bone fragility. *Calcif. Tissue Int.* **53**(Suppl 1), S27–S31.

Stout, S.D. (1983). The application of histomorphometric analysis to ancient skeletal remains. *Anthropos (Greece)* **10**, 61–71.

Stout, S.D. (1986). The use of bone histomorphometry in skeletal identification: The case of Francisco Pizarro. *J. Forensic Sci.* **31**, 296–300.

Stout, S.D. and Lueck, R. (1995). Bone remodeling rates and skeletal maturation in three archaeological skeletal populations. *Am. J. Phys. Anthropol.* **98**, 161–171.

Tommerup, L.J., Raab, D.M., Crenshaw, T.D., and Smith, E.L. (1993). Does weight-bearing exercise affect non-weight-bearing bone? *J. Bone Miner. Res.* **9**, 1053–1058.

Trinkaus, E., Ruff, C.B., Churchill, S.E., and Vandermeersch, B. (1998). Locomotion and body proportions of the Saint-Césaire 1 Châtelperronian neandertal. *Proc. Natl. Acad. Sci. USA* **95**, 5836–5840.

van der Meulen, M.C., Jepsen, K.J., and Mikic, B. (2001). Understanding bone strength: Size isn't everything. *Bone* **29**, 101–104.

Walker, R.A., Lovejoy, C.O., and Meindl, R.S. (1994). Histomorphological and geometric properties of human femoral cortex in individuals over 50: Implications for histomorphological determination of age-at-death. *Am. J. Human Biol.* **6**, 659–667.

Woo, S.L.Y., Kuei, S.C., Amiel, D., Gomez, M.A., Hayes, W.C., White, F.C., and Akeson, W.H. (1981). The effect of prolonged physical training on the properties of long bone: A study of Wolff's law. *J. Bone Joint Surg.* **63A**, 780–787.

Wu, K., Schubeck, K.E., Frost, H.M., and Villanueva, A.R. (1970). Haversian bone formation rates determined by a new method in a mastadon, and in human diabetes mellitus and osteoporosis. *Calcif. Tissue Res.* **6**, 204–219.

13

Bone Remodeling and Age-Associated Bone Loss in the Past: a Histomorphometric Analysis of the Imperial Roman Skeletal Population of Isola Sacra

Helen Cho and Sam D. Stout

1. Introduction

Bone loss is a serious consequence of the aging process in humans and is observed in both modern and archaeological populations. A severe manifestation of bone loss, or osteopenia, can cause mechanical incompetence of the skeletal system and lead to osteoporosis. Osteoporosis is associated with an increase in morbidity and mortality and a decrease in the enjoyment of life. Age-associated bone loss affects all people, regardless of sex, socioeconomic status, and ethnic background. The manifestation of osteopenia and related fragility fractures, however, is highest in modern populations of European descent (Nordin, 1966; Solomon, 1968, 1979; Chalmers and Ho, 1970; Cohn *et al.*, 1977; DeSimone *et al.*, 1989; Luckey *et al.*, 1989; Schnitzler, 1990; Nelson *et al.*, 1991; Baron *et al.*, 1994; Bell *et al.*, 1995; Stini, 1995). Study of the inherent disparities in the incidence and prevalence of osteopenia and osteoporosis between past and modern populations, as well as among modern populations, may reveal biocultural and evolutionary factors related to bone loss and osteoporosis.

The preservation of ancient skeletal remains makes it possible to study them and make inferences about health and disease in past societies. Paleopathologists and osteologists are often able to identify or diagnose pathologies from bone lesions observed in skeletal remains using various macroscopic and microscopic techniques. These lesions and other gross anomalies of the bones are often accompanied by abnormal remodeling dynamics of the skeletal tissue (Ortner and Putschar, 1985), since such changes in bone

Helen Cho • Department of Anthropology, Davidson College.
Sam D. Stout • Department of Anthropology, The Ohio State University.

Bone Loss and Osteoporosis: An Anthropological Perspective, edited by Sabrina C. Agarwal and Sam D. Stout. Kluwer Academic/Plenum Publishers, New York, 2003.

morphology are often due to abnormal bone cell activity. In osteopenic bone, macroporosity and thinner cortices in the skeletal elements are associated with discernible qualitative and quantitative histologic (tissue-level) changes, such as a larger and a higher frequency of resorptive cavities.

Histomorphometry is the quantitative study of discrete morphological structures at the histologic level. Bone histomorphometry can be applied to bone from both present and past populations, provided there is adequate preservation of the integrity of the microstructures, such as osteons. It is a useful method for analyzing age-related changes in bone and the pathophysiology of metabolic skeletal diseases (Stout, 1978; Boivin and Meunier, 1993). Histomorphometric analysis can effectively and directly quantify bone loss at the cellular and tissue level where it occurs. It is used to derive indices of remodeling such as activation frequency and bone turnover rate, which are important for understanding the physiological mechanisms of bone loss.

This chapter will discuss the application of bone histomorphometry to the study of age-related bone loss in past populations. The principles and methodology of histomorphometry for assessing bone loss will be discussed, and its application is illustrated through a review of previous studies of various archaeological samples and the results of a current project involving an Imperial Roman population.

2. Principles and Methodology of Bone Histomorphometry

Age-related bone loss occurs at the tissue level of the skeleton. The manifestation of normal age-associated bone loss is the result of a net bone loss occurring with the metabolic process called remodeling. Remodeling is the major process through which adult bone responds to physiological, environmental, and hereditary influences. Abnormal bone loss results from a "disequilibrium" or "uncoupling" of bone formation and resorption during the remodeling process (Meunier, 1988; Plato *et al.*, 1994). Bone remodeling is a lifelong process, the rate of which generally decreases with increasing age. It involves a chain of cellular events, beginning with the activation of cells that will form a focus of remodeling activity, followed by the resorption and formation of bone by these cells. These organized units of cells are called basic multicellular units of bone remodeling, or BMU's. The coupled sequence of bone resorption and formation produces the basic histomorphological structural units in bone, which in cortical bone are osteons or Haversian systems. The major kinds of cells involved in bone remodeling are osteoclasts and osteoblasts, which resorb old bone and deposit new bone, respectively.

Bone turnover through remodeling is necessary for microfracture/fatigue damage repair and calcium homeostasis, as well as other physiological and mechanical functions (Martin *et al.*, 1998). Even in healthy individuals, the remodeling process results in a net loss in bone, since the exact amount of resorbed bone is not replaced. The uncoupling of the remodeling process can result in a relative increase or decrease in the rates of bone formation or resorption.

Remodeling also occurs in trabecular or cancellous bone where it is somewhat different. For example, the surface to volume ratio of trabecular bone is much higher than that in cortical bone, resulting in a greater turnover rate. The rate of cancellous bone loss is inconsistent with the rate of cortical bone loss, and variability in skeletal remodeling and bone loss exists within an individual skeleton (Frisch and Eventov, 1986; Charnley *et al.*, 1989; Plato *et al.*, 1994; Nordin *et al.*, 1996; Compston, 1999). Due to its faster bone turnover, bone loss is generally observed first in trabecular bone. Bone loss is also greater in trabecular than in compact bone (Ortner and Putschar, 1985). Agarwal (2001a) recently reported finding dramatically different age-related patterns of bone loss and trabecular architecture in three British historical populations as compared to modern populations. This chapter focuses on cortical remodeling, but intra-skeletal variability is an area in need of further exploration.

Bone remodeling rates are essential data in osteoporosis research as they provide information about the disease at the tissue level. Due to the nature of archaeological remains, dynamic remodeling rates cannot be determined. Bone tissue-time markers such as tetracycline used in clinical bone research are not applicable to archaeological specimens for obvious reasons. Although fortuitous tetracycline-like labeling of bone due to certain dietary practices has been reported in bones from archaeological skeletal samples (Bassett *et al.*, 1980), skeletal samples with such labeling are relatively rare and the time controls necessary to estimate dynamic bone remodeling rates are lacking for archaeological samples. Ancient bone histomorphology, therefore, must determine bone remodeling rates indirectly through static indices of bone remodeling. It should be noted that most indices are based upon the identification and measurement of 2–D representations of 3–D microstructures. The problems and errors associated with stereology are beyond the scope of the chapter, and it is suggested that the readers refer to the detailed volume on the techniques and interpretations in bone histomorphometry edited by Recker (1983). Further, in order to insure that histomorphometric data produced from research in various disciplines are comparable, standards of measurements and terminology should be followed. Parfitt *et al.* (1987) outline a recommended standardization of nomenclature in bone histology.

2.1. Cortical Bone Sample Preparation

Quantification of microstructures, such as osteons and Haversian canals, requires that these structures are clearly visible. While modern specimens may not require embedding in plastic resin for cutting and grinding for histological analysis, archaeological samples are usually brittle and fragile and require embedding to ensure structural integrity during preparation. Histomorphometric studies cited in this chapter can be consulted for the specific details of the embedding process and preparation of histological sections of bone. (See also Chapter 12, this volume.)

Histological measurements from cortical bone thin-sections can be accomplished using a grid inserted into the eyepiece of the microscope. Such grids, which are made up of a set of lines and points with specific geometric properties, can be used to calculate surface areas and perimeters of the microstructures (Parfitt, 1983). Several types of grids, also called eyepiece reticules, exist (circular and square grids with differing numbers of lines and points) and the type used depends on the research objective. The grids are superimposed over the bone section in view while relevant measurements are recorded. For examples of the application of such grids to determine cortical bone histomorphometrics, the reader can consult Robling and Stout (2000). Recent advances in digital technology provide image analysis hardware and software that can also be used to assist in the determination of histomorphometric data.

2.2. An Algorithm for Estimating Bone Remodeling Rates in Ancient Skeletal Samples

Although *in vivo* tissue time markers such as tetracycline are used to label bone and measure bone remodeling in clinical settings, an algorithm is available that permits several parameters of bone remodeling to be measured from unlabeled bone. This algorithm, described in Wu *et al.* (1970) and Frost (1987), is applicable to archaeological and paleontological bone (the application of this algorithm to archaeological bone is also discussed in Chapter 12, this volume). It is based upon the principle that an osteon represents the creation of one bone remodeling unit (BRU) in the past. The number of osteons per unit area observed in a cross-section of bone, therefore, represents the visible evidence of past remodeling activity in that area of bone in that individual. This visible evidence includes whole osteons and fragmentary osteons that have been partially obliterated due to subsequent remodeling activity, and is referred to as the osteon population density (OPD).

The algorithm also requires estimating the number of "missing" osteons that have been completely removed by subsequent remodeling activity. Continuous remodeling activity eventually produces an asymptote in OPD where osteonal bone occupies the entire cortex, and each new creation removes evidence for an earlier creation. The number of previously remodeled missing osteons increases exponentially until an asymptote is reached. The total accumulated osteons (AOC), which is the sum of OPD and missing osteons, represents the history of cortical bone remodeling activity in a bone. The derivation of AOC from OPD and its estimated asymptote have been described elsewhere (Frost, 1987; Stout and Paine, 1994; Stout and Lueck, 1995; Abbott *et al.*, 1996).

Activation frequency, or the number of osteons created annually per unit area (i.e., mm^2) of bone, can be estimated from AOC and the chronological age of an individual. Increased bone size and transverse cortical drifts that occur during growth add, replace, and redistribute bone, resulting in the rapid removal of most of the histomorphological evidence for subadult cortical bone remodeling in the adult skeleton. Because of this, the mean tissue age for adult compacta is younger than the chronological age of the individual (for a discussion of subadult bone histomorphometry see Chapter 6, this volume). Wu *et al.* (1970) report that the effective "birth" of adult compacta, the age at which osteon accumulation observed in an adult bone effectively begins, occurs at approximately 12.5 years of age in the middle third of the sixth rib. Activation frequency, therefore, is calculated by dividing the total accumulated osteon creations determined for a bone by its chronological age minus 12.5 years, or the difference between chronological and effective age of the adult compacta.

The mean annual cortical bone formation rate, or the amount of Haversian bone formed per square millimeter of bone per year, is the product of both activation frequency and osteon size (mean osteon area). It represents the average amount of bone formed annually in that bone for that individual. Since it is sometimes impossible to obtain a chronological age for archaeological remains, net bone remodeling rate can be determined in lieu of the annual bone formation rate.

Mean annual activation rates and bone formation rates are general indicators of skeletal health. They can be compared across samples representing different time periods and genetic backgrounds to study population variability in skeletal biology and metabolic bone disease. For an example of the application of this algorithm to several North American archaeological populations, the reader is referred to Stout and Lueck (1995).

2.3. Diagenesis

In histology, adequate preservation of the microstructure of a bone specimen is crucial. Diagenesis, the postmortem and postdepositional changes of the skeletal remains, can alter the chemical composition and/or the microstructure of bones. The type and extent of diagenesis are dependent on the immediate surrounding environment. The environment in which the remains were deposited may serve as an indicator of the type of diagenesis. For example, bones buried in wet environments tend to be exposed to algal growth and exhibit poor histological preservation. Other environments, such as very arid ones, can produce skeletal remains with extremely good histological preservation. (See also Chapter 11, this volume.)

Oftentimes, the microstructural preservation cannot be predicted by the gross appearance of the skeletal remains, and the extent of diagenesis is discernible only after thin ground sections have been prepared (Hanson and Buikstra, 1987; Schultz, 1997; Pfeiffer, 2000). Plant roots and animal activities can destroy the macrostructure of bone, while microorganisms and minerals can damage its microstructure. Plant roots leave impressions and holes which may be mistaken for antemortem damage (Schultz, 1997). Fungi, bacteria, algae, and minerals (leached into bone from the groundwater) that sometimes penetrate bone, and disintegrate and cloud the microstructures are of concern for they can leave the sample unsuitable for histological analysis. For additional information on diagenesis and histomorphological preservation, the reader is referred to Stout (1978), Garland (1993), Herrmann (1993), and Grupe and Dreses-Werringloer (1993).

2.4. Age-At-Death

The effects of aging on the skeleton exhibit considerable phenotypic variability and most osteological aging methods cannot reliably assess age beyond the sixth decade. Individuals over the age of 50 years are usually grouped into the single broad cohort of 50+ years. Therefore, for comparative purposes, the clinical data must be modified to match the age groups reported for the archaeological samples. Since the bone loss associated with severe osteopenia and osteoporosis is usually observed around menopause in females and later in males, comparisons of archaeological data with clinical ones are limited. The derivation of activation frequency and annual bone remodeling rate requires an independent (non-histological) estimate of the age-at-death of the individual. Erroneous osteological age estimation will result in inaccurate estimates of both activation frequencies and bone formation rates that are proportional to the magnitude of the error. Curatorial age estimates are generally given in decades or broader ranges (e.g., 20–29 years). The algorithm for deriving remodeling parameters requires a single estimate of chronological age. Osteological ages, therefore, must be converted to a single age estimate. For example, the chronological age of 25 years can be used for a skeleton whose osteological age is reported to be 20–29 years. In adult remains, this produces only four possible ages (25 years, 35 years, 45 years, and 50 + years), and arbitrarily merging all ages of above 50 years as 50+ will undoubtedly create greater variance than for the younger cohorts.

3. Previous Applications of Histomorphology in Past Populations

It is important to understand the differences that exist in the apparent risk of osteoporosis between modern and past peoples. Although age-associated bone loss has been observed in past populations, the incidence of bone fragility and fractures, which are pathognostic of osteoporosis, appear relatively low in archaeological populations (Agarwal and Grynpas, 1996). However, most ancient bone loss research to date has been conducted using non-Western hunter–gatherer or agricultural populations (Pfeiffer and Lazenby, 1994; Agarwal and Grynpas, 1996). Various methodologies have been employed to measure bone mass and density and cortical bone involution, but we limit our review to cortical bone histomorphometry. The histomorphometric methods outlined above have been applied to several anatomical skeletal sampling sites from archaeological populations representing various geographical areas and time periods.

3.1. African Populations

The main groups that have been studied from Africa are the Sudanese Nubians. Femora from three cultural horizons dating from 0 BC to AD 1300 were subjected to comprehensive quantitative and qualitative histological analyses by Martin and Armelagos (1979, 1985). Results from their histological analyses are consistent with the findings of other studies based upon morphological methods, concluding that Nubian females during this time period began losing bone at an earlier age than their male counterparts or modern populations. Significant bone loss was observed at the endosteal envelope of the Nubian females in the third decade (20–29 years) of life. The young females exhibited faster remodeling rates, and more specifically, increased resorption and slower bone formation rates as indicated by higher frequencies of resorptive spaces and forming osteons, respectively. This remodeling pattern is attributed to a combination of reproductive (multiple pregnancies and prolonged lactation) and nutritional (due to intensification of agriculture) stresses (For a contrasting view of the effects of reproductive factors on the female skeleton, see Chapter 7, this volume.)

Mulhern and Van Gerven (1997) examined sex and age differences in the intact and fragmentary osteon densities, osteon size, Haversian canal diameter, and other derived variables of a late medieval Nubian sample (AD 1250–1450) of femora. They found that females exhibited a significantly higher frequency of fragmentary osteons and a lower frequency of intact osteons, which can be interpreted to mean higher bone remodeling rates. These observed differences between the sexes might also be due, in part, to the fact that females exhibit larger osteon areas than males. Mulhern and Van Gerven (1997) speculate that the sex differences observed in the frequency of the microstructures may reflect sexual division of labor that produced differing mechanical strains on the femora of males and females. Sexual dimorphism for remodeling rates was not observed in this study.

3.2. European Populations

The epidemiology of osteoporosis for modern, urban, western groups reveals them to be especially high-risk populations. Studies of bone loss in the past, however, have been primarily on non-western and pre-industrial archaeological populations. A few bone density studies conducted on European archaeological samples report ambiguous results on osteopenia and related fractures (Bennike and Bohr, 1990; Kneissel *et al.*, 1994; Mays, 1998). Not only is research lacking for archaeological populations of European origin, but previous methods relied primarily on radiography and absorptiometry (Agarwal and Grynpas, 1996).

Two histomorphometric studies involve ancient European populations. The first is a study of variability in osteon size in rib and femora samples from 18th century Huguenots from Spitalfields, London, and 19th century British settlers in Ontario (Pfeiffer, 1998). Osteon size was found to be smaller in the rib than the femur, and there was no correlation found with age and sex. The Spitalfields sample had the largest femoral osteons and the smallest rib osteons when compared to a modern sample of mixed ethnicity from South Africa (white, black, and colored) and the 19th century Canadian sample. The explanation for variability within the same skeletal element is indeterminate but may be due to mechanical, genetic, and/or local factors. Understanding the variability in osteon size is important, as it is an essential parameter of cortical bone remodeling.

In the second study of ancient European skeletal remains, Agarwal (2001a,b) and Agarwal *et al.* (2000) quantified trabecular architecture in British medieval and post-medieval vertebral samples. Age and sex-related changes were examined and compared with modern populations. Sex differences in the trabecular architecture and bone density between modern and archaeological populations were suggested to reflect lifestyle factors, particularly reproductive factors. (See also Agarwal and Stuart-Macadam, Chapter 7 this volume.)

3.3. Native American Populations

The vast majority of histomorphometric studies to date have been conducted on Native American populations from North America and the Arctic. The studies include Pueblo Indian femora from AD 919 to 1600 (Richman *et al.*, 1979; Ericksen, 1980; Iwaniec, 1997), Arikara femora from AD 1550 to 1845 (Richman *et al.*, 1979; Ericksen, 1980), Alaskan Eskimo femora from late 18th to early 20th centuries (Richman *et al.*, 1979; Ericksen, 1980; Iwaniec, 1997), Yupiaq–Inupiaq Eskimo femora from several islands ranging from 700 BC to 19th century (Thompson and Gunness-Hey, 1981; Thompson *et al.*, 1981; Thompson and Cowen, 1984), early Archaic Windover site from 6900 to 8120 BP (Stout and Lueck, 1995), middle Woodland Gibson and Ray sites from 50 BC to AD 400 (Stout, 1983; Stout and Lueck, 1995), late Woodland Ledders site dating to AD 1000 (Stout and Teitelbaum, 1976; Stout, 1983; Stout and Lueck, 1995), and an archaic South American site La Paloma from 7700 to 5000 BP (Stout, 1983; Robling, 1998). (The latter study is reported in greater detail in the chapter by Robling and Stout, Chapter 12 this volume.)

Dietary factors are a common explanation for the differences in intra-cortical remodeling observed among various Native American groups. It has been suggested that the transition from a more diverse intensive foraging to a less diverse agricultural subsistence may have exposed prehistoric people to nutritional stress (Stout, 1983; Pfeiffer and Lazenby, 1994). Stout (1983) compared cortical rib remodeling in three native North American populations, one native South American population, and a modern cadaver sample. The population with the agricultural subsistence base, Ledders, was found to have the highest bone turnover rate compared to the hunting–gathering and modern populations. It is speculated that heavy reliance on maize, which is calcium poor and high in phosphorous, may have triggered a chronic secondary hyperparathyroidism which in turn would increase the cortical remodeling rate.

A more recent histomorphometric study of archaeological agricultural and hunting and gathering societies reports remodeling differences among three Native American populations ranging in antiquity from 8120 BP to AD 1000 (Stout and Lueck, 1995). The remodeling activities are similar between the foraging populations (Archaic Windover site and Middle Woodland Gibson site) who exhibit lower remodeling rates than the agricultural population (Late Woodland Ledders site). When compared to a modern sample from North America, the agriculture-based population was intermediate between the foragers and the modern samples, which exhibited the highest average bone remodeling rates. The authors suggest that the apparent differences in bone remodeling rates might indicate population differences in the age at which the effective age of the adult compacta is reached, rather than, or in addition to actual differences in bone remodeling rates. To a large extent, these differences may reflect genetic and/or behavioral-cultural factors occurring during skeletal development in subadults, rather than entirely the effect of biocultural factors on the skeletal systems of the adults.

Research on other populations also confirms that hunter–gatherer populations exhibit lower bone turnover rates. A comparison of agriculture-based Pueblo and Arikara populations and protein-dependent Eskimos produced interesting results. Bone remodeling in the Eskimo females is highest based upon their higher frequencies of intact and fragmentary osteons, and resorptive spaces (Richman *et al.*, 1979; Ericksen, 1980; Iwaniec, 1997). Ericksen (1980) and Iwaniec (1997) attribute this pattern to a possible combination of greater demands for calcium during pregnancy and lactation in the females, as well as their high protein and low calcium diet. Richman *et al.* (1979) conclude that the high bone remodeling rate in the Eskimo is due to their high protein diet which is associated with accelerated mineral mobilization from bone, metabolic acidosis, increased bone loss, and hypercalciuria; because of the lack of sexual dimorphism in their study, they reject the notion of additional nutritional stress in the Eskimo females due to pregnancy and lactation. A histomorphometric study by Iwaniec (1997) on the effects of dietary acidity on cortical bone remodeling did not find evidence for depletion of bone mineral in response to acid loads using a swine animal model. A retrospective study of two archaeological human populations in the same study found that differences in protein intake did not account for variation in bone remodeling patterns between Inuits, whose diet was high in protein, and Pueblo agriculturalists, whose diet was low in protein and high in carbohydrates. Histomorphometric differences in the femora of these two skeletal populations were observed only between middle aged and older females. Iwaniec (1997) concludes that the histomorphometric differences between the two populations are best explained by the effects of pregnancy and lactation in association with fluctuations in the Inuit diet. The relative importance of the effects of dietary acidity on age-associated bone loss may, therefore, be minimal.

A study of a female Eskimo mummy who died in her sixth decade of life did not corroborate the popular findings that Eskimo populations are more susceptible to earlier onset of age-associated bone loss and osteoporosis (Stout and Teitelbaum, 1976). This mummy's histomorphometric variables were within the values of healthy modern females in the sixth decade. On the other hand, an analysis of the femora and iliac crest samples from two Utqiagvik native Alaskan mummies resulted in femoral cortical thicknesses and trabecular bone volumes significantly lower than U.S. Whites of a comparable age group (Thompson and Cowen, 1984). Both mummies would be classified as osteoporotic by clinical standards.

In a comparison of Canadian Eskimo samples to U.S. Whites, Thompson *et al.* (1981) revealed that the Eskimo had slightly higher osteon frequency in individuals under

35 years old than Whites, but there was no difference in osteon size. No sexual dimorphism in histomorphometrics was observed in the Canadian samples. Remodeling rates were not estimated, but a faster remodeling rate in the Eskimos than in Whites is implied by their higher osteon density. Thompson and Gunness-Hey (1981) also report population differences in osteon density per unit area between Eskimos and Whites. Studies suggest the different remodeling rates between these two groups may be attributable to genetics, diet, and activity patterns, or a combination of these factors. The disparate findings of these studies reinforce the need for developing a better understanding of intra-skeletal variation in bone remodeling and bone loss, and establishing the comparability of different methodologies.

3.4. Other Populations

Histomorphometric studies on archaeological populations from Asia, Australia, and elsewhere remain yet to be done. This may be due to the unavailability of archaeological samples, especially for invasive histological analysis.

A study of Middle Eastern populations involves much older samples than the ones reviewed above. Femoral sections from late Archaic fossils from several Middle Eastern sites have been analyzed for histological age estimation and bone remodeling activity (Abbott *et al.*, 1996). The fossil hominids had a lower OPD, smaller osteons, and a slower activation frequency and bone turnover than recent populations. Abbott *et al.* (1996) speculate that small osteon size could be due to nutritional stress and low bone remodeling is due to high physical strain. But this explanation is inconclusive. In contrast, however, a reexamination of the same fossils by Streeter (1999) found osteon size to not be significantly smaller and remodeling rates that are similar to those determined for other archaeological skeletal remains representing a hunting and gathering mode of subsistence. These results are still consistent with a high activity level model.

4. Present Study: An Example in Histomorphology and Bioarchaeology

The research results presented are based upon the analysis of a preliminary sample of ribs from an Imperial Roman skeletal population. The study represents a unique opportunity to study bone loss in an ancient European sample. Cortical bone histomorphometry and cross-sectional area measurements are used to identify and quantify age-related bone loss. Sex, age, and population differences are the focus of this study.

4.1. Materials

The study sample is from the Isola Sacra necropolis, which is located about 23 km from Rome in southcentral Italy (Figure 13.1). The necropolis is on an island between the ancient cities of Ostia and *Portus Romae* (Figure 13.2). The people of Isola Sacra were inhabitants of *Portus Romae*, an urban city of a major harbor receiving foods and supplies for Rome during its height as an empire. The cemetery was in use during the second and third centuries.

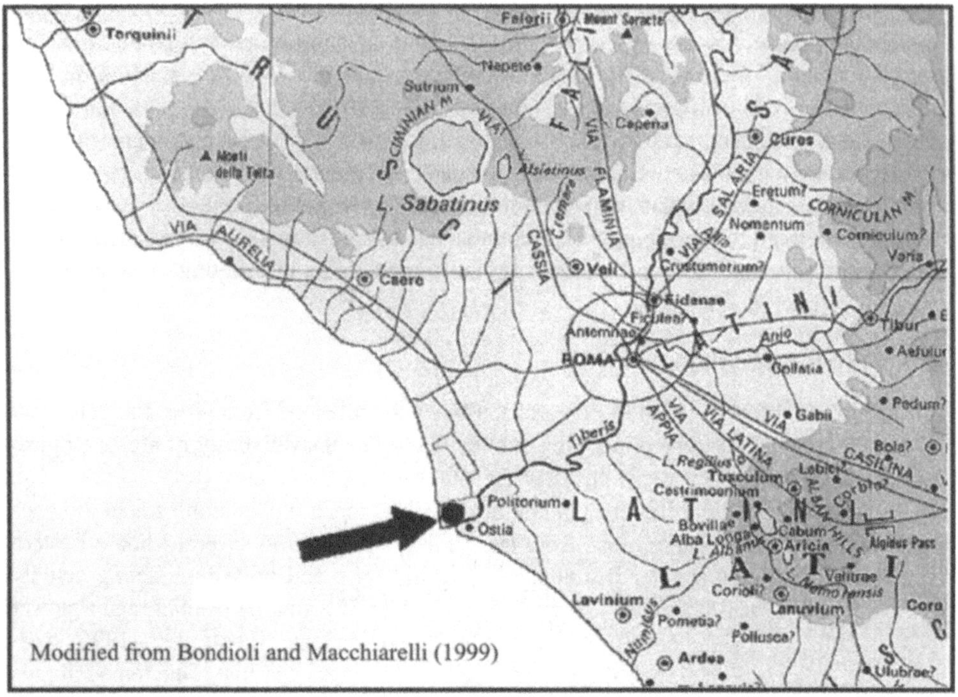

Figure 13.1. Map of southcentral Italy and the location of the Isola Sacra necropolis (arrow).

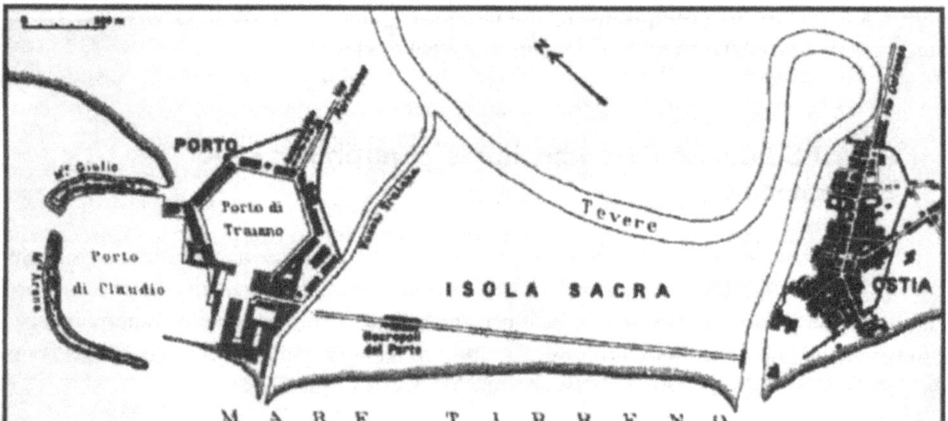

Figure 13.2. The Isola Sacra necropolis.

Excavations of the necropolis began in the 1920s by Guido Calza, an archaeologist, and further excavations took place beginning in 1973 (Bondioli and Macchiarelli, 1999). The types of burials at the necropolis range widely from single burials in amphorae and sarcophagi to multiple interments in monumental house tombs and arcosolea.

Unfortunately, because the excavation notes did not include the locations and associations of the skeletons with particular burials, the assessment of family relations and social status was not possible.

Portus Romae was atypical and unrepresentative of the Classical Period due to its unique position as the Roman port, and the high occurrences of commerce and trade activity. The society was relatively egalitarian, appearing to lack the aristocratic, elite, and political class in social hierarchies observed in other Roman cities (Bondioli and Macchiarelli, 1999). The inhabitants were mainly middle-class traders and merchants of freedmen stock, whose livelihoods were strictly dependent on the commerce and trade relating to the harbor (e.g., traders, merchants, shopkeepers, carpenters, craftsmen).

In addition to the lack of documentation about the identity of the Isola Sacra individuals, there is no clear record of the diets and lifestyles among the middle class, freedmen, freedwomen, and slaves of this port town. Our research is simplified in this aspect. The inhabitants of the Port and their bone biology were not widely influenced by differences in the nutrition and activity that are normally distinguishable among different socioeconomic classes.

This European skeletal sample fills a critical chronological gap in previous bone loss studies of archaeological populations. In addition, Isola Sacra was an urban site, which makes it unique among most archaeological study populations that are typically nonindustrial and agricultural. To date, approximately 2,000 individuals have been excavated and are housed in the Museo Nazionale Preistorico Etnografico "L. Pigorini" in Rome, where multidisciplinary research is actively carried out on the collection. This ongoing and collaborative bioarchaeological research is particularly significant, since compared to the abundant material culture the Romans left behind, their biology and health are surprisingly unknown (Bondioli and Macchiarelli, 1999).

The skeletal element used in this study is the midshaft rib, with a preliminary sample size of 46 individuals (M = 25, F = 21). The osteological ages range from 20 to 50+ years (Table 13.1). Various age estimating methods have been employed by the curators of the collection who have categorized the adult individuals into decades.

The comparative data are derived from modern European American and African American rib samples. European Americans, like modern day Europeans, are one of the most susceptible groups to osteopenic fractures in the United States. African Americans,

Table 13.1. Age and Sex Distributions of the Study and Comparative Samples (M = Male, F = Female, C = Combined)

	Isola Sacra			European American			African American		
Age (years)	M	F	C	M	F	C	M	F	C
20–29	6	5	11	19	2	21	7	7	14
30–39	4	7	11	4	2	6	8	4	12
40–49	8	5	13	6	7	13	13	10	23
50+	7	4	11	23	20	43	45	37	92
Total	25	21	46	52	31	83	73	58	135
Mean age (years)	36.4	33.8	35.2	44.7	57.6	49.5[a]	55.6	54.0	54.3

[a] Seven individuals were of unknown sex and, therefore, the mean age differs from the text.

on the other hand, experience a much lower incidence of fragility fractures. Both modern populations of African ancestry and archaeological populations are reported to exhibit a greater quantity and better quality of bone mass than their modern European counterparts. The modern comparative samples used in this study were previously collected from an African American cemetery, forensic cases, and autopsies (Cho and Stout, 2001).

The European American sample consists of 90 individuals (M = 52, F = 31, unknown = 7) ranging in age from 17 to 102 years with a mean age of 48.6 years. The African American sample is composed of 135 individuals (M = 73, F = 58) with an age range of 17–95 years and mean age of 54.3 years (Table 13.1). The modern samples had known age-at-death records, however, due to the broader age categories available for the Italian archaeological sample, the modern samples were assigned to comparable age groups by decade (i.e., 20–29 years, 30–39 years). Individuals between the ages of 17 and 20 years were placed in the 20–29 year cohort.

4.2. Methods

The cross-sectional area data collected include relative cortical area (Sedlin, 1964) and the parabolic index (Epker and Frost, 1964) for ribs. Relative cortical area, or percent cortical bone, is the ratio of cortical bone to total cross-sectional area. Cross-sectional area measurements of the rib are useful to observe the progression of osteopenia with increasing age and to compare it among populations. The parabolic index is a measure of the optimal distribution of cortical bone around the marrow (bone strength), and has an optimum value of 0.25.

The following histomorphometric variables described by Wu *et al.* (1970), Frost (1987), and Stout and Paine (1994) were measured in the Isola Sacra rib sample: OPD, mean osteon size, mean annual activation frequency, and mean annual bone formation rate. The latter two variables are estimates of the rate at which an individual remodels their cortical bone. Activation frequency and annual bone formation rate were derived by using the median age of the assigned osteological age category (i.e., 25 years for 20–29 year group) for each category.

The analysis and comparison of the Isola Sacra rib data with that for modern European Americans and African Americans was accomplished using the statistical software STATISTICA (StatSoft, Inc., Tulsa, OK).

4.3. Results

The results of the histomorphometric analysis of the rib samples from Isola Sacra are summarized in Table 13.2.

4.3.1. Cortical Area in Isola Sacra

Total subperiosteal area (Tt.Ar), cortical area (Ct.Ar), and endosteal area (En.Ar) are all significantly larger in males than females from Isola Sacra ($p < 0.001$). The relative amount of cortical area (Ct.Ar/Tt.Ar) and the parabolic index, however, do not differ significantly between the sexes ($p = 0.271$ and $p = 0.064$, respectively). When regressed against age, only the parabolic index exhibits a significant decrease (negative slope) with

Table 13.2. Isola Sacra Results (±1SE) (M = Male, F = Female, C = Combined)

	Age categories (years)														
	20–29 (*N* = 11)			30–39 (*N* = 11)			40–49 (*N* = 13)			50+ (*N* = 11)			Total (*N* = 46)		
Variable	M	F	C	M	F	C	M	F	C	M	F	C	M	F	C
Tt.Ar (mm^2)	85.6 ± 13.5	51.0 ± 5.5	69.9 ± 9.2	69.4 ± 2.2	47.4 ± 6.0	54.0 ± 5.4	72.6 ± 8.6	40.6 ± 6.9	61.9 ± 7.5	96.7 ± 9.0	40.9 ± 8.0	76.4 ± 10.5	82.5 ± 5.4	45.6 ± 3.2	65.7 ± 4.3
Ct.Ar (mm^2)	39.6 ± 5.9	20.7 ± 2.5	31.0 ± 4.4	31.5 ± 5.8	20.9 ± 2.1	24.0 ± 2.6	26.5 ± 3.2	16.4 ± 3.8	23.1 ± 2.8	29.7 ± 2.8	16.6 ± 0.7	24.9 ± 2.6	31.3 ± 2.2	19.1 ± 1.2	25.8 ± 1.6
En.Ar (mm^2)	46.0 ± 9.4	30.3 ± 3.9	38.9 ± 5.7	38.0 ± 3.9	26.5 ± 4.5	29.9 ± 3.7	46.1 ± 7.1	24.2 ± 4.1	38.8 ± 5.7	67.1 ± 7.8	24.3 ± 8.1	51.5 ± 8.5	51.2 ± 4.4	26.5 ± 2.4	40.0 ± 3.2
Ct.Ar/Tt.Ar (%)	47.0 ± 4.4	40.6 ± 3.3	44.1 ± 2.9	45.0 ± 6.9	46.1 ± 3.9	45.8 ± 3.2	38.4 ± 4.7	40.3 ± 5.5	39.1 ± 3.5	31.6 ± 3.5	44.7 ± 7.6	36.4 ± 3.9	39.4 ± 2.5	43.3 ± 2.3	41.2 ± 1.7
Parabolic index	0.2 ± 0.01	0.2 ± 0.01	0.2 ± 0.004	0.2 ± 0.002	0.2 ± 0.003	0.2 ± 0.002	0.2 ± 0.01	0.2 ± 0.01	0.2 ± 0.01	0.2 ± 0.01	0.2 ± 0.01	0.2 ± 0.01	0.2 ± 0.004	0.2 ± 0.003	0.2 ± 0.003
OPD (#/mm^2)	15.9 ± 2.0	17.8 ± 1.8	16.8 ± 1.3	22.2 ± 1.9	20.3 ± 1.6	21.0 ± 1.2	21.4 ± 1.3	19.9 ± 1.4	20.8 ± 1.0	21.4 ± 1.9	31.8 ± 2.3	25.2 ± 2.1	20.2 ± 1.0	21.8 ± 1.4	21.0 ± 0.8
On.Ar (mm^2)	0.04 ± 0.004	0.03 ± 0.002	0.03 ± 0.003	0.03 ± 0.002	0.03 ± 0.002	0.03 ± 0.001	0.03 ± 0.003	0.03 ± 0.01	0.03 ± 0.002	0.03 ± 0.002	0.03 ± 0.001	0.03 ± 0.002	0.03 ± 0.002	0.03 ± 0.001	0.03 ± 0.001
Ac.f (#/mm^2/yr)	1.3 ± 0.2	1.5 ± 0.2	1.4 ± 0.1	1.1 ± 0.1	1.1 ± 0.3	1.1 ± 0.2	0.7 ± 0.04	0.7 ± 0.1	0.7 ± 0.04	0.6 ± 0.1	0.9 ± 0.2	0.7 ± 0.1	0.9 ± 0.1	1.1 ± 0.1	1.0 ± 0.1
BFR (mm^2/mm^2/yr)	0.04 ± 0.004	0.1 ± 0.003	0.1 ± 0.003	0.03 ± 0.002	0.04 ± 0.01	0.04 ± 0.01	0.02 ± 0.002	0.02 ± 0.01	0.02 ± 0.002	0.02 ± 0.002	0.02 ± 0.004	0.02 ± 0.002	0.03 ± 0.003	0.03 ± 0.004	0.03 ± 0.002

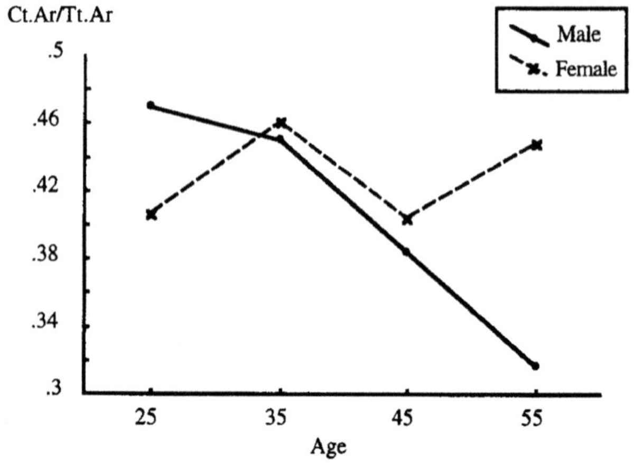

Figure 13.3. Relative cortical area (Ct.Ar/Tt.Ar) for Isola Sacra ribs. Means for males and females plotted against the midpoint for reported osteological ages.

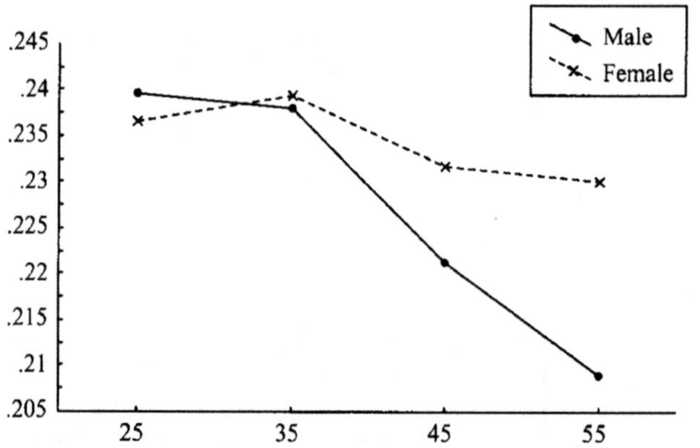

Figure 13.4. Parabolic index for Isola Sacra. Means for males and females plotted against the midpoint for reported osteological ages.

age ($p = 0.002$). When the sexes are considered separately, the results are slightly different. Relative cortical area for males exhibits a small, but significant decrease with age ($p = 0.014$), and the decrease in parabolic index is significant only for males ($p = 0.003$). Relative cortical area decreases steadily in males, while it increases until the fourth decade in females, after which it declines (Figure 13.3). The parabolic index is similar and relatively constant until the fourth decade in males and females, after which it decreases, but at a higher rate in males (Figure 13.4).

4.3.2. Bone Remodeling in Isola Sacra

As expected, there is a significant positive correlation ($p < 0.05$) between the reported osteological ages and OPD (Figure 13.5). When males and females are considered separately, a significant difference is observed, but only for the 50+ year age group

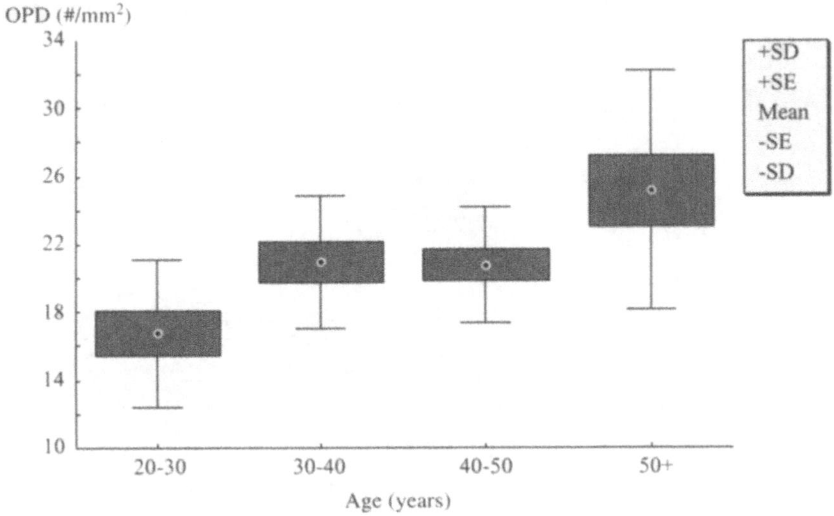

Figure 13.5. Osteon Population Density (OPD) for Isola Sacra ribs. Means and their standard errors and standard deviations for reported osteological ages (decades).

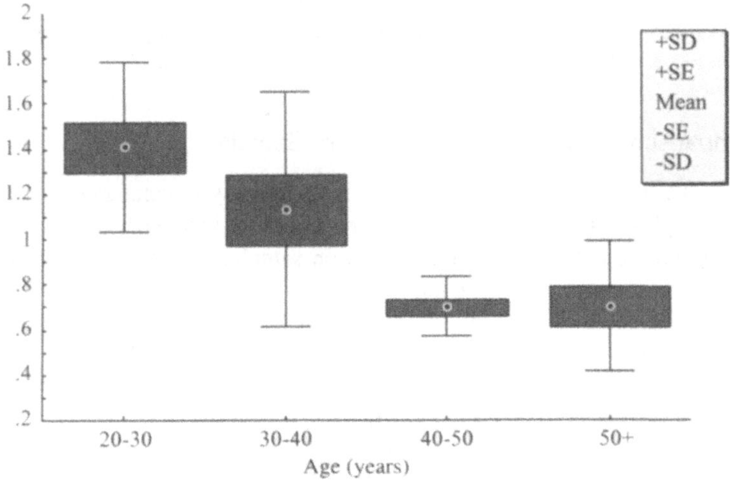

Figure 13.6. Activation frequency (Ac.f) for Isola Sacra ribs. Means and their standard errors and standard deviations for reported osteological ages (decades).

when the average OPD for females is $30.0 \pm 2.05/mm^2$ compared to $20.9 \pm 1.81/mm^2$ for males. The average amount of bone contained within an osteon does not differ between the sexes, and it tends to decrease with age, but this difference is not statistically significant. Both the mean annual rate at which osteons are created (Ac.f), and the mean annual cortical bone formation rate (BFR) decrease with age in males and females (Figures 13.6 and 13.7). Similar to OPD, the Ac.f differs between the sexes only for the 50+ age category. The average amount of bone turned over per unit area of cortical bone (BFR), however, does

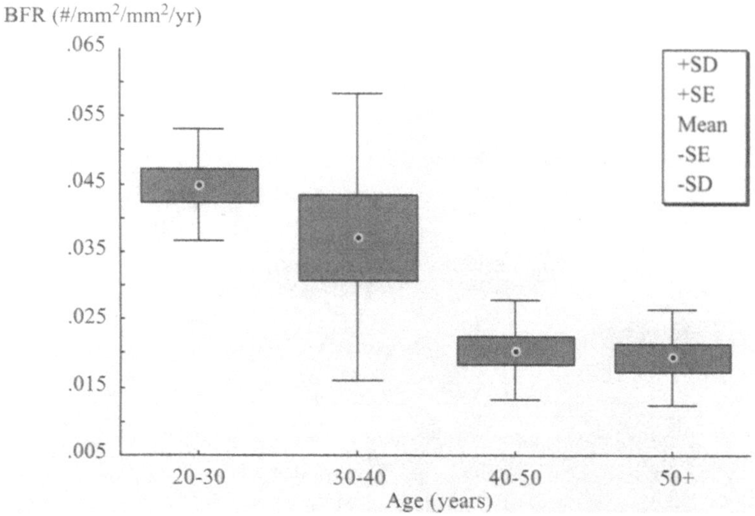

Figure 13.7. Annual bone formation rate (BFR) for Isola Sacra ribs. Means and their standard errors and standard deviations for reported osteological ages (decades).

not differ between males and females for any age group. This similarity in bone formation rates for older males and females, despite a difference in Ac.f, probably reflects the combined effects of the larger osteons and lower OPD's in these male samples.

4.3.3. Comparison of Isola Sacra with Modern Samples

Mean values for each of the variables for Isola Sacra were compared to the modern comparative samples using analysis of covariance and the Scheffé post hoc test to identify significant differences between skeletal population samples. Table 13.3 summarizes the results for Isola Sacra and the two modern comparative samples.

Among the three samples, the modern European American ribs have the largest average subperiosteal area and the modern African Americans the smallest. The differences among the samples, however, are not statistically significant ($p = 0.179$). Absolute rib size, therefore, does not differ among populations or over time.

The amount of cortical area does differ among the samples ($p = 0.019$). Isola Sacra ribs have the greatest mean cortical area (25.7 mm^2) followed by modern European Americans (21.4 mm^2) and modern African Americans (20.9 mm^2). This difference is statistically significant between Isola Sacra and both modern ribs ($p < 0.05$), but not between the two modern samples ($p = 0.898$). The ribs of the people of ancient Isola Sacra, therefore, have a greater average cortical area, compared to either the modern European American or African American samples.

Isola Sacra ribs have smaller marrow cavities (En.Ar) than either of the modern samples. Even though the overall difference in En.Ar among the samples is significant ($p = 0.028$), none of the pair-wise comparisons are statistically significant ($p > 0.05$). These apparent contradictory findings probably reflect the unequal sample sizes and the large amount of variability for marrow cavity size in the samples. Employing a post hoc test that

Table 13.3. Comparison of Mean Histomorphometric Variables (±1 SE)

Variable	Isola Sacra	European American	African American
Tt.Ar (mm^2)	65.73 ± 4.27	69.51 ± 2.39	62.83 ± 1.78
Ct.Ar (mm^2)	25.75 ± 1.62	21.43 ± 0.73[b]	20.92 ± 0.75[b]
En.Ar (mm^2)	39.98 ± 3.22	48.09 ± 2.20[b]	41.91 ± 1.60
Ct.Ar/ Tt.Ar	0.41 ± 0.02	0.33 ± 0.01[b]	0.35 ± 0.01[b]
Parabolic index	0.23 ± 0.003	0.21 ± 0.004[b]	0.21 ± 0.003[b]
OPD (#/mm^2)	20.95 ± 0.81	21.02 ± 0.61	22.54 ± 0.83
On.Ar (mm^2)	0.03 ± 0.001	0.04 ± 0.001[b]	0.03 ± 0.001
Ac.f (#/mm^2/yr)	0.97 ± 0.07	1.17 ± 0.09	0.79 ± 0.03
BFR (mm^2/mm^2/yr)	0.03 ± 0.002	0.05 ± 0.01[b]	0.03 ± 0.001
Net BFR (mm^2/mm^2)	0.72 ± 0.05	1.01 ± 0.08[b]	0.82 ± 0.03

[b] Statistical significance (p <0.05) with Isola Sacra.

is less conservative than the Scheffé test (e.g., Newman–Keuls test) finds the mean En.Ar for Isola Sacra ribs to be significantly smaller than that for the modern European American samples ($p < 0.05$).

Ribs from the site of Isola Sacra also have relatively greater amounts of cortical bone (Ct.Ar/Tt.Ar) than the ribs of either modern European Americans ($p < 0.001$) or African Americans ($p = 0.004$). The relative amount of cortical bone does not differ between the two modern rib samples ($p = 0.474$). It is interesting that the patterns for age-associated change in this measure of bone mass are similar for both European samples. The relative amount of cortical bone peaks during the fourth decade for both the Isola Sacra and modern European American samples, while it exhibits a steady decrease with age for the modern African American sample (Figure 13.8). Isola Sacra ribs also have a higher mean parabolic index than either of the two modern rib samples ($p < 0.005$), with their mean being closest to the optimum value of 0.25. Similar to the results for relative cortical area, the mean parabolic index for the ribs from the African American and European American samples do not differ significantly from each other ($p = 0.673$). These findings, coupled with those for relative cortical area suggest that the ribs of Isola Sacra people are stronger than modern ribs.

The patterns of sexual dimorphism in cross-sectional area measurements of the rib are similar among the three skeletal population samples. As observed for the ribs of both modern skeletal samples, Isola Sacra males have larger total subperiosteal areas, cortical areas, and marrow cavity spaces. Unlike the modern samples, however, the ribs of males and females from Isola Sacra do not have significantly different relative cortical areas ($p = 0.271$). No significant sexual dimorphism was observed for the parabolic indices of any of the three skeletal samples.

A comparison of the histomorphometric variables reveals that average number of osteons that were created per mm^2 (OPD) for Isola Sacra does not differ significantly from either of the modern groups ($p = 0.575$). For all three groups, OPD increases with age (Figure 13.9).

Osteon size differs significantly among the three rib samples ($p < 0.001$). European Americans have the largest mean osteon area, followed by Isola Sacra, and African Americans who have the smallest osteons. Considered individually, this difference is

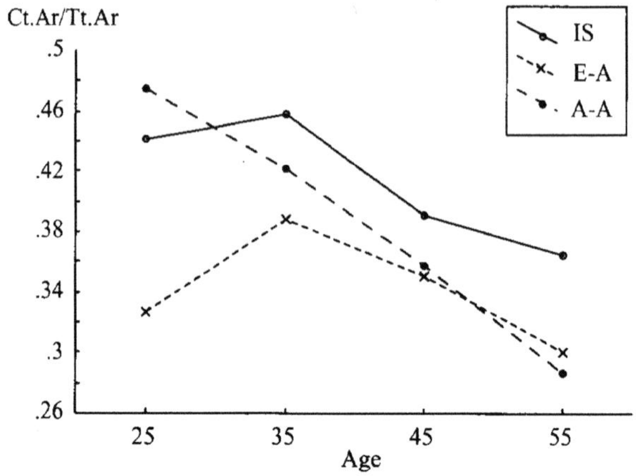

Figure 13.8. Comparison of relative cortical areas (Ct.Ar/Tt.Ar) by age category and sample. Means are for each sample plotted against age. Actual ages for the modern samples have been made equivalent to osteological ages reported for Isola Sacra.

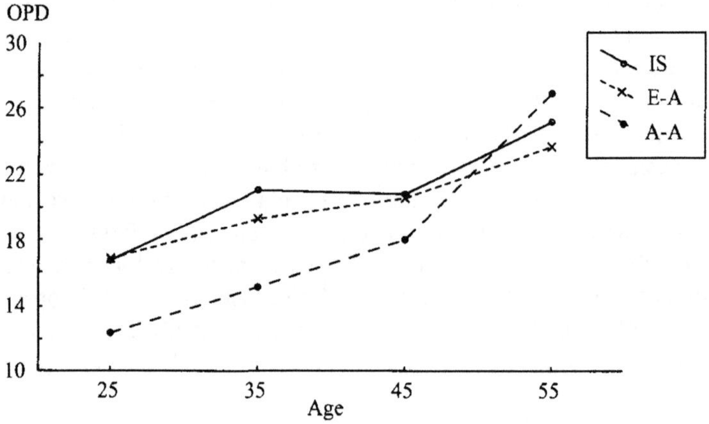

Figure 13.9. Comparison of osteon population density (OPD) by age category and sample.

significant between Isola Sacra and the European Americans ($p < 0.001$), and between the two modern samples ($p = 0.002$), but not between the Isola Sacra and African American ribs ($p = 0.210$). These findings suggest that modern European American ribs exhibit larger osteons than those of ancient Europeans from Isola Sacra, or modern African Americans and that more bone is turned over per basic structural unit during remodeling in modern European American ribs.

Activation frequency (Ac.f), the rate at which osteons are created per mm^2 of cortical bone, is similar among the samples. Both the modern (American) and ancient (Isola Sacra) Europeans create osteons at a higher rate than observed for the modern African American rib sample, but the difference is significant only between European American and African Americans ($p < 0.001$). These findings suggest that bone remodeling units were activated at higher rates in both the modern and ancient European ribs than those of the modern African American sample.

The BFR differs between Isola Sacra and the modern samples ($p < 0.001$). European American rib samples have the highest mean annual cortical bone formation rate at 0.046 $mm^2/mm^2/yr$, followed by Isola Sacra with 0.030 $mm^2/mm^2/yr$. The modern African American rib samples have the lowest mean annual bone formation rate of 0.025 $mm^2/mm^2/yr$. The rates are significantly different ($p < 0.001$) except between Isola Sacra and African Americans ($p = 0.273$).

4.4. Age-Associated Bone Loss in the Imperial Romans

As already noted, it has been reported that modern African Americans and archaeological populations exhibit lower risk of age-associated osteopenia and bone fragility than modern populations of European descent. The results of this study confirm this and suggest that ancient Romans and modern African Americans maintain relatively healthier bone by different mechanisms. Compared to their modern European counterparts, the people of Isola Sacra, who lived some 1,800 years ago, maintained greater bone mass in terms of both absolute and relative cortical area, and they also exhibited lower intra-cortical remodeling rates. Based upon their more optimal parabolic indices, Isola Sacra ribs were also stronger. These findings may indicate that ancient Romans of Isola Sacra produced a greater peak bone mass and/or achieved it at an earlier age. The daily activities in the Roman port such as frequent lifting, carrying, and transporting of grain, foodstuffs, and other goods may have resulted in some individuals attaining and maintaining greater bone mass. In contrast, modern African Americans do not differ from European Americans in terms of the amount of cortical bone, but rather maintain denser bones through reduced intra-cortical remodeling rates and a smaller average osteon size. It is not known whether these findings would hold for bones other than the rib, such as the femur, or other populations and different times.

5. Future Directions

Histomorphometry is a useful approach to investigate and to quantify the progression of osteopenia with increasing age in modern and ancient populations, especially when applied in combination with other measures of bone mass and density. This kind of histological analyses needs to be applied to additional populations that represent different time periods, modes of subsistence, and gene pools. Also, in order to maximize the potential of histological methods, there are several issues that warrant further attention. These include the extent of intra-skeletal variability in bone histomorphometry which will permit greater comparability among different studies, especially of ancient skeletal remains where the availability of bone sampling site is often largely beyond the control of the investigator. New methods of histological analysis need to be explored that will reduce the invasiveness of histological analysis, reduce inter-observer error, and increase the speed and sophistication of analyses. New technologies, such as micro-CT and digital image analysis software should be explored and adapted to histological analyses. Finally, paleopathologists, osteologists, and bioarchaeologists should be encouraged to collect and make available bone samples for histological analysis.

Acknowledgments

We thank Luca Bondioli and Roberto Macchiarelli for permission and assistance in working with the Isola Sacra Necropolis collection.

References

Abbott, S., Trinkaus, E., and Burr, D.B. (1996). Dynamic bone remodeling in later Pleistocene fossil hominids. *Am. J. Phys. Anthropol.* **99**, 585–601.

Agarwal, S.C. (2001a). The influence of age and sex on trabecular architecture and bone mineral density in three British historical populations. Doctoral dissertation, University of Toronto.

Agarwal, S.C. (2001b). The effects of pregnancy and lactation on the maternal skeleton: A historical perspective. An abstract of a paper presented at the seventieth meeting of the American Association of Physical Anthropologists, March 28th–30th, Kansas City, Missouri. *Am. J. Phys. Anthropol.* **32**(Suppl), 30.

Agarwal, S.C., Dumitriu, M., and Grynpas, M.D. (2000). Differences between medieval and modern trabecular bone architecture. An abstract of a paper presented at the 6th–9th meeting of the American Association of Physical Anthropologists, April 10th–15th, San Antonio, Texas. *Am. J. Phys. Anthropol.* **30**(Suppl), 92.

Agarwal, S.C. and Grynpas, M.D. (1996). Bone quantity and quality in past populations. *Anat. Rec.* **246**, 423–432.

Baron, J.A., Barrett, J., Malenka, D., Fisher, E., Kniffin, W., Bubolz, T., and Tosteson, T. (1994). Racial differences in fracture risk. *Epidemiology* **5**, 42–47.

Bassett, E.J., Keith, M.S., Armelagos, G.J., Martin, D.L., and Villanueva, A.R. (1980). Tetracycline-labeled human bone from ancient Sudanese Nubia (AD 350). *Science* **209**, 1532–1534.

Bell, N.H., Gordon, L., Stevens, J., and Shary, J.R. (1995). Demonstration that bone mineral density of the lumbar spine, trochanter, and femoral neck is higher in black than in white young men. *Calcif. Tissue Int.* **56**, 11–13.

Bennike, P. and Bohr, H. (1990). Bone mineral content in the past and present. In C.C. Christiansen and K. Overgaard (eds) *Osteoporosis 1990: Proceedings of the 3rd International Symposium on Osteoporosis*. Osteopress Aps, Copenhagen, pp. 89–91.

Boivin, G. and Meunier, P.J. (1993). Histomorphometric methods applied to bone. In G. Grupe and A.N. Garland (eds) *Histology of Ancient Human Bone: Methods and Diagnosis*, Springer-Verlag, Berlin, pp. 137–156.

Bondioli, L. and Macchiarelli, R. (eds) (1999). *Digital Archives of Human Paleobiology*. E-LISA Sas, Milan.

Chalmers, J. and Ho, K.C. (1970). Geographical variations in senile osteoporosis. *J. Bone Joint Surg.* **52**B, 667–675.

Charnley, R.M., Bickerstaff, D.R., Wallace, W.A., and Stevens, A. (1989). The measurement of osteoporosis in clinical practice. *J. Bone Joint Surg.* **71**B, 661–663.

Cho, H. and Stout, S.D. (2001). Age-associated bone loss in an Imperial Roman population. An abstract of a paper presented at the seventieth meeting of the American Association of Physical Anthropologists, March 28th–30th, Kansas City, Missouri. *Am. J. Phys. Anthropol.* **32**(Suppl), 49–50.

Cohn, S.H., Abesamis, C., Yasumura S., Aloia, J.F., Zanzi, I., and Ellis, K.J. (1977). Comparative skeletal mass and radial bone mass in black and white women. *Metabolism* **26**, 171–178.

Compston, J. (1999). Histomorphometric manifestations of age-related bone loss. In C.J. Rosen, J. Glowacki, and J.P. Bilezikian (eds) *The Aging Skeleton*. Academic Press, San Diego, pp. 251–261.

DeSimone, D.P., Stevens, J., Edwards, J., Shary, J., Gordon, L., and Bell, N.H. (1989). Influence of body habitus and race on bone mass density of midradius, hip and spine in aging women. *J. Bone Miner. Res.* **4**, 827–830.

Epker, B.N. and Frost, H.M. (1964). The parabolic index: A proposed index of the degree of osteoporosis in ribs. *Gerontology* **19**, 469–473.

Ericksen, M.F. (1980). Patterns of microscopic bone remodelling in three aboriginal American populations. In D.L. Brownman (ed.) *Early Native Americans: Prehistoric Demography, Economy, and Technology*. Houton, The Hague, pp. 239–270.

Frisch, B. and Eventov, I. (1986). Hematopoiesis in osteoporosis-Preliminary report comparing biopsies of the femoral neck and iliac crest. *Isr. J. Med. Sci.* **22**, 380–384.

Frost, H.M. (1987). Secondary osteon population densities: An algorithm for estimating the missing osteons. *Yrbk. Phys. Anthropol.* **30**, 239–254.

Garland, N.A. (1993). An introduction to the histology of exhumed mineralized tissue. In G. Grupe and A.N. Garland (eds) *Histology of Ancient Human Bone: Methods and Diagnosis*. Springer-Verlag, New York, pp. 1–16.

Grupe, G. and Dreses-Werringloer, U. (1993). Decomposition phenomenon in thin sections of excavated bones. In G. Grupe and A.N. Garland (eds) *Histology of Ancient Human Bone: Methods and Diagnosis*. Springer-Verlag, New York, pp. 27–36.

Hanson, D.B. and Buikstra, J.E. (1987). Histomorphological alteration in buried human bone from the Lower Illinois valley: Implications for paleodietary research. *J. Archaeol. Sci.* **14**, 549–563.

Herrmann, B. (1993). Light microscopy of excavated human bone. In G. Grupe and A.N. Garland (eds) *Histology of Ancient Human Bone: Methods and Diagnosis*. Springer-Verlag, New York, pp. 17–26.

Iwaniec, U.T. (1997). Effects of dietary acidity on cortical bone remodeling: A histomorphometric assessment. Doctoral dissertation, University of Wisconsin-Madison.

Kneissel, M., Boyde, A., Hahn, M., Teschler-Nicola, M., Kalchhauser, G., and Plenck, Jr., H. (1994). Age- and sex-dependent cancellous bone changes in a 4000y BP population. *Bone* **15**, 539–545.

Luckey, M.M., Meier, D.E., Mandeli, J.P., Dacosta, M.C., Hubbard, M.L., and Goldsmith, S.J. (1989). Radial and vertebral bone density in white and black women. *J. Clin. Endocrinol. Metab.* **69**, 762–770.

Martin, R.B., Burr, D.B., and Sharkey, N.A. (1998). *Skeletal Tissue Mechanics*. Springer-Verlag, New York.

Martin, D.L. and Armelagos, G.J. (1979). Morphometrics of compact bone: An example from Sudanese Nubia. *Am. J. Phys. Anthropol.* **51**, 571–578.

Martin, D.L. and Armelagos, G.J. (1985). Skeletal remodeling and mineralization as indicators of health: An example from prehistoric Sudanese Nubia. *J. Hum. Evol.* **14**, 527–537.

Mays, S.A., Lees, B., and Stevenson, J.C. (1998). Age-dependent bone loss in a medieval population. *Int. J. Osteoarchaeology* **8**, 97–106.

Meunier, P.J. (1988). Assessment of bone turnover by histomorphometry in osteoporosis. In B.L. Riggs and L.J. Melton III (eds) *Osteoporosis: Etiology, Diagnosis, and Management*. Raven Press, New York, pp. 317–332.

Mulhern, D.M. and Van Gerven, D.P. (1997). Patterns of femoral bone remodeling dynamics in a medieval Nubian population. *Am. J. Phys. Anthropol.* **104**, 133–146.

Nelson, D.A., Feingold, M., Bolin, F., and Parfitt, A.M. (1991). Principal components analysis of regional bone density in black and white women: Relationship to body size and composition. *Am. J. Phys. Anthropol.* **86**, 507–514.

Nordin, B.E.C. (1966). International patterns of osteoporosis. *Clin. Orthop.* **45**, 17–30.

Nordin, B.E.C., Chatterton, B.E., Schultz, C.G., Need, A.G., and Horowitz, M. (1996). Regional bone mineral density interrelationships in normal and osteoporotic postmenopausal women. *J. Bone Miner. Res.* **11**, 849–856.

Ortner, D.J. and Putschar, W.G.J. (1985). *Identification of Pathological Conditions in Human Skeletal Remains*. Smithsonian Institution Press, Washington, D.C.

Parfitt, A.M. (1983). Stereological basis of bone histomorphometry; theory of quantitative microscopy and reconstruction of the third dimension. In R.R. Recker (ed.) *Bone Histomorphometry: Techniques and Interpretation*. CRC Press, Inc., Boca Raton, pp. 53–88.

Parfitt, A.M., Drezner, M.K., Glorieux, F.H., Kanis, J.A., Malluche, H., Meunier, P.J., Ott, S.M., and Recker, R.R. (1987). Bone histomorphometry: Standardization of nomenclature, symbols, and units. *J. Bone Miner. Res.* **2**, 595–610.

Pfeiffer, S. (1998). Variability in osteon size in recent human populations. *Am. J. Phys. Anthropol.* **106**, 219–227.

Pfeiffer, S. (2000). Paleohistology: Health and Disease. In M.A. Katzenberg and S.R. Saunders (eds) *Biological Anthropology of the Human Skeleton*. Wiley-Liss, Inc., New York, pp. 287–302.

Pfeiffer, S.K. and Lazenby, R.A. (1994). Low bone mass in past and present aboriginal populations. In H.H. Draper (ed.) *Advances in Nutritional Research*, Vol. 9. Plenum Press, New York, pp. 35–51.

Plato, C.C., Fox, K.M., and Tobin, J.D. (1994). Skeletal changes in human aging. In D.E. Crews and R.M. Carruto (eds) *Biological Anthropology and Aging: Perspectives on Human Variation over the Life Span*. Oxford University Press, Inc., New York, pp. 272–300.

Recker, R.R. (ed.) (1983). *Bone Histomorphometry: Techniques and Interpretation*. CRC Press, Inc., Boca Raton.

Richman, B.A., Ortner, D.J., and Schulter-Ellis, F.P. (1979). Differences in intracortical bone remodeling in three aboriginal American populations: Possible dietary factors. *Calcif. Tissue Int.* **28**, 209–214.

Robling, A.G. (1998). Histomorphometric assessment of mechanical loading history from human skeletal remains: The relation between micromorphology and macromorphology at the femoral midshaft. Doctoral dissertation, University of Missouri-Columbia.

Robling, A.G. and Stout, S.D. (2000). Histomorphometry of human cortical bone: Applications to age estimation. In M.A. Katzenberg and S.R. Saunders (eds) *Biological Anthropology of the Human Skeleton*. Wiley-Liss, Inc., New York, pp. 187–213.

Schnitzler, C.M., Pettifor, J.M., Mesquita, J.M., Bird, M.D.T., Schnaid, E., and Smyth, A.E. (1990). Histomorphometry of iliac crest bone in 346 normal black and white South African adults. *Bone Miner.* **10**, 183–199.

Schultz, M. (1997). Microscopic investigation of excavated skeletal remains: A contribution to paleopathology and forensic medicine. In W.D. Haglund and M.H. Sorg (eds) *Forensic Taphonomy: The Postmortem Fate of Human Remains*. CRC Press, Inc., Boca Raton, pp. 201–222.

Sedlin, E.D. (1964). The ratio of cortical area to total cross-section area in rib diaphyses: A quantitative index of osteoporosis. *Clin. Orthop.* **36**, 161–168.

Solomon, L. (1968). Osteoporosis and fracture of the femoral neck in the South African Bantu. *J. Bone Joint Surg.* **50B**, 2–13.

Solomon, L. (1979). Bone density in ageing Caucasian and African populations. *Lancet* December 22/29, 1326–1329.

Stini, W. (1995). Osteoporosis in biocultural perspective. *Annu. Rev. Anthropol.* **24**, 397–421.

Stout, S.D. (1978). Histological structure and its preservation in ancient bone. *Curr. Anthropol.* **19**, 601–604.

Stout, S.D. (1983). The application of histomorphometric analysis to ancient skeletal remains. *Anthropos* (Greece) **10**, 60–71.

Stout, S.D. and Lueck, R. (1995). Bone remodeling rates and skeletal maturation in three archaeological skeletal populations. *Am. J. Phys. Anthropol.* **98**, 161–171.

Stout, S.D. and Paine, R.R. (1994). Bone remodeling rates: A test of an algorithm for estimating missing osteons. *Am. J. Phys. Anthropol.* **93**, 123–129.

Stout, S.D. and Teitelbaum, S.L. (1976). Histomorphometric determination of formation rates of archaeological bone. *Calcif. Tissue Res.* **21**, 163–169.

Streeter, M.A. (1999). Histomorphometric analysis of Pleistocene hominid fossil bone. Masters thesis, University of Missouri-Columbia.

Thompson, D.D. and Cowen, K.S. (1984). Age at death and bone biology of the Barrow mummies. *Arctic Anthropol.* **21**, 83–88.

Thompson, D.D. and Gunness-Hey, M. (1981). Bone mineral-osteon analysis of Yupik-Inupiaq skeletons. *Am. J. Phys. Anthropol.* **55**, 1–7.

Thompson, D.D., Slater, E.M., and Laughlin, W.S. (1981). Bone core analysis of Baffin Island skeletons. *Arctic Anthropol.* **18**, 87–96.

Wu, K., Schubeck, K.E., Frost, H.M., and Villanueva, A. (1970). Haversian bone formation rates determined by a new method in a mastodon, and in human diabetes mellitus and osteoporosis. *Calcif. Tissue Res.* **6**, 204–219.

Index

Actinomycetes, 184, 185
Activation frequency
in African Americans, 224–225
of basic multicellular units (BMUs), 10, 193
definition of, 210
estimation of, 210
in European Americans, 224–225
in fossil hominids, 215
histomorphic measurement of, 162
in Imperial Roman population, 224–225
Adaptation
functional, 121–131
as homeostasis, 121
mechanisms of, 122–125
genetic, 130–131
somatic *versus* evolutionary, 130–131
African-American men, prostate cancer in, 83
African Americans
activation frequency in, 224–225
bone density in, 83
bone mass in, 51, 52
bone mineral density in, 50
bone quality in, 218
bone size in, 52
bone turnover in, 51
calcium excretion in, 54
cortical bone formation rate in, 225
cortical bone remodeling rate in, 223–224
dietary calcium intake in, 54
hip fractures in
correlation with hip axis length, 55
incidence rates, 48
osteon size in, 223, 224, 225
volumetric bone mineral density in, 51
African-American women
body mass index in, 53
proximal femoral structure in, 56–57
African women, bone remodeling in, 212
Age determination, of bone, 211
Algae
effect on bone microstructure, 211
as postmortem bone loss cause, 183–184
Alkaline phosphatase, lactation-related turnover in, 110
Aluminum, as osteomalacia cause, 38
Amenorrhea, lactation-related, 105–106, 112
Animal models, of lactation, 110–111
Anisotropy, 39
Anthropometrics. *See also* Body mass index (BMI); Body size
as peak bone mass determinant, 93–94
Antlers, growth cycle of, 11
Apoptosis
of osteoblasts, 11
of osteoclasts, 11, 13
Archaeological bone specimens
biomechanical analysis of, 189–205
bone geometry analysis, 190–192
bone microstructure analysis, 192–196
mechanical loading history, 190–196
bone density measurement in
areal *versus* volumetric, 167
with dual energy x-ray absorptiometry, 166–168
bone loss measurement in
in cortical bone, 160–162
in trabecular bone, 162–165
bone remodeling rates in, 209
algorithm for, 210
calcium carbonate content of, 159
cortical
cortical histomorphometric analysis of, 161–162
metacarpal radiogrammetric analysis of, 160–161
diagenesis in, 35–36, 158–159, 211
fractures in, 159
hip fractures in, 159–160
histomorphometric analysis of, 173–174, 189–205, 207–228
in African populations, 212, 217–218
age-at-death determination in, 211
bone remodeling algorithm for, 210
definition of, 208
in European populations, 212–213, 217
in Imperial Roman population, 215–225
in Native American populations, 213–215
principles and methodology of, 173–174, 208–209
intravitam bone loss causes in, 174–180
postmortem bone loss causes in, 180–186
trace element analysis of, 36
Arizona Bone Density Study, 69–85
Arthropods, as postmortem bone loss cause, 183, 184
Asian Americans, hip fractures in, 55–56

Back-scattered electron imaging, 34
Bacteria
effect on bone microstructure, 211
as postmortem bone loss cause, 183, 184
Basic multicellular units (BMUs), 6–11
activation frequency of, 10, 193
bone remodeling function of, 6–11, 20–21
conservation mode, 21, 22
disuse mode, 21–22
cancellous, 7–8
cortical, 7

Bacteria *contd.*
hydrogen ion movement in, 8
in irreversible bone loss, 11, 12, 13
life span of, 11
origination of, 9, 10, 11
in physically-active individuals, 192–193
progression of, 9, 10, 11
structural organization of, 6–8, 13, 123
termination of, 9, 11
Beam theory, 190
Bending rigidity, of long bones, 190–192
Biomechanical analysis, of preserved skeletal remains
bone geometry analysis, 190–192
bone microstructure analysis, 192–196
mechanical loading history, 190–196
Biomechanical factors. *See also* Mechanical loading; Strain
in peak bone mass, 93
Bisphosphonates
action mechanism of, 38
effect on bone mineralization, 38
effect on bone quality, 34
Blacks. *See also* African Americans; Africans; African women
bone strength in, 57
hip bone mineral density in, 57
Black women, vitamin D levels in, 66
Blood pressure, vitamin D-related regulation of, 143
BMD. *See* Bone mineral density
Body composition
age-related changes in, 81–83
components of, 53
estimation of, 81–82
fracture risk relationship, 68–69
in older males, 81–83
Body mass, estimation of, 192
Body mass index (BMI)
age-related changes in, 71, 72, 74–77
percentage of body fat relationship, 74, 76, 77
total body potassium level relationship, 81
Arizona Bone Density Study data, 69–85
body surface area relationship, 81–82
bone density relationship, 76, 82
computation of, 52
cortical bone density relationship, 78, 79
effect of lean body mass on, 81
ethnic/racial factors in, 53
fracture risk relationship, 48–49
low, as osteoporosis risk factor, 65
in older males, 72, 74–77, 78, 79
Body size
bone mineral density relationship, 51–52
cortical bone remodeling relationship, 129–130
gender differences in, 132
Body surface area, as body mass index indicator, 81–82
Bone. *See also* Cortical bone; Trabecular bone
load-bearing, function of, 26
in paralyzed limbs, 24
primary function of, 5
relationship with muscle, 128
structural bone, 5
metabolic bone, 5
weight of, 128, 130
Bone *contd.*
effect of bone remodeling on, 128–129
evolutionary aspects of, 131
Bone architecture. *See also* Bone geometry
dual-energy x-ray absorptiometric measurement of, 47
ethnic/racial factors in, 47–62
as fracture risk predictor, 49
genetic factors in, 130
Bone cells. *See also* Osteoblasts; Osteoclasts
supracellular organization of, 4
Bone density
Arizona Bone Density Study of, 69–85
body mass index relationship, 76, 82
bone strength relationship, 39
in children, ethnic/racial factors in, 50
comparison with other tissue density, 128
correlation with vitamin D serum levels, 66
in diabetes mellitus, 67
ethnic/racial factors in, 50–51, 68
evaluation of, 34
in fractures, 79
gender factors in, 66
mineralization profile histograms of, 34
in osteoporosis, 64
osteoporotic fracture relationship, 39
peak
bone strength relationship, 68
development of, 64
gender factors in, 66, 72
periosteal expansion and, 68
during pregnancy, 106, 107
in animal models, 111
Bone density loss
age-related, 80–81
gender factors in, 71, 72, 80, 81
in males, 68
mechanical factors in, 68–69
in older males, 71, 72, 73
weight reduction-related, 64
Bone density measurement
areal *versus* volumetric, 167
with dual energy x-ray absorptiometry (DEXA), 47, 48, 50, 166–168
with optical/photo densitometry, 166
with quantitative computed tomography, 50
in whole bone, 165–168
Bone fatigue, 129–130. *See also* Fatigue damage
Bone formation, 3. *See also* Bone modeling; Bone remodeling
during pregnancy, 106, 107
animal models of, 110
rate of, 4
Bone fragility. *See also* Bone strength
in archaeological populations, 211–212
bone weight relationship, 135
determinants of, 39–40
genetic factors in, 131–132
Bone geometry, 55–57
cross-sectional, 56–57
hip axis length, 55–56
mechanical loading relationship, 190–192
in prehistoric populations, 196–203

Bone gla-protein, lactation-related turnover in, 110
Bone growth, continuous nature of, 4
Bone length, and biomechanics, 192
Bone-lining cells (BLCs), 123–124, 125
Bone loss
in African archaeological populations, 212
age-related, 11, 19–31, 33
in archaeological bone, 157–172
bone resorption depth in, 14–15
disordered bone remodeling-related, 11–15
estrogen deficiency-related, 26
gender factors in, 80
irreversible, 11–13
muscle weakness-related, 26
1960 paradigm of, 19, 20, 26–27
reversible, 11
sedentary lifestyle-related, 15
testosterone deficiency-related, 26
Utah paradigm of, 19–24
bone remodeling-related, 4, 11–14
cancellous, 14
cancer-related, 179–180, 181, 182
on endocortical surface, 25
in European archaeological populations, 212–213
Haversian, 25
maternal, 105–106
microscopic analysis of
in intravitam bone loss, 174–180
methods and techniques in, 173–174
in postmortem bone loss, 180–186
in older males
hormonal factors in, 66, 67, 85
rate of, 66, 80–81
osteomyelitis-related, 179, 180
as osteoporosis cause, 39
on periosteal surface, 25
postmenopausal, mechanostat and, 134–135
postmortem causes of
algae, 183–184
arthropods (insects), 184, 185, 186
bacteria, 183, 184
fungi, 183–184, 185
larvae, 184, 185, 186
plant roots, 183
protozoa, 183, 184
during pregnancy, nutritional stress-associated, 112
sedentary lifestyle-related, 189
on trabecular surface, 25
Bone loss measurement
in archaeological bone
in cortical bone, 160–162
in trabecular bone, 162–165
in trabecular bone
with image analysis, 163–164
with energy dispersive low angle x-ray scattering analysis, 165
Singh (radiographic) index of, 163
with stereometric analysis, 164–165
with visual examination, 162–163
in whole bone, 165–168
Bone loss rate, 14, 35, 65
aging-related, 14–15
bone turnover rate relationship, 14
gender differences in, 66
postmenopausal, 65, 105
Bone marrow
remodeling mediator mechanism in, 25
types of, 5
Bone marrow cavity, of subadult rib, 95, 96, 97
Bone mass
definitions of, 50
effect of calcium nutrition on, 53–54
effect of parity on, 108
endocrinological factors in, 66–67
ethnic/racial factors in, 47–62, 51
during lactation, 109
peak
age-related bone loss relationship, 92–93
biomechanical factors in, 93–94
development of, 63–64, 93
ethnic/racial factors in, 93
factors determining, 93–94
gender differences in, 66
genetic factors in, 93
hormonal factors in, 93
nutritional factors in, 93
relationship with muscle mass, 53
Bone metabolism, hormonal factors in, 66, 67
Bone mineral content (BMC), 50
development of, gender differences in, 133, 134
lactation-related decrease in, 110
normal, 158
Bone mineral density (BMD)
areal, 50
body size relationship, 51–52
bone strength relationship, 26
effect of dietary calcium on, 53–54
effect of estrogen on, in males, 66, 67
effect of female reproductive factors on, 112, 114–115
lactation, 107, 112
parity, 107–108
pregnancy, 106, 107
effect of physical fitness on, 94
ethnic/racial factors in, Hip Structure Analysis of, 56–57
fracture risk relationsip, 48–49
as hip fracture risk factor, 55
measurement of
with dual-energy x-ray absorptiometry, 33
normal, 158
in osteoporosis, 33
volumetric/true, 50
Bone mineralization
age-related increase in, 40
determination of, 34, 36
disease-associated changes in, 36–37
effect of diagenesis on, 36
effect of trace elements on, 37–38
fetal, 105

Bone modeling, 4
  as bone strength mechanism, 21
  formation and resorption drifts in, 20, 21
  osteoblasts in, 123
  osteoclasts in, 123
Bone porosity
  age-related increase in, 24–25, 34–35
  histomorphic measurement of, 161–162
  intracortical, 126
Bone quality, 33–44
  definition of, 33–34
  determination of, 34
  effect of parity on, 115
  osteoporotic fracture relationship, 51
  in past populations, 168
  during pregnancy, 111
Bone remodeling
  by basic multicellular units, 6–11, 20–21
    activation frequency, 10, 193
    conservation mode, 21, 22, 25
    disuse mode, 21–22, 25
  as bone loss cause, 4, 11–14
  in calcium homeostasis, 127
  cancellous, 4, 208–209
    bone multicellular units in, 9
  comparison with hematopoiesis, 10–11
  conservation-mode, 21, 22
    located next to bone marrow, 25
  definition of, 4
  disordered, 11–15
  disuse-mode, 21
  effect of strain on, 15
  effect on skeletal weight, 128–129
  endosteal, 125
  fatigue damage repair function of, 127, 128, 132
  function of, 6–11, 20–21
  hemiosteonal, 7–8
  hormonal effects in, 10
  in Imperial Roman population, 220–225
  intensity of, 10
  of long bone diaphyses, 77
  microdamage repair function of, 39
  in Native American populations, 213–215
  osteoblasts in, 123
  osteoclasts in, 123
  osteonal, 7–8, 35, 125
  purposes of, 5–11
  responsive *versus* permissive, 128–129
  skeletal maintenance function of, 126–131
  as skeletal weight reduction mechanism, 130
Bone remodeling rate
  in archaeological bone, 209
    algorithm for, 210
  effect of protein diet on, 214
Bone resorption, 3
  depth of, 14–15
  nocturnal increase in, 6
  during pregnancy, 106, 107
  rate of, 4
  tumorous osteoclastic, 179–180, 181, 182
Bone size
  bone strength relationship, 129–130
  ethnic/racial factors in, 52
Bone strength
  bone cross-sectional geometry-based, 56–57
  bone density relationship, 39
  bone mineral density relationship, 26
  bone modeling-related, 21
  bone size relationship, 129–130
  definition of, 63
  effect of muscle strength on, 22, 23
  genetic factors in, 131–132
  in Imperial Roman population, 225
  peak bone density relationship, 68
  strain relationship, 23
Bone strength indices (BSIs), 26
Bone turnover
  calcium homeostasis and, 208
  ethnic/racial factors in, 51
  factors affecting, 65–66
  during lactation, animal models of, 110
  for microfracture/fatigue repair, 208
  during pregnancy, 106–107, 111
  seasonal fluctations in, 65–66
Bone turnover rate
  bone loss rate relationship, 14
  in fossil hominids, 215
  histomorphic measurement of, 162
  in hunter-gatherer populations, 214
Breast cancer
  breast-feeding-based prevention of, 114
  vitamin D-based prevention of, 143
Breast-feeding
  as breast cancer prophylaxis, 114
  duration of, 111–112
  health benefits of, 114
  as vitamin D deficiency cause, 109

Caffeine, effect on peak bone mass, 93
Calcaneus fractures, 69
Calciotropic hormones, during lactation, 110
Calcium
  absorption of
    intestinal, 67, 114
    during lactation, 108
    during pregnancy, 106
  availability during pregnancy, 114
  effect on hip fracture rate, 53–54
  effect on peak bone mass, 93
  excretion of
    ethnic/racial factors in, 66
    during lactation, 114
  homeostasis of
    during pregnancy, 110
    role of bone remodeling in, 127
    role of bone turnover in, 208
  intestinal absorption of, 67, 114
  intestinal transport of, 140, 142
  maternal-fetal transfer of, 105
  prehistoric humans' intake of, 144
  as prostate cancer risk factor, 83–84

Calcium *contd.*
Recommended Dietary Allowances for, 145
renal conservation of, 114
serum content of, 82, 83
sources of, 145
Calcium carbonate, archaeological bone content of, 159
Calcium demand, effect on cortical bone porosity, 6
Calcium nutrition
effect on bone mass, 53–54
variability of, 144–145
Cancellous bone, *see also* Trabecular
marrow of, 5
remodeling of, 4, 208–209
basic multicellular units in, 9
cycle of, 12
resorption of, 13
Cancellous bone density, during lactation and pregnancy, 115
Cancellous bone loss, 14, 208–209
lactation-related, 109
in animal models, 110
pregnancy-related, in animal models, 110
rate of, 14
Cancer. *See also* specific types of cancer
as bone loss cause, 179–180, 181, 182
Cardiac output, during pregnancy, 114
Chaldeans, bone mass in, 50
Children, bone density in, 50
Chinese, bone mass in, 52
Chinese women, bone mineral density in, 53–54
Cholecalciferol. *See* Vitamin D_3
Cholecystokinin, during lactation, 114
Cholesterol
cutaneous synthesis of, 140, 141
functions of, 141
Chylomicrons, 142
Collagen type 1 alpha (COLIA 1), 68
Colles' fractures, 158, 175
Colon (large bowel) cancer, vitamin D-based prevention of, 143
Computed tomography (CT)
quantitative, 26, 50
of trabecular bone, 163, 164
Copper, 38
serum content of, 82, 84
Cortical area
in Imperial Roman population, 218–225
of subadult rib, 95, 96, 97
Cortical area:total cross-sectional area (PCA), 77–78, 79
Cortical bone
archaeological
histomorphometric analysis of, 161–162
in Imperial Roman population, 218–225
metacarpal radiogrammetric analysis of, 160–161
bone loss measurement in, 160–162
with cortical histomorphometry, 161–162
with metacarpal radiogrammetry, 160–161
microstructure of, effect of mechanical loading on, 192–196
porosity of, 126
age-related increase in, 24–25
Cortical bone *contd.*
preparation for histomorphometric analysis, 209
of the rib, 95, 96, 97, 98
shape of, 125
in subadult bone, 95, 96, 97
turnover rate in, 5, 39
Cortical bone density
age-related decrease in, 71, 77–78, 79
correlation with body mass index, 78, 79
in older males, 71
Cortical bone formation, mean annual rate of, 210
Cortical bone loss
age-related, 92
rate of, 14, 65
Cortical bone remodeling, 123
body size relationship, 129–130
effect of mechanical loading on, 192–196
in Native American populations, 213
in subadult rib, 91–92, 97–98
osteon population density in, 97–98
Cortical bone remodeling rate, algorithm for, 210
Cranial bones, 24
Cross-sectional moment of inertia (CSMI), 56

Dairy products, as calcium source, 145
7-Dehydrocholesterol, 140, 141, 145
Densitometry, optical/photo, 166
Density fractionation technique, 34, 36–37
Diabetes mellitus
bone density in, 67
vitamin D-based risk reduction for, 143
Diagenesis, 35–36, 158–159
definition of, 158
effect on histomorphometric findings, 211
1,25-Dihydroxyvitamin D
in bone resorption and formation, 142
in calcium transport, 140
during lactation, 110, 114
during pregnancy, 106
in animal models, 111
synthesis of, 139, 140, 141
normal rate of, 142
in tissue, 143
tissue effects of, 142–143
Dual-energy x-ray absorptiometry (DEXA), 47, 48
for bone density measurement, 166–168
for bone mineral density measurement, 33
of hip axis length, 55
use in Hip Structure Analysis, 56

Effector cells, 123. *See also* Osteoblasts; Osteoclasts
Endocortical surface, bone loss on, 25
Endosteal apposition, in metacarpal cortex, 132, 133
Endosteal envelope, as bone loss site, 14
Endosteal expansion
age-related changes in, 98
during puberty, 95
in subadult rib, 95
Energy dispersive low angle x-ray scattering analysis (EDLAXS), of trabecular bone, 165

Energy requirements, estimation of, in older populations, 81–82
Ergocalciferol. *See* Vitamin D_2
Eskimos (Inuit), 52, 213, 214–215
Estradiol, postpartum levels of, 110–111
Estrogen
effect on bone metabolism, in males, 66, 67, 85
effect on endosteal bone formation, 132
effect on mechanostat, 133–134, 136
effect on osteoblasts, 113
during lactation, 110–111, 114
during pregnancy, 110–111, 114
effect of calcium homeostasis on, 110
effect on bone turnover, 106
Estrogen deficiency
as bone loss cause, 26
as disuse-pattern osteopenia cause, 25
effect on osteoclast apoptosis, 13
as osteoporotic fracture cause, 175
Estrogen receptor genotype, 68
Ethmoid bones, 24
Ethnic/racial factors. *See also* specific ethnic/racial groups
in body mass index, 53
in bone architecture, 47–62
in bone density, 50–51
in bone mass, 47–62, 51
in bone size, 52
in bone turnover, 51
in calcium excretion, 66
in hip fractures, 48–49, 57, 64
effect of dietary calcium on, 53–54
in osteoporosis rate, 49–50
in osteoporotic fractures, 57
bone geometry and, 55–56
in peak bone mass, 93
in rickets, 147
European Americans
activation frequency in, 224–225
cortical bone formation rate in, 225
cortical bone remodeling rate in, 223–224
osteon size in, 223–224
European archaeological populations, bone loss in, 212–213
Evolution
of bone fatigue response, 130
of female reproductive patterns, 111
of 25-hydroxyvitamin D serum concentrations, 149, 150
of menopause, 135, 136
Evolutionary adaptation, 130–131
Exercise, load-bearing, 94

Falls, aging-related increase in, 15
Fatigue damage, bone remodeling repair of, 127, 128, 132
Fatigue fractures, 193
Fatigue life, 129–130
Fatigue strength, 129–130
Female skeleton, effect of reproductive patterns on, 105–119
in ancient African populations, 212
animal models of, 110–111, 115
in Eskimo (Inuit) populations, 214
evolutionary evidence for, 111
health benefits of, 114–115
historical evidence for, 111–113, 115
lactation, 105–106, 108–110, 113–114
parity, 107–108
pregnancy, 106–107, 113–114
Femoral neck
anteversion of, genetic factors in, 130–131
bone density in, 66
bone mineral density in, effect of parity on, 107–108
fractures of, 66
Femoral shaft, fractures of, 65
Femur
age-related porosity increase in, 24–25
bending rigidity of, 191
biomechanical analysis of, in archaeological bone, 196–203
fatigue life of, 129–130
inflammation-related osteolytic changes in, 179
osteon size in, 213
pregnancy-related bone loss in, 106
proximal
bone mass loss in, 66
ethnic/racial differences in, 56–57
fractures of, age factors in, 65
in hip axis length measurement, 55
Ward's Triangle of, 163
rachitic, 122
second moments of area (SMA) of, 191–192
strength of, 26
Fetus, bone mineralization in, 105
Fish, as vitamin D source, 148
Fluoride
effect on bone mineralization, 37–38
effect on bone quality, 34
as osteoporosis treatment, 37
Fracture healing, 3
Fracture rate, gender factors in, 85
Fractures
age factors in, 65
in archaeological bone, 159
bone density associated with, 79
Colles', 158, 175
fatigue, 193
genetic factors in, 65
of the hip
in African Americans, 48, 55
in archaeological bone, 159–160
ethnic/racial factors in, 48–49, 55–56, 57, 64
gender factors in, 57
incidence of, 159
overweight as risk factor for, 52
parity as risk factor for, 108
in postmenopausal women, 65
testosterone levels associated with, 67

Fractures *contd.*
incidence of, 48, 65
microstrains associated with, 124
osteoporotic, 47, 158
in archaeological bone, 159, 211–212
bone density relationship, 39
bone geometry relationship, 55–56
bone quality relationship, 33–34, 51
ethnic/racial factors in, 51, 55–56
gender factors in, 64
incidence of, 105
mechanical factors in, 39
microdamage as risk factor for, 39, 40
during pregnancy, 106
risk prediction for, 33
sedentary lifestyle-related, 189, 203
trabecular, 162
peri- or postmortem examination of, 160
postmenopausal, 135
stress, mechanisms of, 126
ulnar, in archaeological bone, 177, 178
vertebral, gender differences in, 40, 66
vertebral crush, 158, 175
in archaeological bone, 159
Frontal bone, 24
Functional adaptation, of the skeleton, 121–131
as homeostasis, 121
mechanisms of, 122–125
subnormal, 125, 127
supernormal, 125, 126, 127
Fungi
effect on bone microstructure, 211
as postmortem bone loss cause, 183–184, 185
provitamin D synthesis in, 141

Galileo Galilei, 128
Gastrin, during lactation, 114
Gastrointestinal tract, lactation-associated blood flow to, 114
Genetic adaptation, 130–131
Genetic factors. *See also* Ethnic/racial factors
in bone architecture, 130
in bone fragility, 131–132
in bone strength, 131–132
in peak bone mass, 93
Gla-protein, lactation-related turnover in, 110
Glucagon, during lactation, 114
Growth, skeletal, hormonal factors in, 132
Growth factors, 6
Growth spurt, bone remodeling effects during, 6

Haversian canals, age-related decrease in number of, 92
Haversian surface, bone loss on, 25
Haversian systems
age-related increase in, 34
in osteoporotic bone, 175, 176, 177, 178, 179
Height, gender-related loss in, 66–67
Hematopoiesis, comparison with bone remodeling, 10–11
Hemiosteons, 7, 123
Hip axis length, 55–56
Hip fractures
in African Americans, 48, 55
in archaeological bone, 159–160
ethnic/racial factors in
bone geometry and, 55–56
effect of calcium nutrition on, 53–54
gender factors in, 57
incidence of, 48, 159
ethnic/racial factors in, 48–49, 64
osteoporotic, 57
overweight as risk factor for, 52
parity as risk factor for, 108
in postmenopausal women, 65
testosterone levels associated with, 67
Hip Structure Analysis, 56–57
Hispanic-American women, hip fractures in, 55–56
Hispanics
dietary calcium intake in, 54
hip fracture incidence rates in, 48–49
obesity in, 52
Histomorphometric analysis, 207–228
age-at-death determination in, 211
bone remodeling algorithm for, 210
cortical, 161–162
definition of, 208
effect of diagenesis on, 211
of European populations, 212–213, 217
of Imperial Roman population, 215–225
bone remodeling, 220–222
comparison with modern populations, 222–225
cortical area, 218–225
methodology for, 218
osteological age, 217
of Native American populations, 213–215
Paloma, Peru study, 196–203
principles and methodology of, 173–174, 208–209
of the subadult rib, 91–101, 94–99
cortical area, 95, 96, 97, 98
cross-sectional area, 95–97
intracortical bone remodeling and, 91–92, 97–98
marrow cavity, 95
osteon population density, 97–98
total subperiosteal area, 95, 96
Homeostasis
of calcium
during pregnancy, 110
role of bone remodeling in, 127
role of bone turnover in, 208
functional adaptation as, 121
physiologic, 122
Hominids, histomorphometric analysis of, 215
Hormones
effect on bone remodeling, 10
effect on peak bone mass, 93
Howship's lacunae, 179, 180, 181, 182, 186
Hueguenots, 213
Hunter-gatherer populations, 213–214, 215
25-Hydroxylase, 140
1,25-Hydroxyvitamin D_3, 67
cell diffusion of, 142
receptors for, 67–68

25-Hydroxyvitamin D, 139
cell diffusion of, 142
in osteomalacia, 142
in rickets, 142
role in paracrine mechanisms, 143, 144
serum concentrations of
during human evolution, 149, 150
in modern humans, 146–147, 150
in nonhuman primates, 145, 146, 150
in Paleolithic humans, 146, 147, 150
synthesis of, 139, 140
as vitamin D nutritional status indicator, 139, 141, 142
25-Hydroxyvitamin D-1-hydroxylase, 143, 144

Iliac crest bone, lactation-related increase in, 110
Image analysis, of trabecular bone, 163–164
Imperial Roman population, histomorphometric analysis of, 215–225
bone remodeling, 220–222
bone strength, 225
comparison with
African Americans, 217–218, 222, 223, 224–225
European Americans, 217, 218, 222, 223–225
cortical area, 218, 219, 220, 222, 225
methodology for, 218
osteological age, 217
Indians, obesity in, 53
Inflammatory processes, as bone loss cause, 179
Inner ear ossicles, 24
Insects, as postmortem bone loss cause, 183, 184
Insulin, during lactation, 114
Inuit (Eskimos), 52, 213, 214–215
Iodine deficiency, 144
Isola Sacra necropolis, histomorphometric analysis of, 215–225

Japanese, hip fracture incidence in, 64

Kidney, 25-hydroxyvitamin D synthesis in, 140

Lactase, 148
Lactation, 108–110. *See also* Breast-feeding
as amenorrhea cause, 105–106, 112
animal models of, 110–111
bone maintenance during, 105
bone mass during, 109
bone mineral density during, 107, 108–109, 112
calciotropic hormones during, 110
calcium absorption during, 108
cancellous bone density during, 115
cardiovascular changes during, 114
estrogen levels during, 114
health benefits of, 114, 115
hormonal changes during, 114
as maternal bone loss cause, 105–106
in medieval populations, 112–113
oxytocin levels during, 114
prolactin levels during, 114
urinary excretion of calcium during, 114
Larvae, as postmortem bone loss cause, 184, 185, 186
Lead, 38
Lean body mass, 52, 53
bone component of, 82
development of, gender differences in, 133–134
effect on body mass index, 81
as osteoporosis risk factor, 65
Liver
lactation-associated blood flow to, 114
vitamin D metabolism in, 140, 142
Loading. *See* Mechanical loading
Long bones
bending rigidity of, 190–192
bone mass in, 66
bone remodeling of, 77
Lumbar spine, bone mineral density in, during lactation, 109

Malnutrition, as osteoporosis risk factor, 64
Mammary glands, lactation-associated blood flow to, 114
Manganese, 38
Mean wall thickness (MWT), 161–162
Mechanical loading
bone geometry-based analysis of, 190–192
bone geometry relationship, in prehistoric populations, 196–203
bone microstructure analysis of, 192–196
effect on intracortical remodeling, 192–196
effect on phenotype, 189
mechanostat model of, 192–193
strain-dependent signals in, 21
subnormal, 125, 127
supernormal, 126, 127
synergistic interaction with estrogen, 134
whole-bone strength adaptation to, 23–24
Mechanical properties, of bone, in osteoporotic fractures, 39
Mechanosensor, 123
Mechanostat, 15, 192–193
effect of estrogen on, 133–134
effect on bone fragility, 131
effect on bone strength, 23
during menopause, 134–135
in responsive remodeling, 128, 129
sexual dimorphism and, 132
strain-regulating function of, 124–125
Menarche, onset age of, 111–112, 113
Menopause
evolution of, 135, 136
mechanostat set point during, 134–135
onset age of, 111–112, 113
Menstrual cycles, average number of, 111–112
Metabolic bone, function of, 5
Metacarpals
gender-related and age-related changes in, 132, 133
radiogrammetry analysis of, 160–161
Metastases, as bone loss cause, 179–180, 182
Microdamage, in bone, 39, 40
effect on bone remodeling rate, 192–193
physical activity-related, 192–193
Microhardness testing, 34
Microradiography, 35
for bone quality determination, 34

Microstrains, 124
Milk, vitamin D fortification of, 147
Milk consumption, in adult humans, 145, 148
Mineralization profile, 34, 40
Minerals. *See also* specific minerals
  dietary, effect on peak bone mass, 93
Modeling threshold, 21, 22, 23
Multiple sclerosis, vitamin D-based control of, 143
Mummies
  bones from, 36
  Eskimo (Inuit), 214
Muscle, relationship with bone, 128
Muscle strength, effect on bone strength and bone bank, 22, 23
Muscle weakness
  as bone loss cause, 26
  as disuse-pattern osteopenia cause, 25

Nasal bones, 24
National Health and Nutrition Examination Surveys (NHANES), 52, 54
Native Americans, histomorphometric studies of, 213–215
Natural selection, for skin color, 147–148, 149
Neanderthals
  osteoporosis in, 177–179
  skeletal differences with modern humans, 131
Nubians, 212
Nutritional factors, in peak bone mass, 93
Nutritional stress, as pregnancy-related bone loss cause, 112

Obesity
  definition of, 52
  ethnic/racial factors in, 52–53
Older adults
  calcium requirements in, 150
  vitamin D deficiency in, 150
  vitamin D supplementation in, 144
Older males
  body composition in, 68–69, 81–83
  body mass index in, 72, 74–77, 78, 79
  bone density in, 71, 72, 73
  bone loss in
    hormonal factors in, 66, 67, 85
    rate of, 66, 80–81
  cortical area:total cross-sectional area (PCA) in, 77–78, 79
  prostate cancer in, 83–84
Optical/photo densitometry, 166
Ossicles, of inner ear, 24
Osteoarthritis, spinal bone density in, 64
Osteoblasts
  aging-related death of, 14
  apoptosis of, 11
  in bone formation, 13–14
  as bone matrix component, 124
  in bone modeling, 20–21, 123
  in bone remodeling, 123
  functions of, 3, 4
  life span of, 11
  mechanostat regulation of, 15
Osteocalcin, during pregnancy, 111
Osteoclasts
  apoptosis of, 11, 13
  in bone modeling, 123
  in bone remodeling, 123
  formation of, 10
  functions of, 3, 4
  life span of, 11
  mechanostat regulation of, 15
  role in bone modeling, 20–21
Osteocytes
  apoptosis of, 125
  definition of, 123
  effect of strain on, 125
  formation of, 11
Osteogenesis imperfecta, 131
Osteological age, determination of, 211
Osteomalacia
  aluminum-related, 38
  as female pelvic deformity cause, 147–148, 149
  25-hydroxyvitamin D levels in, 142
  during pregnancy, 148
  vitamin D-based prevention of, 143
Osteomyelitis, as bone loss cause, 179, 180
Osteonal population density, 161–162
Osteon fragments, 193, 194
Osteon population density, 97–98
  calculation of, 193–195
  definition of, 210
  femoral, 200
  in fossil hominids, 215
  in Imperial Roman population, 220–221, 222, 223
  in rib, 200
Osteons
  as bone matrix component, 124
  double, 35
  formation of, 6
  mineralization of, 35
  secondary, 4, 193
  structure of, 124
Osteon size, 97, 193
  in African Americans, 223, 224, 225
  in ancient European populations, 213
  in European Americans, 223–224
  in fossil hominids, 215
Osteopenia
  disuse-pattern, 24, 25
  in older adult females, 98
  as osteoporosis cause, 65, 207
  as pathological fracture cause, 160
Osteopenic bone, histologic changes in, 208
Osteoporosis
  animal models of, 37
  in archaeological bone, 157, 211–212
  bone loss relationship, 39
  in bones of mummies, 214
  calcium-related prevention of, as prostate cancer risk factor, 84, 85
  cyclic physiologic, 11
  definition of, 33, 47, 63–64, 105, 158
  diagnostic criteria for, 33

Osteoporosis *contd.*
  in Europeans, 212
  fluoride treatment for, 37
  as fracture risk factor, 33
  inactivity/immobilization-related, 177–179
  incidence of, 159
  malnutrition-related, 64
  in men, 84, 85
  osteopenia-related, 65, 207
  pregnancy-related, 106
  primary
    idiopathic, 175
    postmenopause, 175
  rheumatoid arthritis-related, 64
  risk factors for, 33, 65–69
  secondary, in archaeological bone, 177–180
  senile, 175, 176
  type II (age-related), 33, 158
  type I (postmenopausal), 33, 158
  vitamin D_3 administration in, 67
  vitamin D-based prevention of, 143
  vitamin D deficiency-related, 149
  vitamin D insufficiency-related, 142
  vitamin K_2 administration in, 67
Osteoporosis rate, ethnic/racial factors in, 49–50
Oxytocin
  during lactation, 114
  during pregnancy, 114

Paget's disease, 131
Paleolithic humans, 25-hydroxyvitamin D serum concentrations in, 145, 146
Paloma, Peru, skeletal remains study in, 196–203
Paracrine mechanisms, in vitamin D nutrition, 143, 144
Paralyzed limbs, bone in, 24
Parathyroid gland, suppression of, 142
Parathyroid hormone, 65, 66, 67
  in bone resorption and formation, 142
  in 1,25-dihydroxyvitamin D synthesis, 141
  during lactation, 110, 114
  during pregnancy, 106, 108
Parathyroid hormone-related protein, 110
Parietal bone, 24
Parity, 107–108
  average, 111
  effect on bone quality, 115
  in medieval populations, 112–113
Pelvis
  female, osteomalacia-related deformity in, 147–148, 149
  gender-related mechanical loading in, 200–201
Periosteal apposition, 40
  in metacarpal cortex, 132, 133
  in subadult ribs, 98
Periosteal expansion
  age-related changes in, 98
  in subadult ribs, 98
Periosteal surface
  bone loss on, 25
  effect of testosterone on, 132
Phenotype, effect of mechanical loading on, 189
Phosphorus
  effect on peak bone mass, 93
  lactation-related increase in, 114
Photodecomposition, of vitamin D, 141
Physical activity
  as bone microdamage cause, 192–193
  effect on bone geometry, in prehistoric populations, 196–203
  effect on fracture risk, 54
Plant roots
  effect on bone microstructure, 211
  as postmortem bone loss cause, 183
Plants, provitamin D synthesis in, 141
Pneumonia, vitamin D-based resistance to, 143
Polynesians, 130–131
Portus Romae, 215, 219
Potassium, total body levels of, 81
Postmortem examination, of fractured bone, 160
Potassium
  serum, 82, 83
  urinary, 82
Postmortem bone loss, 180–186
Pregnancy
  blood flow during, 114
  bone density during, 106, 107
    in animal models, 111
  bone loss during, 106
    nutritional stress-associated, 112
  bone maintenance during, 105
  bone mineral density during, 106, 107
  bone turnover during, 106–107
  calcium homeostasis during, 110, 114
  cancellous bone density during, 115
  cardiac output during, 114
  osteomalacia during, 148
  osteoporosis during, 106
  osteoporotic fractures during, 106
  parathyroid hormone levels during, 108
  trabecular bone loss during, 106
Prehistoric humans
  dietary calcium intake in, 144
  25-hydroxyvitamin D serum concentrations in, 145, 146
Preosteoclasts, 10
Previtamin D, 141
Primates, nonhuman
  age-related bone loss in, 64
  female reproductive patterns in, 111
  25-hydroxyvitamin D serum concentrations in, 145, 146, 150
  lactation in, 110–111, 115
  pregnancy in, 110–111
  rickets in, 145
  vitamin D metabolism in, 141
  vitamin D requirements in, 145
Prolactin
  during lactation, 114
  during pregnancy
    effect of calcium homeostasis on, 110
    effect on bone turnover, 106
  pregnancy-related increase in, 114

Prostate cancer
in African-American men, 83
calcium as risk factor for, 83, 84, 85
vitamin D-based prevention of, 143
Protein, dietary
effect on bone remodeling rate, 214
effect on peak bone mass, 93
Proteoglycans, genetic coding for, 131–132
Provitamin D, 141

Race. *See also* Ethnic/racial factors
American Anthropological Association's position on, 49–50
Radial shaft, pregnancy-related bone loss in, 106
Radiogrammetry, metacarpal, 160–161
Radiographic analysis, of trabecular bone, 163–164
Radius bone
age-related cortical thinning of, 77, 78
bone density in, 68–69
bone mineral density in, effect of parity on, 107–108
ratio of cortical area:total cross-sectional area, 77–78 79, 85
Ratio of cortical area:total cross-sectional area, 77–78 79, 85
Remodeling threshold, 21, 22, 23
Renal conservation, of calcium, 114
Reproductive capacity, effect of vitamin D deficiency on, 147–148, 149
Reproductive patterns, female
evolution of, 111
skeletal effects of
in ancient African populations, 212
animal models of, 110–111, 115
in Eskimo (Inuit) populations, 214
evolutionary evidence for, 111
health benefits of, 114–115
historical evidence for, 111–113, 115
lactation, 105–106, 108–110, 113–114
in nonhuman primates, 111
in non-industrialized human populations, 111–112
parity, 107–108
in postindustrialized human populations, 111, 112
pregnancy, 106–107, 113–114
Rheumatoid arthritis, 64
Rib
biomechanical analysis of, in archaeological bone, 196–203
histomorphometric analysis of, in Imperial Roman population, 217–225
mean tissue age estimation of, 194
osteons of, 194
subadult, histomorphometry of
cortical area, 95, 96, 97, 98
cross-sectional area, 95–97
intracortical remodeling, 97–98
marrow cavity, 95
osteon population density, 97–98
total subperiosteal area, 95, 96
Rickets
ethnic/racial factors in, 147
25-hydroxyvitamin D levels in, 142
in nonhuman primates, 145
Rickets *contd.*
as pelvic deformity cause, 147–148, 149
untreated, 147–148
vitamin D-based prevention of, 143

Sarcopenia, 25
Second moments of area (SMA), 190–192, 198
Sedentary lifestyle
as bone loss risk factor, 15, 189
as osteoporotic fracture risk factor, 203
Sensor cells, 123–124
Sex hormone binding globulin, 67
Sexual dimorphism, relationship to the mechanostat, 132
Singh (radiographic) index, 163
Skeletal growth, hormonal factors in, 132
Skeleton
functional adaptation of, 121–131
as homeostasis, 121
mechanisms of, 122–125
weight of, 130
effect of bone remodeling on, 128–129
evolutionary aspects of, 131
Skin
cholesterol synthesis in, 140, 141
vitamin D synthesis in, 140, 141, 142, 144, 145
Skin cancer, skin pigmentation and, 147
Skin color
effect on vitamin D synthesis, 146–147
natural selection for, 147–148, 149
Smoking, as osteoporosis risk factor, 65
Soil erosion, as postmortem bone loss cause, 180, 182
Somatic adaptation, 130–131
Somatostatin, during lactation, 114
South African blacks, bone turnover in, 51
Sphenoid bone, 24
Spinal fractures, 68
Spine, bone mineral density in, effect of parity on, 108
Spitalfields, London, 213
Stereometric analysis, of trabecular bone, 164–165
Steroids, effect on female bone structure, 113
Strain, in bone, 124–125
bone strength relationship, 23
effect on bone remodeling, 15
effect on cortical remodeling, 192
in long bone cortices, 190
modeling threshold for, 21, 22, 23
remodeling threshold for, 21, 22, 23
role in stress fractures, 126
Structural bone, remodeling of, 5–6
Subperiosteal surface, in bone remodeling, 77
Sun City/Tucson Longitudinal Study, 69–85
Sunlight
effect on serum 25-hydroxyvitamin D concentrations, 146–147
inverse correlation with cancer risk, 84
role in vitamin D synthesis, 141, 144

Tachysterol, 141
Testosterone
effect on bone metabolism, 66, 67, 85
effect on periosteal bone formation, 132

Testosterone deficiency
as bone loss cause, 26
as disuse-pattern osteopenia cause, 25
as osteoporotic fracture cause, 175
Testosterone replacement therapy, 66
Tetracycline, as bone marker, 209, 210
Tissue
1,25-dihydroxyvitamin D synthesis in, 143
effect of 1,25-dihydroxyvitamin D on, 142–143
Total accumulated osteon creations (AOCs), 193–195, 210
Trabeculae, 162
Trabecular bone, *see also* Cancellous bone
architecture of, 125
in medieval populations, 213
distribution of, 162
microstructure of, during pregnancy, 107
in osteoporosis-related fractures, 162
as percentage of skeletal mass, 162
remodeling of, 208
thickness of, during lactation and pregnancy, 111, 115
turnover rate in, 39
Trabecular bone loss, 209
age-related, in medieval females, 112, 113
measurement of
with image analysis, 163–164
with energy dispersive low angle x-ray scattering analysis, 165
Singh (radiographic) index of, 163
with stereometric analysis, 164–165
with visual examination, 162–163
during pregnancy, 106
rate of, 65
structural factors in, 68–69
Trabecular surface, bone loss on, 25
Trace element analysis, of archaeological bone, 36
Trace elements, effect on bone mineralization, 37–38
Tuberculosis, vitamin D-based prevention of, 143
Tumors, as bone loss cause, 179–180, 181, 182
Turbinate bones, 24
Ulnar fractures, in archaeological bone, 177, 178
Ultraviolet light
role in vitamin D metabolism, 146–147
role in vitamin D_2 synthesis, 139, 140
role in vitamin D_3 synthesis, 141
Utah paradigm, of skeletal physiology, 19–24

Vertebral bodies, age-related density decrease in, 39
Vertebral crush fractures, 158, 175
in archaeological bone, 159
Vertebral fractures, gender differences in, 40, 66
Vertebrates, vitamin D requirements in, 141
Vinci, da, Leonardo, 129
Vitamin D, 139–154
absorption of, 141–142
as 1,25-dihydroxyvitamin D substrate, 139, 140
effect on intestinal calcium absorption, 67
metabolism of, 142
in older adults, 150
oral intake of. *See also* Vitamin D supplementation
in nonhuman primates, 145
photodecomposition of, 141
prostate cancer-suppressing activity of, 84
Recommended Daily Allowance (RDA), 142, 149–150
role in disease prevention, 143, 144
serum levels of
correlation with bone density, 66
seasonal fluctuations in, 65–66
synthesis of, 146
age-related decrease in, 141
effect of skin color on, 146–147
in skin, 140, 141, 142, 144, 145, 146–147
Vitamin D deficiency. *See also* Osteomalacia; Rickets
breast-feeding-related, 109
definition of, 142–144
effect on bone mineral density, 37
effect on reproductive capacity, 147–148, 149
in older adults, 150
as osteoporosis cause, 149
skin color and, 147–148
Vitamin D-binding protein, 141–142
Vitamin D genotype, 67–68
Vitamin D insufficiency, 142, 149, 150
Vitamin D supplementation
in the elderly, 144
as fracture prophylaxis, 144
Vitamin D supplements, sources of, 141
Vitamin D_2, synthesis of, 139, 140
Vitamin D_3, 67, 139
Vitamin K_2, 67
Volume effect, on bone strength and fatigue life, 129–130

Ward's Triangle, 163
Water erosion, as postmortem bone loss cause, 180, 182
Weaning
age of
in medieval populations, 113
natural, 111
maternal bone loss recovery following, 109–110, 115
Weight, of bone, 128, 130
effect of bone remodeling on, 128–129
evolutionary aspects of, 131
Weight reduction, effect on bone density, 64
Wheat Bran Fiber Colon Cancer Prevention Study, 81, 82
Whole bone, measurement of, 165–168
Wolff, Julius, 122
Wolff's Law, 34, 122, 190
World Health Organization
obesity definition of, 52
osteoporosis definition of, 64
osteoporosis diagnostic criteria of, 33
Wrist fractures, age factors in, 65

X-ray powder diffraction, 166

GPSR Compliance

The European Union's (EU) General Product Safety Regulation (GPSR) is a set of rules that requires consumer products to be safe and our obligations to ensure this.

If you have any concerns about our products, you can contact us on ProductSafety@springernature.com

In case Publisher is established outside the EU, the EU authorized representative is:

Springer Nature Customer Service Center GmbH
Europaplatz 3
69115 Heidelberg, Germany

Batch number: 10704039

Printed by Printforce, the Netherlands